The Respiratory Therapist's Legal Answer Book

Anthony L. DeWitt, RRT, CRT, JD, FAARC
Attorney at Law
Bartimus, Frickleton, Robertson & Obetz, PC
Jefferson City, Missouri

JONES AND BARTLETT PUBLISHERS
Sudbury, Massachusetts
BOSTON   TORONTO   LONDON   SINGAPORE

World Headquarters

Jones and Bartlett
Publishers
40 Tall Pine Drive
Sudbury, MA 01776
978-443-5000
info@jbpub.com
www.jbpub.com

Jones and Bartlett
Publishers Canada
6339 Ormindale Way
Mississauga, ON L5V IJ2
CANADA

Jones and Bartlett
Publishers International
Barb House, Barb Mews
London W6 7PA
UK

Jones and Bartlett's books and products are available through most
bookstores and online booksellers. To contact Jones and Bartlett
Publishers directly, call 800-832-0034, fax 978-443-8000, or visit our
website www.jbpub.com.

Substantial discounts on bulk quantities of Jones and Bartlett's
publications are available to corporations, professional associations,
and other qualified organizations. For details and specific discount
information, contact the special sales department at Jones and Bartlett
via the above contact information or send an email to
specialsales@jbpub.com.

Production Credits
Chief Executive Officer: Clayton Jones
Chief Operating Officer: Don W. Jones, Jr.
President, Higher Education and Professional Publishing: Robert W. Holland, Jr.
V.P., Sales and Marketing: William J. Kane
V.P., Design and Production: Anne Spencer
V.P., Manufacturing and Inventory Control: Therese Bräuer
Publisher: Jack Bruggeman
Production Manager: Amy Rose
Associate Production Editor: Dan Stone
Editorial Assistant: Kylah Goodfellow McNeill and Katilyn Crowley
Marketing Manager: Emily Ekle
Associate Marketing Manager: Laura Kavigian
Composition: Graphic World
Cover Design: Anne Spencer
Printing and Binding: Malloy, Inc.
Cover Printing: Malloy, Inc.

Library of Congress Cataloging-in-Publication Data
DeWitt, Anthony L.
  The respiratory therapist's legal answer book / Anthony L. DeWitt.--1st ed.
      p. ; cm.
  ISBN 0-7637-3440-3 (hardcover : alk. paper)
  1. Respiratory therapists--Legal status, laws, etc.--United States. I. Title.
  KF2915.T45D49 2006
  344.7304'12--dc22
                                            2005007392

Printed in the United States of America
09 08 07 06 05   10 9 8 7 6 5 4 3 2 1

Dedication

This book is dedicated to the most wonderful woman in the world, my wife, Ginger DeWitt. No man in the history of the world has been as lucky as I have in finding an angel to live with here on earth. Every word, every bit of advice, everything good in this book owes its life and existence to this wonderful woman who brought me into her arms and made the world right by doing so.

Table of Contents

Preface

When I was asked to write a book about Respiratory Care and the law, I literally didn't know where to start. My original thought was for a quick and easy guide to legal issues therapists might face. This idea lasted only so long as it took me to write down the topics I needed to cover, however, and the publisher wanted a longer text that could be used in Respiratory Care Programs. When I sat down to write the volume of material, I quickly saw that this would be a daunting task.

I promised myself to write at least 10 pages a day. Some days I would write 40 pages, and some days only 10, but every day I wrote something until, 700 pages of manuscript later, this work was done.

This has been a labor of love. It is my hope that it is worthwhile and helpful for therapist, student and educator alike. And if you, the reader, have questions, I do hope you will write and ask me at lawbook@aldewitt.com.

Acknowledgments

I wish to thank the following people for their help with this text. Jack Bruggeman, who asked me to write the book for the publisher. Rebecca Bean, RRT, and David Bach, RRT, who, through their courage and friendship, have taught me all I know about managing people and respiratory care. Ray Masferrer, Sam Giordano, and Bill Dubbs at the American Association for Respiratory Care, who have gone out of their way to help me with issues related to the profession.

Introduction

HOW TO USE THIS BOOK

This book contains more information than most therapists will ever need about the court system, lawyers, law, and litigation. But I have erred on the side of including material rather than excluding the material because when you want information, you should be able to find it. This book is meant to fill that need.

Generally, when you have a question about the process of how a case is tried or handled through the courts, or need to understand the basic workings of the justice system, Chapter 1 is there. It is a complete guide to the federal and state courts in the United States. It is meant to provide a basic and fundamental understanding of the court system, to allow anyone to quickly figure out how the process of suing or being sued works.

Chapter 2 discusses patient rights and how those rights are defined by common law and statute. Important clinical subjects like informed consent and patient autonomy are discussed in detail.

In Chapter 3 we look at the important things that every therapist needs to know about the law of contracts. The chapter looks at the common law of contracts (what constitutes a valid and binding contract) as well as the statutory law of contracts (what the Uniform Commercial Code does). Common contract situations, like employment contracts and insurance contracts, are set out in detail, as are warranties. The chapter features the three most important rules of contract law for therapists.

Employment Law is one of the most important topics covered in this book. Both sides of the spectrum are covered in Chapters 4, 5, and 6. Employee rights are laid out in exacting detail in Chapters 4 and 5, and Chapter 6 discusses employment law from the standpoint of the employer. If an employee had a question about his rights, he would check Chapter 5, and if a manager wanted some guidance in a particular situation, he would look in Chapter 6.

The basic tenets of tort law are laid out in Chapter 7. In this chapter, the entire spectrum of tort law (except medical malpractice) is presented, along with the policy issues inherent in these types of cases. The chapter examines three types of tort actions: intentional torts, negligent torts, and "strict liability" torts. This chapter provides the fundamentals to understanding the information presented in Chapter 8, dealing with medical negligence.

Chapter 8 is meant to be the most important part of this book in that, in most instances, the legal problem that most therapists are sure to face one day or another is the issue of personal liability for medical negligence. The chapter examines the issues of medical negligence in detail. What constitutes negligence? How is it proved in a court? What factors go into the patient's decision to sue a provider? Chapter 8 answers these questions and more.

In every hospital or health care organization, the subject of Risk Management is often understated and misunderstood. Few therapists understand what the Risk Manager does, and what the function of the Risk Management department is. Chapter 9 explains the process and why it is so important to therapists. It also provides guidance for therapists who own their own businesses in terms of minimizing risks and thinking like a risk manager.

Because Medicare has taken over more of the role of paying for medical care in the United States, health care law has become more and more a subject governed by statute. The federal statutes that govern health care law, including the Antikickback Statute and the False Claims Act, are laid out in Chapter 10 on Health Care Law.

Since therapists are an inventive bunch, Chapter 11 discusses how to protect your own business from disaster by incorporating or forming a business association. Therapists are urged to get good legal advice in setting up a corporation or limited liability company so as to avoid the pitfalls that come with having a company simply prepare the paperwork for you.

Chapter 12 focuses on the civil law for individuals. While a therapist might rightly be most worried about being sued for malpractice, the topics covered in this chapter, including the federal Consumer Protection and Credit Protection statutes, are vital to understanding what rights a therapist has in his own right. How does bankruptcy work? What laws protect my ATM card? How would I know if I had a cause of action for any of the torts in Chapter 7? The answers to these questions are found in Chapter 12.

Like the chapter on medical malpractice, Chapter 13 deals with, among other things, medical negligence. The focus of the chapter is not on the negligence, but on the process of litigation. In other words, while Chapter 8 talks about medical negligence, Chapter 13 talks about the process of litigation. How should you structure your relationship with your lawyer? What is the difference between fact witnesses and expert witnesses? What should you do if you are subpoenaed? How do you prepare for a deposition? All this information, as well as some of the rules that govern the conduct of lawyers in litigation are presented.

Criminal law is the topic discussed in Chapter 14, and it is a topic I would hope most therapists would never need. The goal of the chapter is to give quick advice to someone facing criminal charges, or otherwise involved as a victim in the criminal process. It is a quick guide to the law of search and seizure and what the police can and cannot do when they question a suspect. It is not meant as specific advice in a specific situation, but as general information to assist someone who might be suspected of a criminal offense.

Hopefully anyone reading this book already has a family lawyer, which is every bit as important as having a family doctor. Chapter 15 details the process of finding such a lawyer, and how to find lawyers who specialize in specific areas of the law. It examines the differences between small and large law firms, and discusses the process of hiring an attorney, as well as what questions to ask.

Chapter 16 briefly examines the relationship between law and ethics in health care. It focuses on placing the patient first and on applying the golden rule as a yardstick in measuring your own ethical compliance. It also provides some guidance in how to resolve ethical conflicts.

It is my fervent hope that the readers of this book will take away several things from their reading. First, the law is a difficult and complex subject where common sense often has nothing to do with the outcome. Second, any time a therapist faces a situation where her legal rights are threatened, where her property is at issue, or where her livelihood is in jeopardy, a knowledgeable and compassionate attorney is not a luxury, it is a necessity. Finally, I hope therapists understand that the law grows and changes, and the only person who can truly offer advice to them about how to proceed in any legal situation is an attorney who knows the specific situation. What is written in this book will change over time. That principle, however, will not.

CHAPTER 1

The Courts and the Law— Essentials You Need to Know

"Rightful liberty is unobstructed action according to our will within limits drawn around us by the equal rights of others."

Thomas Jefferson

A. THE LEGAL SYSTEM

This book is, most importantly, about a legal system that very few people really know very much about, or understand. It is difficult to adequately describe "the legal system" in a book that isn't filled with legal jargon, because the legal system tries very hard to make itself difficult to understand. It is a system filled with nuance. There is seldom one right answer. The law is an area where shades of grey, not blacks and whites, dominate. The law differs in each state. Procedural rules that guide courts are different from state to state. Statutes vary significantly from state to state.[1]

When lawyers write books for each other, telling them how to try a case, or how to handle a certain type of legal situation, they generally stay away from the substance of the law because they assume that other lawyers know this information. But a book for clinicians can't make that kind of assumption. Thus, a full explication of the law as it pertains to respiratory care depends, at the outset, upon an understanding of the structure and history of the legal system.

---

[1]Several years ago some brilliant legal scholars got together and drafted model laws and certain "uniform" statutes that have been enacted in almost all of the fifty states. These "uniform" laws, however, quickly became jumbled when courts in different states began interpreting the clear language of the statutes differently in each jurisdiction. There is very little clarity in the law, and that is one of the main reasons why lawyers exist.

B. OVERVIEW

Someone once observed that the American legal system is the worst thing ever invented, except for all the others. The American system is fraught with its problems. First, it is poorly understood. Fewer than half the adults reaching voting age understand how law is really made, how courts reach decisions, and what each branch of government contributes to the process. The awful part is that through high school and college courses in "Civics" or "Government," many people have terrible misconceptions about how government actually operates.

More importantly, while most people who watch television have a basic understanding of the criminal justice system, those same people are completely ignorant of the civil justice system in this country, except in the context of "frivolous lawsuits" and "runaway juries." Sure, they've heard of lawsuits and litigation, but only in the context of a spilled coffee case and the cases the media label as "frivolous" or "junk."

Fortunately, most people live and die without their life or their death becoming the basis for a lawsuit of any kind. That is a good thing, because lawsuits are not, as some would have you believe, a ticket to the lottery. A lawsuit is much more like a ride through a haunted house at Halloween. People generally don't understand the legal system because the system, as mentioned, makes it difficult. Also, good people, who are well-intentioned but uninformed, have built many myths into the legal system. Those myths crumble when they are confronted with the harsh realities of the law. The purpose of this book is to try to eliminate some of those myths, and to help the respiratory therapist understand her role in the justice system.

1. How Many Legal Systems Are There?

There are two legal systems in the United States—one at the state level and one at the federal level. The two systems more or less compete with each other for cases, but only in the loosest sense.

Jurisdiction means the power of a court to hear or decide a case. Under the United States Constitution, only the Supreme Court of the United States has the power to hear cases between states. Under the constitutions of most states, local district or "circuit" courts have jurisdiction over claims between individuals.

Criminal courts acquire jurisdiction based on where the wrong was committed, and what body of law—state or federal—was broken.

What Cases Do State Courts Handle?

State courts are courts of limited jurisdiction. They can only try cases inside the borders of their state, and usually can only apply the law of their state or the federal government.[2] These courts handle two broad kinds of cases: civil and criminal.

A state court criminal case enforces the criminal law of the state. For example, each state's law forbids murder. When a state prosecutor files a criminal charge of murder, he does that in a state court. Similarly, whether a state highway patrolman or a city police officer issues a driver a ticket for a moving violation, that action is tried in the state court system.[3]

The second broad class of cases, civil cases, involves all lawsuits that do not involve criminal acts. This includes contract cases, employment law, tort actions (like malpractice), and actions brought in the probate courts under a person's will. Generally, if the issue is the protection of the public through the imposition of fines or punishment, that is a criminal case. A civil case, federal or state, is a case designed to vindicate the rights of private parties (including the government) to damages or to attain the resolution of a controversy.

While a state prosecutor can only file an action in state court, and a federal prosecutor can file only in federal court, a civil plaintiff has the right to choose whether to file a case in the state or federal court. But because the federal courts are courts of "limited jurisdiction" a plaintiff can only file her action in the federal courts if the federal court has jurisdiction.

What Cases Do Federal Courts Handle?

Like their state counterparts, federal courts are courts of limited jurisdiction. Federal criminal cases must arise from a federal criminal statute. Civil cases can be predicated on either the residence of the parties or the body of law involved in the case. Under the doctrine known as "federal question" federal courts can try civil cases that "arise under" a federal statute (e.g., when a plaintiff complains that a collection agency violated the Fair Debt Collection Practices Act) or the federal constitution (e.g., where a prisoner

---

[2]This is not always true. Sometimes a state court can apply another state's law depending on the situation. But a state always uses its procedural law regarding how the case is tried.

[3]Although it may be tried in a magistrate court, municipal court, or some lower form of court than those where serious criminal cases are heard.

complains that getting crunchy peanut butter violates his right to be free from cruel and unusual punishment under the Eighth Amendment).

Under a doctrine known as "diversity jurisdiction" a federal court can acquire jurisdiction where the controversy involves the citizens of different states and where the amount of money at issue is more than $75,000. So, if a person living in Iowa sued a person in Missouri, they could sue in federal court if they were asking for more than $75,000 in damages. Another way that federal courts acquire jurisdiction is through "removal." Removal allows a defendant to take a case from state court into federal court if all the defendants in the action are from another state, or if the action is based on federal law.[4]

A medical negligence action is normally an action that can only be brought in state court because it is an issue of state law, committed to the jurisdiction of the state courts. Federal courts usually will not hear state medical malpractice cases unless the defendant has moved to a different state.[5] Medical malpractice generally does not arise under a federal law, although there is an exception to that rule too. Where the plaintiff makes a claim that the defendant violated the Emergency Medical Treatment and Active Labor Act, 42 USC § 1395dd, the case may be brought originally in state court, but can be removed to federal court because the federal statute is pleaded as the basis for the trial court's jurisdiction.

Federal courts can apply state laws, and state courts can apply federal laws, but how those courts decide what law to apply and the processes they engage in to make those decisions is beyond the scope of this book. Suffice it to say that no therapist ever wants to end up in either a federal or a state court.

Who Has the Ultimate Say on State and Federal Law?

While this can be a bit confusing, the state supreme courts of each and every state are the final word on what is the law of that state. If a law is passed in Kentucky outlawing a particular type of handgun, and the Kentucky Supreme Court decides that the statute violates the constitution of Kentucky, that court is the final decision-maker with respect to that issue.

---

[4]Most federal courts are not thought of as "plaintiff friendly" and usually the last thing a plaintiff wants is to take his case into federal court. Often plaintiffs will be sure to sue someone in their own state just to avoid "removal."

[5]There is an exception where the malpractice occurred at a federal facility. When a state malpractice action is filed against federal physicians or against a federal health care entity like the Veterans Administration, the action is heard in federal court pursuant to the Federal Tort Claims Act. The FTCA, however, does not permit a jury and relies instead on a federal judge.

Only the Supreme Court of Kentucky can tell us what the Kentucky Constitution and Kentucky statutes mean.

If the issue, however, concerns any federal constitutional rights, then only the United States Supreme Court has the right to make a **final** determination on the issue of law. In most cases the state supreme courts decide these issues, and only in rare instances are they reviewed by the United States Supreme Court.

Suppose the State of Kentucky passes a law limiting the rights of patients to sue for malpractice. Let's assume further that the case is tried before a circuit court, and the circuit court applies the law and refuses to let the patient sue. Let's further assume that the citizen appeals that ruling on the basis of both the Kentucky and United States Constitutions to the Kentucky Supreme Court. That court's decision that the law is constitutional under the Kentucky Constitution is made once and for all by the Kentucky Supreme Court.

Let's suppose, however, that the plaintiff challenged the law on the basis of the United States Constitution, and the Supreme Court of Kentucky held against him. He still has a right to appeal that decision (since it involves federal constitutional law) to the United States Supreme Court. If that court were to take jurisdiction of the case, and decide that the statute violated the federal guarantees of equal protection and due process, the U.S. Supreme Court's ruling would be the final word on those federal constitutional questions.

C. SOURCES OF LAW

1. What Does the Legislative Branch Do?

If you ask the average man on the street the question "who makes the laws," you would most likely get "Congress" or "The State Legislature" as the answer. Many people mistakenly think the law is made **only** by the legislature in their state, or is made **only** by the Congress in the federal system. If you believe that, sit down, take a deep breath, and relax. Your reality is about to change.

Congress and legislatures do make law, but they are not the only body of lawmakers in the state. Although it seems like a truth you've been taught since sixth grade civics class, the truth is that law is not a static creation of the legislature. And while the statement that the law is made by the legislature is true, as far as it goes, there is an entirely different area of the law that isn't

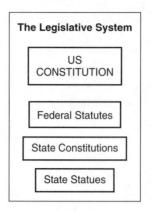

Figure 1-1 The U.S. Legislative System. The United States Constitution is supreme over all other forms of state law. A federal law valid under the constitution is supreme over the law or constitution of any state under the Supremacy Clause of the United States Constitution. The state constitution is supreme over the state statutes and any municipal ordinances.

made by the legislature or the congress that controls your daily life. That law is called "the common law."

The constitution of the state in which you live, and the United States Constitution make up the "organic" law of the United States. The United States Constitution is supreme over all the states, and the state constitutions are supreme over the individual states.

The relationship of state and federal laws can be shown graphically. See Figure 1-1.

If the state passed a law that said that convicted felons gave up their right to counsel, that law would be contrary to the Sixth Amendment of the United States Constitution, and that state law would be unconstitutional and unenforceable against a felon.

If the federal government, however, through Congress, were to pass a law that restricted access to Missouri courts, the only "organic" law that would apply would be the federal constitution, because the federal government cannot be restrained by the state governments.[6]

---

[6]The reason is that the Supremacy Clause of the federal constitution makes federal law supreme over state law whenever there is a conflict between the two.

Importantly, the concept that many people don't understand is that the act of Congress or the act of the state legislature that becomes law doesn't mean that the only place a person goes to interpret the law is that particular piece of legislation. Quite the contrary is true. Whenever the law is "tested" in the courts, the body of law that develops through interpretation becomes as important as the statute itself. This "decisional" law—that part of the lawmaking process that regards the interpretation and construction of laws passed by the various lawmaking bodies—is sometimes called "case law" and becomes the other place where "law" is "made."

Courts may announce tests that they will use in later cases to decide these issues. These tests are likely made up on the basis of the facts of the case, and are not grounded in any particular statute or regulation. Thus, while the statute may provide general guidance, to really know "what the law is," one must look at the cases to see how courts have interpreted the statute.

2. What Does the Executive Branch Do?

The executive branch of government also has a role in the lawmaking process. The executive branch is charged with approving laws sent from the legislative bodies. This form of oversight is one of the many checks and balances built into the system. But the executive branch is also charged with enforcing the law. Not only does the executive branch have the option of signing or not signing legislation, and the option of imposing a veto, but it also has considerable discretion in how it enforces the laws.[7]

Once a law is passed, the executive branches of the state and federal government, although charged with upholding and enforcing the law, do not have to do so. For example, while the Federal False Claims Act empowers the Department of Justice to investigate every claim of fraud and abuse brought to it by a whistleblower, in fact many of the claims are never thoroughly investigated, and as a result, thousands are dismissed by the federal government. This is because the executive branch is said to have "discretion" over what laws to enforce and what laws not to enforce.

---

[7]One good example here is immigration law. During the first four years of the Bush Administration the Immigration and Naturalization Service imposed fines on employers of illegal aliens only 13 times across the entire country. Obviously the statute that provides for fines for people who employ undocumented and illegal aliens is not being enforced as it was written.

The executive branch has the power and duty to set priorities about law enforcement. Under former Attorney General Janet Reno, health care fraud was the number two target of the Justice Department, right behind violent crime. Under Attorney General John Ashcroft, terrorism and terrorism prevention was the primary focus of the Justice department. Since a prosecutor has discretion about which cases to bring and which ones to leave alone, the executive branch has a great deal to do with how law gets made.

3. What Does the Judicial Branch Do?

The judiciary's role is more definite in the lawmaking process, and more pointed. "It is distinctly the province of the courts to say what the law is." When Justice Marshall wrote that in *Marbury v. Madison,* 1 Cranch 137, 163 (1803),[8] he defined the power of "judicial review" that gives courts the right to pass on whether a law violates the constitution.

Courts are entrusted to hear cases brought by adverse parties. In the criminal law system that means the state (or the "people" when the cause is brought by the federal government) is one interested party, and the defendant is another.

The adverse parties try their case in court. In court there are two kinds of fact finders. The first, and most important, is a jury. A jury is provided at common law for all cases at criminal law and most civil cases. Certain cases (like divorce cases, injunctive relief cases, cases brought against the government, and appeals) are tried to judges as the finders of fact. In every case there is a judge who is the person who applies the law to the facts.

For example, in a civil case the question may well be whether a person who ran a stop sign was negligent, and whether he caused or contributed to the cause of the damage to the plaintiff. The jury has to decide the ultimate facts (Was he negligent? Did the negligence cause the damages?). The judge has to decide the legal issues (Can the plaintiff admit the statements of the defendant after the accident?). The judge also has to apply the law to the facts that the jury finds. So if a jury finds damages of $100,000, the court must issue a judgment for that amount, unless the law requires a different result.

For example, in a car accident case in Kansas, if the jury awards damages of $5,000,000 for pain and suffering to a man rendered paraplegic by a drunk driver, the judge, without telling the jury, will reduce that amount of non-economic

---

[8]Cases from the 1800s often do not have a US or SCT citation.

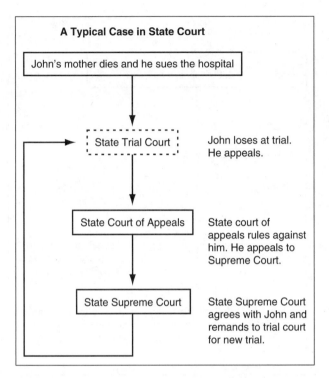

A Typical Case in State Court

John's mother dies and he sues the hospital

State Trial Court   John loses at trial. He appeals.

State Court of Appeals   State court of appeals rules against him. He appeals to Supreme Court.

State Supreme Court   State Supreme Court agrees with John and remands to trial court for new trial.

Figure 1-2 A somewhat typical case in State Court.

damages to $250,000 because that is what the law requires. That is the judge's role in the judicial system—to fairly and impartially apply the law, and to en-sure that both parties have a fair trial.

In the event one party or the other thinks the trial court made an error in how it decided issues during the case, or how it applied the law after the jury found the facts, they can appeal. The appeal is decided by a panel of judges who issue a written opinion. That opinion becomes binding precedent, and the next time a similar case comes up before the court, they may use the facts from that case to argue in favor of their position. A typical case in state court is shown in Figure 1-2.

A similar result occurs in the federal system whenever there is a trial. In most cases, a trial will result in a verdict, and that verdict can be appealed. Usually about 95% of all federal cases are finally decided (meaning, the

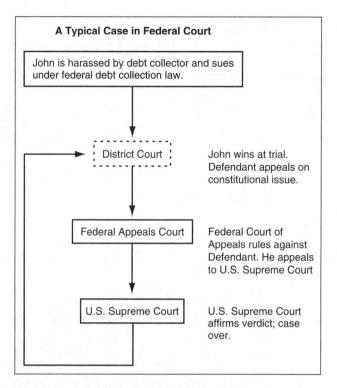

Figure 1-3 A typical case in Federal Court.

appeal ends) at the Court of Appeals level.[9] The Supreme Court of the United States is not an "error correcting" court so much as it is a court that sets binding precedent. The Supreme Court grants "certiorari" (which means a directive for the lower court to send up the file) only when the lawsuit presents an issue of great public interest or importance. For example, the election of the president in 2000 reached the United States Supreme Court from the Florida Supreme Court by virtue of its public interest and importance, and because of the impact on the federal political system. The issue of federal law decided by the Florida Supreme Court would never have merited Supreme Court review otherwise.

A typical trip through the federal court system is shown in Figure 1-3.

---

[9]There are 11 federal circuit courts of appeal, and the federal circuit court of appeals in Washington D.C.

Usually the state and federal systems operate independently of one another. The State Supreme Court, owing to the "Supremacy Clause" of the constitution, is obligated to obey the decisions of federal courts.[10] For example, when the chief judge of the Alabama Supreme Court recently refused to honor a directive from the 11th Circuit Court of Appeals, he was ignoring the Supremacy Clause. Judge Moore was directed to remove the Ten Commandments from his courtroom, and he disobeyed that federal order. The federal court enforced its order by dispatching United States Marshals to remove the statue. As federal marshals stood ready to remove the offending display, the State Supreme Court met. The State Supreme Court's other judges overruled the chief judge, and the display was moved into a closet. Ultimately, the Chief Justice was removed from the Alabama Supreme Court because he had taken an oath to preserve, protect, and defend the Constitution of the United States, and in refusing to obey an order of a superior court, he violated that oath.

Normally, the United States Supreme Court gets involved in state law cases only if there is an issue of importance involving a federal law or the U.S. Constitution. For example, if John, in the example in Figure 1-2, had appealed to the State Supreme Court on the basis of some evidentiary error made by the trial court, and the State Supreme Court held against him, the United States Supreme Court would be unlikely to hear the case on appeal because the law of evidence in the state courts is a matter of state law. However, if John had appealed because he said the trial court denied him due process of law, a federal constitutional issue, he could appeal the case to the United States Supreme Court.

Every year, literally thousands of people appeal their cases to the United States Supreme Court. Fewer than one percent reach the stage where a brief is submitted to the Court. This is because the Court does not view its role as one of correcting errors made in lower courts unless and until those courts create confusion in the law.

4. Where Can the Law Be Found?

If you frequently tire of hearing people say that "the law says . . ." and you want to prove them wrong, where do you go to find an answer? The process is complicated (in many ways, needlessly so) by the way the courts and

---

[10]Where both the federal government and the state government have passed a law relating to a particular topic (e.g., nursing home administration), the federal law is said to "preempt" the state law because the U.S. Constitution Supremacy Clause says that federal law trumps state law.

legislative systems work. The legislature passes a law. The courts cannot only declare it in violation of the constitution, they can "construe" it—or interpret it according to their views as to what is desirable or appropriate in a given situation. As facts change, the law changes. This creates issues for knowing exactly how the law might affect any particular issue.

Sometimes the legislature hasn't spoken on an issue, and the matter becomes one of "common law."

a) What Is the "Common Law"?

Before the invention of a legislative body, rules were handed down by the King and interpreted by the King's Courts. Sometimes the King's Courts were simply too harsh on the common folk, and so the Court of the Chancery developed. These chancery courts were courts of equity—or fairness—and they were more interested in reaching the right result in a situation and doing "justice" than they were in following the strictest dictates of the King.

When the United States was formed, we "borrowed" the "common law" of England, including not only the cases interpreting the dictates of the King, etc., but also, the law of equity. But the courts in the United States did not just accept everything in English law. Rather, they picked what they considered to be the best and when the courts couldn't find an English case, they simply decided the case on their own notions of fair play and justice.[11] This history of the early courts in America is rich, and well worth reading.[12] There are numerous scholarly articles on the subject.[13]

---

[11]See, e.g., Hall, The Common Law: An Account of Its Reception in the United States, 4 Vand. L.Rev. 791, 796 (1951) ("Whether we emphasize the imitation by the colonists of the practices of English local courts or whether we say the early colonial judges were really applying their own common-sense ideas of justice, the fact remains that there was an incomplete acceptance in America of English legal principles, and this indigenous law which developed in America remained as a significant source of law after the Revolution").

[12]See, e.g., Reinsch, English Common Law in the Early American Colonies, at 7 (finding that the colonists developed their own "rude, popular, summary" system of justice despite professed adhesion to the common law); C. Hilkey, Legal Development in Colonial Massachusetts, 1630-1686, p. 69 (1967) (emphasizing Biblical and indigenous sources); Radin, The Rivalry of Common-Law and Civil Law Ideas in the American Colonies, in 2 Law: A Century of Progress 404, 407-411 (1937) (emphasizing natural law and Roman law); Goebel, King's Law and Local Custom in Seventeenth Century New England, 31 Colum. L.Rev. 416 (1931) (finding that the early settlers imported the law and procedure of the borough and manor courts with which they had been familiar in England).

[13]See Jones, The Common Law in the United States: English Themes and American Variations, in Political Separation and Legal Continuity 95-98 (H. Jones ed. 1976) (Jones) (acknowledging that a true common-law system had not yet developed in the early colonial period); Stoebuck, Reception of English Common Law in the American Colonies, 10 Wm. & Mary L.Rev. 393, 406-407 (1968).

While equitable law is based on principles of fairness, common law is judge-made law. As referenced earlier, judges have the power to effectively "write" the common law. As men and machines began to dominate commerce and industry, the law adapted with it. England's common law of the 1700s knew nothing of automobiles. It understood that people hauled goods, and sometimes people, in wagons and coaches, but it could not foresee the day when someone would put a motor inside a coach and drive it along a road. The common law in the 1700s developed rules for what happened when two horse-drawn coaches collided on a street. But because those collisions were often the product of animals as much as men, the rules didn't apply perfectly to the situation of a Model T colliding with another Model T. Judges had to write those new rules relying on the old ones. Judges similarly had to adapt the rules of transportation when the first "iron horse" struck a bold path across the United States.

In short, the law that governs our relationships today, the law that protects us from assaults and batteries, that makes it possible for us to recover for our injuries after a bad car accident, and imposes liability on negligent clinicians, has arisen by the common law adapting old principles to new and changing times.

The common law will change between the time this book is written and the time it is printed. It normally changes in small ways, and every now and then, like the Massachusetts Supreme Court's decision in the gay marriage case, all at once. When the common law changes in ways that the people do not like, they are not without a remedy. When the common law must itself be changed, it is the duty of the legislative body to make that change.

But the common law is the creation of the courts, not the legislature, and courts guard their right to declare this law very jealously.

b) What Are State Statutes?

When a state legislature passes a bill, it becomes a state statute. State statutes are collected into volumes, and there is no standard numbering system between the states. Each act passed by the state legislature and signed by the Governor (or, when vetoed, when that veto is overridden) becomes a state statute and is added to the volumes. In Missouri that job falls to the Indexer of Statutes.

Almost any good law library has a collection of state statutes. A good library also maintains an "update service" and obtains changes to the statutes as they are written.

Statutes can be simple and clear or they can be wildly confusing. One would think that a state legislature could learn to write simple, short, declarative sentences, but this would be giving most legislative bodies way too much credit. The fact is that state statutes are often very confusing and often have very confusing cross-references to "this section" and "this chapter" that make reading them a very difficult exercise.

c) How Are Federal Statutes Different?

Like state statutes, federal statutes can be simple or confusing.[14] When an act is passed by the Congress and signed by the President, that act becomes an official statute of the United States. The Congressional Printing Office compiles the United States Code and places similar sections in similar chapters. For example, statutes dealing in any significant way with Medicare or Social Security are in Chapter 42. Statutes imposing criminal penalties for violations of the law are in Chapter 18. Banking is found in Chapter 31 of the United States Code, and Taxes in Chapter 26.

Like state statutes, most good law libraries have a copy of the United States Code. It can also be accessed on line at http://uscode.house.gov/search/criteria.php.

d) What Are State Regulations?

In nearly every state in the United States the Secretary of State (or some other office of the state government) is in charge of compiling a list of all the state's regulations on a given subject. The regulations governing the State Respiratory Care Board will be found in this compilation, as will the regulations setting appropriate vaccination standards and curriculum standards for public and private high schools.

Just because a state statute exists, setting out the basics of a law, doesn't mean that the state statute is the only place a person needs to look to figure out what the law says or means.

For example, in Missouri, the Merchandising Practices Act specifies what practices are deceptive and unlawful marketing practices. The Attorney

---

[14]The Federal Tax Code is found in Chapter 26 of the United States Code. Pick any section in the Tax Code and read through it. If you know what you've read when you're finished, you are in the top 0.05% of the country.

General, however, is permitted to issue regulations interpreting this law. The Attorney General's regulation says:

> *(1) Deception is any method, act, use, practice, advertisement or solicitation that has the tendency or capacity to mislead, deceive or cheat, or that tends to create a false impression.*

Thus, state regulations are the place a person goes to look to determine if the agency assigned the responsibility of enforcing a particular statute has written any guidelines to assist the public in enforcing those statutes.

e) How Are Federal Regulations Different?

Like their state counterparts, the federal regulations are the body of "interpretative law" of the federal government. When Medicare elected to go to a prospective payment system for hospital care, the statute was amended to provide basic guidelines for how hospitals would get payments.

The real work, however, was done when those statutes were turned into Medicare guidelines and regulations interpreting the statute written. The Centers for Medicare and Medicaid Services (now CMS and formerly Health Care Financing Administration) wrote thousands of pages of guidelines for how the new program would be implemented.

f) What Is the Importance of State Constitutions?

In each state the "organic law"—or the law that serves as the foundation for that state's statutes, regulations, and court decisions—is the state constitution. Most states have a specific "bill of rights" spelled out in their state constitutions, and some have dizzying methods of amendment. In some states the amendments to the constitution outweigh and outnumber the actual text of the constitution, making any principled analysis of the constitution difficult even for the most seasoned attorney.

The constitution sets out the branches of government, how the government is elected, and the relative duties and powers of the government. In Nebraska they have a unicameral legislature (in other words, only one lawmaking body instead of a senate and a group of representatives). In other states, like Louisiana, the state constitution abandons the "common law" found in other United States jurisdictions in favor of "civil law" holdings from France and Europe. How a state sets up its government is important only from the standpoint that all the citizens' rights in that state are found in that document, and are interpreted in concert with it.

g) Where Does the Federal Constitution Fit In?

The entire United States Constitution and all the amendments are found in Appendix A of this book. The Constitution is the single most important legal document in the United States. All of the rights of the citizens are in one way or another found in that document and the numerous court decisions interpreting it.

The federal Constitution is supreme. No state constitution, federal law, state law, or city ordinance may contravene the United States Constitution. The United States cannot enter into a treaty that violates the Constitution. It is the final source of law, and the bedrock upon which the United States Supreme Court issues its opinions.

If a state constitution, state statute, federal statute, municipal ordinance, or state or federal regulation in some significant way intrudes onto the ground of the United States Constitution, it is going to be void. The Federal Constitution trumps all other forms of statutory or common law.

h) Where Are Court Decisions Found?

Throughout this book, and indeed, in almost any book discussing the law, you'll find references to cases in a rather peculiar form of legal shorthand. What exactly does 323 S.E.2d 244 really mean? It means volume 323 of the South Eastern Reporter, Second Edition, at page 244.

There are several different court opinion reporter systems. Cases that appear in the state courts and state appellate courts are found in the "regional reporters." These include the Atlantic Reporter, The Northeastern Reporter, the Northwestern Reporter, the Southern Reporter, the Southwestern Reporter, the Pacific Reporter, the Atlantic Reporter, and the Northern Reporter. These are abbreviated as follows:

Reporter	Abbreviation
Southern	So.
Northern	No.
Northeastern	NE
Southeastern	SE
Southwestern	SW
Northwestern	NW

Reporter	Abbreviation
Atlantic	Atl.
Pacific	Pac.
California[15]	Cal. Rptr.

These reporters cover different dates, and some have first, second, and third series. Thus 50 S.W.3d 201 refers to volume fifty of the Southwestern Reporter, Third Series, at page 201.

In addition to the state reporters there are federal reporters. These include the Federal Supplement (F.Supp.), the Federal Reporter (F.), The Federal Rules Decisions (FRD), and the Supreme Court Reporters (U.S. or SCT). Thus, 150 U.S. 201 refers to volume 150 of the U.S. Reporter, page 201. Like the state reporters, the federal reporters have second and third series. Thus 201 F.Supp.2d 101 is the two-hundred-first volume of the Federal Supplement, Second Set, page 101.

These reporters can be found in almost any good-sized law library, and in many college and county libraries. County Courthouse law libraries also will have copies of these reporters.

5. What Happens When a Lawsuit Is Filed?

Criminal cases are discussed in Chapter 13. This section focuses on the civil law and damages lawsuits because those are the types of lawsuits most therapists are likely to face.

Lawsuits are filed by paying a filing fee and placing the documents into the court system. What happens before, during, and after a lawsuit is important to understanding the legal system and how it works.

a) What Must a Lawyer Do Before Filing?

Before any lawsuit is filed, the attorney must do a complete investigation of the facts, circumstances, and controlling legal authority in order to present a valid claim. When a bad event happens, usually the last thing people think about is calling an attorney. When they do get around to contacting a lawyer, the thing that usually brings them in is the distinctly uneasy feeling that they are not being told the whole story.

Lawyers are required by Rule 11 in the federal courts (and by similar rules of practice in nearly every other court) to initiate an investigation into the

---

[15]California has so many courts of appeals, and so many court decisions, that it has its own reporter for its cases.

claims of their client before they begin a lawsuit. The law requires that a lawyer not simply take every word of his client at face value. A lawyer must find other supporting information in order to prosecute an action on behalf of a client.

Normally an investigation means gathering the public records of the matter, and examining them. In the case of a medical liability issue, it means getting the medical records and examining them for evidence of negligence. Sometimes, however, the records do not support a finding of negligence, and the additional investigation needs to be done.

Importantly, lawyers often make decisions about cases that have absolutely nothing to do with the law or whether a patient has been the victim of negligence. Many lawyers are simply concerned with how much money the case might bring them. When a lawyer is so focused, often they will decline cases that do not meet their predefined level of damages.

Sometimes, a lawyer will find enough evidence to prosecute a negligence case, but decline to pursue it because he isn't sure he can win the case in front of a jury. In other instances, the amount of damages might be so slight that a client who wins a verdict won't have anything left over. These are sound reasons not to take a case.

But a lawyer's decision on whether to take a case starts with his investigation. After he completes the investigation, he usually reports back to the client that the case is either going forward, or is being declined.

If an attorney makes a decision to prosecute the action, the next thing he has to do is draft a petition (or, in federal court, a complaint) that sets out the basis for his client's claims against the defendant or defendants.

b) What Is a Petition or Complaint?

The petition is the heart of the case against the defendant, or, in the case of multiple parties, the defendants. The petition sets out the facts of the case, the legal theory of recovery, and the type and sometimes the amount of damages.

Beginning with the names of the parties who are suing, and moving on to the names of the parties who are being sued, the complaint or petition sets out in numbered paragraphs the who, what, when, where, and sometimes the why of the lawsuit. An example petition for Wrongful Death can be found in Appendix B-1.

In some states all a plaintiff must do is put the defendant on notice about the basic facts of the lawsuit. That is the policy of the federal courts as well. But in many state courts a plaintiff must "plead facts" that show he is entitled to relief.

c) What Is an Answer?

The defendant in a lawsuit is required to file an answer to the petition. The answer usually admits certain facts (like the name and address of the company, the names and addresses of the plaintiffs, and so forth), but denies the bulk of the petition. Most answers include one of the following statements:

- Defendant admits paragraph 9.
- Defendant denies paragraph 10.
- Defendant is without sufficient information to either admit or deny paragraph 11, and so denies the same.

Anything that the defendant admits in his answer to the petition is deemed admitted for the purposes of any trial, and the plaintiff does not need to prove that fact. Sometimes, however, a defendant won't want to file an answer to the petition, and will file a pleading that asserts a technical defense by motion.

Defendants also may plead a counterclaim (that is, a right to recover from the plaintiff, for example, on an unpaid medical bill) or a cross-claim. A cross-claim says that if the jury holds the defendant liable, it must examine the conduct of the cross-defendant to determine if the cross-defendant breached any duties to the primary defendant.

Suppose Mary Doe files a medical malpractice lawsuit against Dr. Jones. She claims that Jones did not properly supervise her care at the hospital. Dr. Jones believes that he did everything possible, but could not have foreseen that the therapist assigned to care for Mary would increase her PEEP to 25 cm H_2O and cause her to develop a pneumothorax. Dr. Jones files a cross-complaint against Our Lady of Perpetual Billing saying that if the plaintiff recovers against the doctor, then the doctor should be able to recover against the hospital.

The hospital finds that Richard Roe, the therapist who was on duty that night and set the PEEP level too high without a physician's order, has been terminated from employment. They bring a cross-claim against him stating that if they are liable, he is liable under the doctrine of indemnity. This is how cross-claims work.

Defendants also get a chance to plead any affirmative defenses. An affirmative defense is a defense that the defendant bears the burden of proof on. In other words, if the defendant proves the facts of the defense, then the defendant is entitled to judgment. A therapist's judgment is an affirmative defense. If, in the judgment of the therapist, the patient required 5 cm of

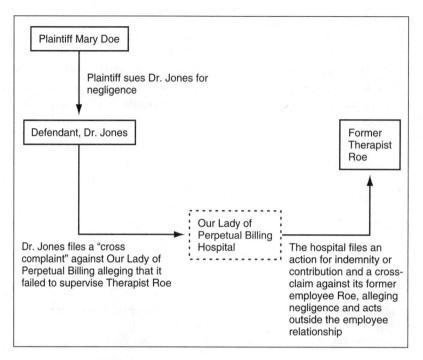

Figure 1-4 A Cross-Claim Situation

PEEP, but unknown to the therapist the patient had a pneumothorax, the exercise of judgment—even though later facts showed that judgment to be wrong—is protected by "the judgment defense." The therapist has the burden of pleading any affirmative defenses.

An example Answer to a Petition is found in Appendix B-2.

d) What Is Discovery?

Discovery is open and equal access to the facts and witnesses under rules that permit both sides to keep their legal theories secret, but disclose the evidence they intend to present.

It may seem unfair to make the sides give away the evidence that they plan to use at trial. But the policy behind it is a sound one. Ninety-five percent of cases settle before trial because discovery shows up the weaknesses and strengths of the various cases.

Trial attorneys have several tools they use to discover information about the other side's case. Interrogatories are written questions that must be answered under oath by the other side. Requests for Production are made under the rules and require a party with access to, or control over, a document to turn that document over to the other side. Depositions are long examinations taken under oath and recorded by a court reporter for the purpose of finding out what a witness knows about a particular case. In cases where a piece of property or a location is involved, attorneys may request to inspect and photograph the area.

Most of the legal wrangling in a case occurs in discovery. Discovery battles sometimes become so heated that lawyers lose their common sense. When that happens, courts step in and impose rules that limit the attorney's behavior.

(1) What Are Interrogatories?

Interrogatories are used by trial attorneys to get a baseline of information about a party and to use that information to find other information. They usually contain instructions for answering, and then, in numbered paragraphs, sometimes with subparagraphs, ask the answering party a series of questions under oath. For an example of interrogatories see Appendix B-4.

(2) What Are Requests for Production?

Requests for Production are used by trial attorneys to get records and other tangible information. For example, the plaintiff may want the original medical records, and the defendant may want to inspect the part of the airplane that plaintiff says failed. They usually contain instructions for answering, just like interrogatories and then, in numbered paragraphs, sometimes with subparagraphs, ask the producing party to provide information. For an example of Requests for Production see Appendix B-5.

e) What Is the Purpose of a Deposition?

Depositions are interrogations under oath in front of a court reporter. They are conducted under rules different than those of a court of a law. A lawyer can ask a question in a deposition that he could never ask in a court of law (for example: Have you ever been arrested?). There is no judge present, so the questions are taken down by the court reporter along with the objections made by the lawyers. If the court rules on the objection at some later point in time, the court can either allow the question to be heard by the jury, or strike it from the deposition.

The idea behind a deposition is to get the witness committed to the story they are going to tell at trial, and to try and find out what information they knew and what information they didn't. Depositions can be used at trial if the witness doesn't show up, or in some cases, if the witness dies before trial. In some cases they are taken before the patient even files a lawsuit. An example deposition is found in Appendix B-7.

f) What Are Motions for Summary Judgment?

A motion for summary judgment is a request to the court to rule on the case on the legal issues instead of the factual issues. The trial court judge is responsible for ruling on the legal matters, and if there is a disputed issue of fact, must send the matter to the jury.

In a motion for summary judgment the issues are usually complex. Normally a defendant will ask for summary judgment on the issue of liability based on a failure of the plaintiff to prove some fact it claims is necessary to the case. The plaintiff may move to eliminate certain defenses. The court decides if the evidence is sufficient to let the case move to a jury trial. That is the entire purpose of a motion for summary judgment.

g) What Happens in a Jury Trial?

Ultimately, of course, the goal of every trial lawyer is to be ready for the day when it becomes necessary to walk into the courtroom and try the case to a civil jury.

Like the pre-trial area, trials contain a variety of stages and steps that have a very different impact on the end result.

(1) What Is Jury Selection (Voir Dire)?

Voir dire literally means "to speak the truth" and it has come to be known among trial lawyers as the most important part of the trial. Legal commentators on CNN, Fox News, and ABC all agreed that the selection of the jury in the OJ Simpson case was the turning point in that case. When a jury can be selected that contains the same biases as one of the parties, generally that party has the advantage.

In voir dire the lawyers have a chance to inquire of the jurors about their biases, prejudices, and feelings. They find out if the jurors know any of the parties, and if they have any biases or prejudices that will keep them from deciding the case fairly. An excerpt from *voir dire* can be found at Appendix B-8.

(2) How Does Plaintiff Submit His Case?

In the plaintiff's case the plaintiff lays out his case against the defendant. The plaintiff's case begins with an opening statement, sometimes mistakenly called "opening argument" by the media. The opening statement is not supposed to contain any argument. Rather, it is a road map to the plaintiff's case. The plaintiff states what he intends to prove, and how he intends to do that.

Opening statement is mandatory, and failure to make an opening statement that includes all the elements of the plaintiff's case can result in dismissal of the lawsuit. So opening statement is something that lawyers spend a lot of time preparing.

Next, the plaintiff examines its witnesses. Plaintiff's counsel brings the witnesses to the stand and examines them carefully. Frequently this means that the plaintiff will get the opportunity to examine the defendant directly about his or her failures in the case.[16]

(3) How Does Defendant Submit His Case?

Technically, the defendant does not have to put on a case. He gets the right to cross-examine during the plaintiff's case, and if the plaintiff has not proved his case, the defendant can stand on the evidence in the case and ask the jury for a verdict.

In most cases, however, the defendant produces its own witnesses and examines them under oath so as to help the jury understand the issues in the case. If it has pleaded an "affirmative defense" in its answer, it may have to prove those issues to prevail in front of the jury, and so the defendant will have an opportunity to present its witnesses and tell its story when its turn comes.

(4) Does Plaintiff Get Rebuttal?

After the defense presents its case the plaintiff gets a chance at rebuttal and may call additional witnesses to challenge the defense version of

---

[16]Unlike a criminal trial, where a defendant has a right not to testify, in a civil trial the defendant has no right not to testify. While the defendant may invoke his Fifth Amendment rights if his testimony will likely result in revealing matters that will result in his being charged with a crime, any answer he gives using the Fifth Amendment may be considered an admission of the ultimate fact by a civil jury.

things. At the close of this testimony, the parties prepare to argue their cases to the jury.

(5) What Are Jury Instructions?

After the last of the evidence has been submitted, if the court determines that the plaintiff has made a submissible case, the court instructs the jurors on what facts they must find in order to bring in a verdict for one side or the other.

These "jury instructions" are written based on the law and are designed to help jurors decide the case.

(6) What Is Closing Argument?

In closing argument the party with the burden of proof (plaintiff in civil cases, state in criminal cases) gets to go first. It lays out its case and argues about what happened and why. Normally courts are constrained to limit closing argument to no more than one hour, although in certain exceptional cases, or cases where volumes of evidence have been submitted, the time may be longer.

Once the plaintiff finishes, the defendant has an opportunity to refute the arguments of the plaintiff and argue for no verdict against his client. Once the defense rests, then the plaintiff (or the state in criminal cases) gets one more chance to rebut what the defendant said on closing. Then the case is submitted to the jury.

(7) What Happens in Jury Deliberation and Who Renders the Verdict?

When the jury decides the case, they issue a verdict, and that verdict lays out not only whether a party is liable or not, but if they are, how much the damages are. In some cases the trial court may cut back that amount if a proper after-trial motion is made.

h) How Do Appeal Procedures Work?

If one party or the other is aggrieved by the judgment, they can take an appeal to the court of appeals, or, in some instances, directly to the state supreme court. If the case is tried in federal court, the appeal goes directly to the Circuit Court of Appeals.

The appeals court asks for a copy of the trial transcript (all the testimony given, including the objections that were made) and a copy of the legal file (all the documents filed with the court during the trial and before). It then asks for "briefs" written by lawyers discussing the relevant points of law applicable to the case. These briefs may be short or they may extend for hundreds of pages in complex litigation.

If the case is heard at the intermediate court of appeals (or the Circuit Court of Appeals in the federal system) there is still an appeal to the state supreme court (or United States Supreme Court in the federal system). Once those courts decide the issue, however, the case is final.

D. KEY POINTS

- There are two court systems in the United States.
- The federal court system is primarily for enforcing federal criminal laws and for certain specific types of civil lawsuits.
- State courts enforce state laws.
- Sometimes state and federal courts have overlapping jurisdiction.
- A state supreme court is the final word on state law; the United States Supreme Court is the final word on federal law.
- The role of the courts is to say what the law is.
- The role of the legislature is to write statutes.
- The role of the executive branch of government is to enforce the law and to set priorities for how cases are brought and handled.
- The plaintiff must begin his case with an investigation.
- The investigation is for the purpose of determining if the case has a factual and legal basis.
- After investigating, the plaintiff may file an action in state or federal court.
- The defendant either may answer the petition or may file motions to dismiss or other "pre-trial" motions.
- The case proceeds next into discovery where both sides share information about the other, and about the strengths of their case.
- At some point before trial there may be an attempt to settle the case.
- 95% of all cases settle before trial.
- When a case cannot settle, there may be "dispositive motions" like Summary Judgment filed.
- If the case goes to trial it begins with jury selection.
- After jury selection parties make opening statements.
- After opening statements evidence is presented by the plaintiff, and later, by the defense.

- The case is submitted to the jury and the jury judges the facts.
- The judge applies the law and renders a judgment.
- If one party or the other is unhappy with the outcome they can appeal.
- Appeals courts decide cases and make binding precedent that has the force of law.
- Appeals courts construe the statutes and regulations, and have the power to declare statutes unconstitutional.
- Lawyers are important and protect the legal rights of clients by understanding the legal system and using the protections built into the system to benefit clients.

E. SUMMARY

There are federal and state courts. Federal courts tend to apply federal law, and hear only certain types of cases. State courts are capable of hearing cases under both state and federal law. Whether a case is brought in federal or state court, the law they apply comes from several sources:

- United States Constitution (supreme over all other law)
- Federal Statutes (supreme over state statutes and state constitutions)
- State Constitutions (supreme over state laws)
- State Statutes (provide the law that governs in a particular state)

State court systems may also have district and municipal courts that are inferior to state courts that handle things like traffic tickets and small claims, but those courts are beyond the scope of this book.

While legislative bodies like state legislatures and congress may write statutes, how those statutes are applied, interpreted, and construed varies with the facts of each case. Each case is set down and recorded so as to serve as precedent for cases that follow.

CHAPTER 2

The Essential Guide to Patient's Rights

"Above all, our nation must develop uniform national standards so that health plans can compete on quality, not just cost; and so that health care consumers can judge for themselves. This is the best way to assure quality health care for all Americans."

President Clinton, March 13, 1998

A. INTRODUCTION

Patients are the reason therapists exist. It is the patient who comes through the hospital door and asks for care that determines the assignments and activities of the Respiratory Care or Cardiopulmonary department.

An understanding of the legal consequences of medical error, as well as an understanding of some of the basics of health care law begins with an analysis of the patient and her rights in her own health care. This chapter sets out those rights a patient has under both the state and federal law that governs health care. It examines the sources of common law rights, and the specific rights that are provided by statute.

Rights—as opposed to privileges—are entitlements that every person has simply by virtue of their existence. The founding fathers expressed them broadly as the rights to life, liberty, and the pursuit of happiness. The Constitution attempted to identify the important ones in the Bill of Rights, but remembered to set out that rights not enumerated were nonetheless retained by the people. The United States Supreme Court has held that there are certain rights that exist by virtue of "penumbras" in the Constitution.

These penumbral rights (penumbra means "the gases of the spirit") are rights usually created or set apart by court decisions (see Chapter 1). One of those rights is the right to privacy, from which the right to refuse medical treatment originates.

This chapter looks at the rights of patients. It examines the rights of the patient in the context of health care.

B. WHAT ARE THE SOURCES OF HEALTH CARE RIGHTS?

Every person has basic human rights—what Thomas Jefferson called the right to "life, liberty, and the pursuit of happiness." Those rights are natural rights that every man and woman has. In addition to those natural rights, the Constitution gives each person additional rights. Some of those rights are set out in the Bill of Rights (see Appendix A) as well as the other amendments to the Constitution.

In addition to the rights guaranteed under our system of "ordered liberty" every patient has specific statutory rights that arise either out of federal or state law. The problem is, most patients do not know what they are. As a result, they do not ask for information or assistance to help them gain those rights, unless and until a lawyer steps in and advises them that their rights were violated.

Because lawyers may view a deprivation of rights, even an unintentional deprivation, as a serious matter, it is important for therapists to know what rights a patient has. If a lawyer alleges you violated them, you could be on the hook for damages.

C. WHAT IS THE CONSUMER BILL OF RIGHTS?

The Advisory Commission on Consumer Protection and Quality in the Health Care Industry was appointed by then President Clinton on March 26, 1997, to "advise the President on changes occurring in the health care system and recommend measures as may be necessary to promote and assure health care quality and value, and protect consumers and workers in the health care system." As part of its work, the President asked the Commission to draft a "consumer bill of rights" for health care.

This "consumer bill of rights" is a good starting point for a discussion of individual patient rights. The rights enumerated in the Committee's report are not the only rights a patient has. But they are an important starting point in analyzing patient rights.

1. What Is a Patient's Right to Information Disclosure?

Every patient should have access to his own information about his health care condition. That basic right is what allows patients to make informed decisions.

In putting together their recommendations, the President's panel suggested that all consumers have the right to know the level and extent of specialty preparation of each of their primary caregivers. Most informed health care consumers know whether their physician is board-certified or not, and how much general experience the provider has. The document stops short of mandating the disclosure of information, but simply states that consumers have a right to know the information.

As such, the government suggested that disclosure was voluntary, and not mandatory. In other words, if a patient asks his provider about the level and extent of training he has, that provider should give a truthful answer. But the provider is under no duty to volunteer the information to the client.

Similarly most state and federal laws that mandate information disclosure to patients do so as a voluntary act with but a few exceptions. The Health Insurance Portability and Accountability Act, HIPAA, mandates that health care providers disclose certain information to all patients, including the information that the patient may have a surrogate decision-maker, and that the patient may designate those who can receive information about the patient's care. Only HIPAA truly _mandates_ a disclosure of any particular information to the patient. Most other statutes merely state that the patient should be informed.

New York State stands alone as an important exception to that rule. Public Health Law (PHL) 2803 (1)(g) Patient's Rights, 10NYCRR, 405.7,405.7(a)(1), 405.7(c) mandates nineteen specific rights for a hospital patient in New York State. Among those rights are the right to:

- Understand and use the statutory rights. If for any reason you do not understand or you need help, the hospital MUST provide assistance, including an interpreter.
- Receive treatment without discrimination as to race, color, religion, sex, national origin, disability, sexual orientation, or source of payment.
- Receive considerate and respectful care in a clean and safe environment free of unnecessary restraints.
- Receive emergency care if you need it.

•••

- A no smoking room.
- Receive complete information about your diagnosis, treatment and prognosis.

• • •

- Refuse to take part in research. In deciding whether or not to participate, you have the right to a full explanation.
- Privacy while in the hospital and confidentiality of all information and records regarding your care.
- Participate in all decisions about your treatment and discharge from the hospital. The hospital must provide you with a written discharge plan and written description of how you can appeal your discharge.
- Review your medical record without charge. Obtain a copy of your medical record for which the hospital can charge a reasonable fee. You cannot be denied a copy solely because you cannot afford to pay.

New York's statutory requirement goes beyond simply giving the patients certain rights. It mandates disclosure of these rights to the patient, and provides a booklet for hospitals and health care providers to use in informing patients about these rights.

The law provides that patients have a right to make decisions about their care. But those decisions can only be made when a caregiver provides proper information to a patient about the clinical situation, and provides enough information for the patient to make an informed choice. This is the doctrine of informed consent.

2. What Is "Informed Consent" and Why Does It Matter?

The doctrine of informed consent played a major role in one of the most important patient's rights cases ever decided by the U.S. Supreme Court. In *Cruzan v. Director, Missouri Department of Health,* 497 U.S. 261 (1990) (see Appendix C-3), the Supreme Court held that the right to bodily integrity was one of the many basic rights that were so fundamental that they did not need to be spelled out in the Constitution.

The doctrine of informed consent means that a patient must be told sufficient information to make a reasonable choice about the procedure. That means that they must be told not only the benefits, but any risks or potential harms that may come to them as a result. The law requires that all the information a reasonable person would want to know about the procedure must be given for the consent to be considered "informed."

3. What Is a Consumer's Right to Choose a Health Care Plan?

The President's Commission wanted to make sure that patients and their family members knew what kinds of choices they had in health care. The general concept of the Bill of Rights was to encourage choice in health care decision-making. Although this Bill of Rights includes the right to choice, from a practical standpoint it is a right without many teeth attached.

Consumers are, more often than not, wedded to the health plan chosen by their employer, and most of those plans obtain savings and discounts primarily by using particular physicians, hospitals, and laboratory services. A plan member still has "choice" in that he or she can use any hospital and any physician they choose. In most cases, however, the health care plan penalizes the use of non-plan providers by capping the amount paid at 70% or 80% of the bill, leaving the consumer to pick up a sizeable portion of the bill. As a result of this economic disincentive, most plans effectively leave the individual consumer with little real choice.

4. Does a Patient Have a Right to Emergency Care?

One place where a consumer frequently has little choice is in the area of emergency services. Ambulances frequently take patients to the closest medical facility and, as a result, many patients don't get to choose where they go. Each patient has a right to receive emergency care under both the common law and a special federal statute, the Emergency Medical Treatment and Active Labor Act (EMTALA). (See Appendix I.)

5. What Is EMTALA?

The Emergency Medical Treatment and Active Labor Act, 42 USC § 1395(dd) was a statute passed by Congress after the CBS News program 60 Minutes ran a story about patient dumping in Texas hospitals. The 60 Minutes story was cited in the Congressional Record and in several cases interpreting the statute as the reason Congress passed the law. That statute provides, in relevant part, as follows:

42 USC Sec. 1395dd   **Examination and Treatment for Emergency Medical Conditions and Women in Labor**

(a) Medical screening requirement

In the case of a hospital that has a hospital emergency department, if any individual (whether or not eligible for benefits under this subchapter) comes to the emergency department and a request is made on the individual's behalf for examination or treatment for a medical condition, the hospital must provide for an appropriate medical screening examination within the capability of the hospital's emergency department, including ancillary services routinely available to the emergency department, to determine whether or not an emergency medical condition (within the meaning of subsection (e)(1) of this section) exists.

(b) Necessary stabilizing treatment for emergency medical conditions and labor

(1) In general

If any individual (whether or not eligible for benefits under this subchapter) comes to a hospital and the hospital determines that the individual has an emergency medical condition, the hospital must provide either—

(A) within the staff and facilities available at the hospital, for such further medical examination and such treatment as may be required to stabilize the medical condition, or

(B) for transfer of the individual to another medical facility in accordance with subsection (c) of this section.

Congress passed the Emergency Medical Treatment and Active Labor Act to deal with what used to be (and in some locations, still is) a common problem in hospital care. Certain hospitals (predominantly those serving wealthier, white communities) were "dumping" their uninsured or underinsured patients on community hospitals that were obligated to treat everyone. This dumping took the form of refusing admission or care to patients without insurance or means of paying for treatment. As a result patients died or suffered serious complications that could have been prevented by emergency medical treatment.

Congress' response to this patient dumping problem, as discussed in the case just referenced, is to require that a hospital that offers emergency medical services must provide a basic screening examination, and stabilizing treatment within the abilities of the hospital.

Under EMTALA, the screening exam must be sufficient to detect life-threatening conditions, but the degree of examination is limited by the capabilities of the hospital. Thus, if a patient presents at the emergency room of a 45-bed community hospital with chest pain, the degree of his screening examination offered to detect an emergency medical condition might well be basic vital signs and a 12-lead EKG, particularly where the hospital does not have a 24-hour laboratory that can run emergent cardiac enzymes.

On the other hand, a patient presenting at a 350-bed community hospital would most likely be entitled to the same examination but with access to emergency cardiac enzymes, chest radiography, and other basic emergency testing.

EMTALA has spawned a great deal of litigation because it does not adequately define many of the terms it uses (like "screening examination") and terms that it does define are not defined in a workable manner. For example, EMTALA defines "stabilized," but courts have added their own unique twists to what that term means.

EMTALA provides important statutory rights precisely because patients can sue for damages if they are denied access to health care. It is important for health care professionals to be aware of EMTALA's many provisions and the ways the courts have enforced the rights under EMTALA.

6. Does the Patient Get to Participate in Treatment Decisions?

The principle behind EMTALA and the New York State statute mandating information disclosure is to guarantee meaningful access to health care. In order to be meaningful, patients must not only understand their rights, and the information their health care providers give them, but they must be able to act on that information and make their own informed decisions about patient care.

Every person has a right to control what happens to them, within certain limits. The contours of the right of autonomy, or the right to participate in health care decisions as defined by the President's Commission, should be fairly easy to discern, but they are not. There are few hard and fast rules in the law, but from cases and decisions we can make certain judgments.

Autonomy means the ability to make decisions about what happens to you, and each patient has that right. Patients can, however, lose that right under certain conditions. For example, a competent individual facing a diagnosis of lymphoma can make the principled decision not to receive treatment for the disease, even though the normal course of the disease will claim his life. He has the right to refuse treatment.

Generally a patient has the right to control his or her own destiny, and make decisions about his or her treatment unless one of the following conditions exists:

- He is unconscious.[1]
- He is declared mentally incompetent.
- He presents a danger to himself and others and requires immediate psychiatric treatment.
- He is unable to communicate his or her desires.
- He is under age 18 and his parent consents to the treatment.

A patient of sound mind may lawfully refuse treatment. That means a patient who is of sound mind and who doesn't want to receive a nebulizer treatment can refuse it. A therapist presented with such a refusal should be sure to document it.[2] Under no circumstance should the clinician press forward and try to "muscle" a treatment onto a weak or debilitated patient. That is battery.

Mike is an 8-year-old who presents to the Emergency Room with aphasia, drooling, high fever, and crowing respirations. The ER physician orders an IPPB treatment. A therapist places a mask over the patient's face, and begins the treatment. The patient resists forcefully, and the mother asks the caregiver to stop. "I have to follow doctor's orders," says the therapist.

Does a physician's order trump a patient's right to self-determination? Absolutely not; unless the patient is considered incompetent and has been so declared by competent authority, they retain their right to refuse care. In the case of a minor, that right can be asserted only through a parent or guardian. In the case above, the therapist stopped after a few more breaths when the patient voided on him out of abject fear. The patient was ultimately trached for epiglottitis, and a large malpractice verdict was thereby narrowly avoided.

7. What Is an Advanced Directive?

Simply put, an advanced directive is a guideline that allows health care team members to know a patient's wishes and to act on them. Unfortunately, the advanced medical directive is subject to abuse and manipulation. Many

---

[1]Keep in mind that a living will or a durable health care power of attorney may provide a means of the competent individual expressing an opinion about treatment even when he or she may be unconscious. However, to have effect, the caregiver must know of the documents.

[2]A frequent defense in medical negligence cases is that the patient was not compliant with the plan of care, and that any harm, if it resulted at all, resulted from the negligence of the patient in not complying with the plan of care. For this reason any time a patient refuses care, the clinician should document it.

nursing homes automatically request that patients be labeled as Do Not Resuscitate, a form of making an advanced directive. In so doing, the nursing homes often equate this non-resuscitation order with a non-treatment order, and these patients die, not from a natural disease process, but from neglect and dehydration.

In furthering the patient's right to autonomy, perhaps the most underused tool is the "advanced directive."[3] Although federal regulations now require hospitals to discuss advanced directives, lawyers have done a poor job of assisting most clients in preparing for the process of making important health care decisions.

All high risk surgical and medical patients, particularly those with chronic obstructive pulmonary disease, should be instructed to bring a health care advanced directive with them anytime they come to the hospital, and some thought should be given to having them file one with the hospital Medical Records department in order to ensure it is always available.

There are two types of advanced directives. A living will[4] merely states the patient's wishes with regard to health care decisions. A living will may suggest to health care providers under what circumstances the patient might want advanced cardiac life support, mechanical ventilation, and other invasive treatments furthering hydration and nutrition. It may also suggest when it would be appropriate to withhold these things.

Importantly, the living will is not binding on anyone, including a physician. As a statement of the patient's intent, the physician may still feel free, using his best judgment, to act in a manner contrary to the patient's expressed wishes. For this reason it is important for patients to discuss this document with their physician and get that physician's commitment to follow the document, if that is the only document they care to execute.

8. Can a Patient Let Someone Else Decide for Them?

Often patients can look down the road, particularly in a case of a terminal disease, and know that at some point they will not be able to make decisions on their own. When this occurs, they can and often do appoint someone else to make decisions for them. But the durable power of attorney—the

---

[3]For purposes of simplicity, we use the term "advanced directive" as a catch-all for documents that are designed to inform health care providers or empower friends or relatives to make health care decisions. Advanced directives include living wills and durable powers of attorney for health care.

[4]A poorly named document that is in fact nothing like a will.

document that provides for a surrogate decision-maker—should not be thought of as simply a tool for managing terminal illness. Every hospitalized patient should have such a document in the event of an emergency.

a) What Is a Durable Power of Attorney?

A "power of attorney" involves two people: the patient (or principal) and the surrogate decision-maker (or agent). Because the power of attorney gives the agent the power to act as though they were the principal, and generally, to do anything that the patient might lawfully do for himself, these powers must be carefully drafted and even more carefully assigned. This is especially true for the **durable** power of attorney for health care.

A power of attorney is durable if it survives the incompetency (but not the death) of the principal.[5] A durable health care power of attorney allows an individual named in the document to make health care decisions on behalf of the principal, even if those decisions will ultimately bring about the death of the principal.

An important limitation of a durable power of attorney (or any power of attorney, for that matter) is that the agent can only act on behalf of the principal in accordance with the principal's wishes. So, for example, if a durable power of attorney gives the agent power to write checks on the principal's account, that power can only be exercised with the permission of the agent.

The agent is in what is called a "fiduciary" relationship with the principal. The agent must carry out the principal's instructions, and may not act for his or her own behalf. Thus if the agent uses the power of attorney to loot the incompetent person's bank account, they have breached their duty, and may be subject to a lawsuit.

b) What Is a Guardianship or Conservatorship?

While a durable health care power of attorney is an important tool, it is not the end of the discussion when it comes to patient autonomy. A guardian is more or less a court-appointed durable power of attorney, except that every-

---

[5]At common, law powers of attorney expired whenever a principal became unable to revoke the power. The law, to protect those who might be abused by errant relatives, stated that a power of attorney could not be used when the patient was not able to consent to its continued use. The legislative response was to create the "durable" power of attorney, which outlasts the incompetence of the principal. All powers of attorney, however, expire on the death of the principal, and no person may act on behalf of a decedent under a power of attorney.

thing the guardian does must be approved by the court that appoints him. The guardian has the power to make health and welfare decisions. A conservator is an individual who is charged with preserving the financial assets of the patient.

If a clinician suspects that a patient is being abused, neglected, or improperly denied medical care by either a power of attorney or an individual acting as the health care decision-maker, they have an option. Almost every state court system has a provision that allows an "interested party" (in this case, most likely the hospital) to file a petition for guardianship.

c) How Do I Get an Advanced Directive?

Although a health care power of attorney or a living will cannot always forestall the problems that erupt among relatives, an advanced directive can be used to focus all the parties on what the patient really wants. They are a good first step in unifying the family when end-of-life decisions must be made.

There are several good ways to get one. The best way is to see an attorney and have the document drafted for your individual and special needs. This means a document that limits the powers of the person holding the power of attorney to only those powers necessary to carry out the tasks. Some durable powers of attorney are too broad, giving access to business records and receipts, financial institutions, and stock accounts. The person making health care decisions may not need this access, or may wrongly take advantage of it.

If an attorney cannot be found to draft such an instrument, many state bar organizations have Advanced Directives available. A copy of the free form available from the Missouri Bar is shown as Appendix D. Note there is no guarantee that this form would be suitable in any other state.

In addition to the above, several pieces of software assist the layman in drafting a durable power of attorney for health care or advanced directive. The most powerful of these is Broderbund's *Family Lawyer,* available for $29 direct from the manufacturer. While only a lawyer can draft a durable power of attorney or living will for someone else, the *Family Lawyer* program lets individuals draft their own, at considerable savings, and purports to be valid in each of the fifty states.[6]

---

[6]Neither the author nor the publisher recommends any software for any particular use or purpose. The most satisfactory way to have a durable power of attorney or any other legal document prepared is to see an attorney in your jurisdiction.

9. Can Health Care Providers Discriminate?

Adhering to patients' wishes (within the bounds of ethics), providing them with accurate and understandable information, and ensuring that they have adequate access to emergency procedures regardless of their ability to pay, and regardless of their race, religion, or skin color, are more than simply goals. They are federal law.

No therapist makes a determination of whether to treat a patient on the basis of sex, religion, color, or national origin. But sometimes hospitals or private clinics might engage in such behavior. When they do, they could find themselves subject to litigation.

Hospitals are at special risk because of the Hill-Burton Act. Hill-Burton provided funds to hospitals in order to help them build and expand. In return it required that the hospitals provide certain amounts of indigent care. Although most hospitals now no longer accept these funds, in many states they may still be bound by the Act.

In 1994, voters in California approved Proposition 187, a ballot measure that was intended to deny to illegal immigrants many government services. One of the governmental services that the drafters of that proposition had in mind to deny was health care. Proposition 187 included language that forbade hospitals from providing publicly funded health care, but did so in a particularly badly drafted way. In *League of United Latin American Citizens v. Wilson*, 908 F.Supp. 705, the federal district court in California struck down the denial of health care services to Hispanics and illegal immigrants saying it violated federal law.

In short, any denial of health care predicated on someone's age, sex, religion, skin color, national origin, or immigration status is a violation of the basic right to access for health care.

10. What Rights Does a Patient Have to Confidentiality?

There are few rights more precious and more sacrosanct than the right of a person to keep information about their medical condition private. Every therapist is expected to respect the wishes of the patient and maintain his or her medical confidences.

a) What Are the Basic Rights to Confidentiality?

The President's Commission set out the sixth right to health care privacy as follows:

I. Confidentiality of Health Information

Consumers have the right to communicate with health care providers in confidence and to have the confidentiality of their individually identifiable health care information protected. Consumers also have the right to review and copy their own medical records and request amendments to their records.

Although the statement above brings together most of the rights a patient has under state and federal law, those rights have greater force under the Health Insurance Portability and Accountability Act, or HIPAA.

b) What Is HIPAA?

When Congress passed the Kennedy-Kassebaum HIPAA statute, the aim was to improve information privacy in the emerging field of electronic medical records. Under regulations published by Health and Human Services related to the Health Insurance Portability and Accountability Act, new standards were implemented and the field of medical privacy became needlessly complicated. HIPAA established some statutory definitions and goals related to the privacy of medical information, and let HHS set the regulations governing access to health information. The result has been to create a full employment act for health care lawyers.

The volumes of regulations under HIPAA are so complex and so deeply cross-referenced that their discussion here in terms of the statutes or the actual language used would be beyond the scope of this text. Suffice it to say that HIPAA creates certain medical privacy rights.

c) HIPAA Patient Protections

The new privacy regulations ensure a national uniform standard of privacy protections for patients by limiting the ways that health care providers can use a patient's personal medical information. The regulations protect medical records and other individually identifiable health information, whether it is on paper, in computers or communicated orally.

Access to Medical Records. Patients should be able to see and obtain copies of their medical records and request corrections if they identify errors and mistakes. Health plans, doctors, hospitals, clinics, nursing homes, and other covered entities generally should provide access to these records within 30 days and may charge patients for the cost of copying and sending the records.

Notice of Privacy Practices. Covered health plans, doctors, and other health care providers must provide a notice to their patients how they may use personal medical information and their rights under the new privacy regulation. Doctors, hospitals, and other direct-care providers generally will provide the notice on the patient's first visit following the April 14, 2003, compliance date and upon request. Patients generally will be asked to sign, initial, or otherwise acknowledge that they received this notice. Health plans generally must mail the notice to their enrollees by April 14, 2004, and again if the notice changes significantly. Patients also may ask covered entities to restrict the use or disclosure of their information beyond the practices included in the notice, but the covered entities would not have to agree to the changes.

Limits on Use of Personal Medical Information. The privacy rule sets limits on how health providers may use individually identifiable health information. To promote the best quality care for patients, the rule does not restrict the ability of doctors, therapists, and other providers to share information needed to treat their patients. In other situations, though, personal health information may not be used for purposes not related to health care, and covered entities may use or share only the minimum amount of protected information needed for a particular purpose. In addition, patients would have to sign a specific authorization before a covered entity could release their medical information to a life insurer, a bank, a marketing firm, or another outside business for purposes not related to their health care.

Prohibition on Using Medical Information for Marketing. The final privacy rule sets new restrictions and limits on the use of patient information for marketing purposes. Pharmacies, health plans, and other covered entities must first obtain an individual's specific authorization before disclosing their patient information for marketing. At the same time, the rule permits doctors and other covered entities to communicate freely with patients about treatment options and other health-related information, including disease-management programs.

Stronger State Laws Control. The new federal privacy standards do not affect state laws that provide additional privacy protections for patients. The confidentiality protections are in addition to any state law providing privacy protections. Those laws would still apply. When a state law requires a certain disclosure—such as reporting an infectious disease outbreak to the public health authorities—the federal privacy regulations would not preempt the state law. All Confidential Communications Protected. Under the privacy rule, patients can request that their providers take reasonable steps to ensure that their communications are confidential. For example, a patient could ask a doctor to call his or her office rather than home, and the doctor's office should comply with that request if it can be reasonably accommodated.

Consumers May File Complaints. Consumers may file a formal complaint regarding the privacy practices of a covered health plan or provider. Such complaints can be made directly to the covered provider or health plan or to HHS' Office for Civil Rights (OCR), which is charged with investigating complaints and enforcing the privacy regulation. Information about filing complaints should be included in each covered entity's notice of privacy practices. Consumers can find out more information about filing a complaint at http://www.hhs.gov/ocr/hipaa or by calling (866) 627-7748.

d) Health Plans and Providers

The privacy rule requires health plans, pharmacies, doctors, and other covered entities to establish policies and procedures to protect the confidentiality of protected health information about their patients. These requirements are flexible and scalable to allow different covered entities to implement them as appropriate for their businesses or practices. Covered entities must provide all the protections for patients cited above, such as providing a notice of their privacy practices and limiting the use and disclosure of information as required under the rule. In addition, covered entities must take some additional steps to protect patient privacy:

Providers Must Maintain Written Privacy Procedures. The rule requires covered entities to have written privacy procedures, including a description of staff that have access to protected information, how it will be used, and when it may be disclosed. Covered entities generally must take steps to ensure that any business associates who have access to protected information agree to the same limitations on the use and disclosure of that information.

Providers Must Provide Employee Training and Privacy Officer. Covered entities must train their employees in their privacy procedures and must designate an individual to be responsible for ensuring the procedures are followed. If covered entities learn an employee failed to follow these procedures, they must take appropriate disciplinary action.

Providers May Comply with Public Responsibilities. In limited circumstances, the final rule permits—but does not require—covered entities to continue certain existing disclosures of health information for specific public responsibilities. These permitted disclosures include: emergency circumstances;

identification of the body of a deceased person, or the cause of death; public health needs; research that involves limited data or has been independently approved by an Institutional Review Board or privacy board; oversight of the health care system; judicial and administrative proceedings; limited law enforcement activities; and activities related to national defense and security. The privacy rule generally establishes new safeguards and limits on these disclosures. Where no other law requires disclosures in these situations, covered entities may continue to use their professional judgment to decide whether to make such disclosures based on their own policies and ethical principles.

Equivalent Requirements for Government. The provisions of the final rule generally apply equally to private sector and public sector covered entities. For example, private hospitals and government-run hospitals covered by the rule have to comply with the full range of requirements.

What does HIPAA really mean for health care providers? Under the Health Insurance Portability and Accountability Act (HIPAA), patients have certain rights to their medical information, and have the right to designate who sees that information. Most hospital admission forms allow all employees with a patient care mission to see the patient's medical record. However, a patient may withhold that permission in some cases. Of course, if a patient were to withhold that permission, the hospital might have a reason to refuse further treatment. Providing information to someone not designated to receive it can result in civil and sometimes criminal penalties.

Consider, for a moment, a physician who posts a chest radiograph on the internet discussion list aimed at his colleagues. The film itself does not contain any identifying data. However, the discussion of the radiograph and the illness contain enough information to identify a particular hospital where the patient was admitted, the general age and sex of the patient, as well as her particular diagnoses. Is the physician treading on dangerous ground?

Certainly a chest radiograph is a part of the medical record, and is protected from disclosure to persons without an interest in the management of the patient. Publishing the information, if it leads to a breach of the patient's privacy, can be problematic.

For this reason whenever a therapist discusses a patient in an online forum, the therapist should either have the patient's permission, or alternately, not release any information from which the patient might be identified.

Another right not commonly known, but included in HIPAA, is the patient's right to examine and correct her medical records. Under HIPAA, a

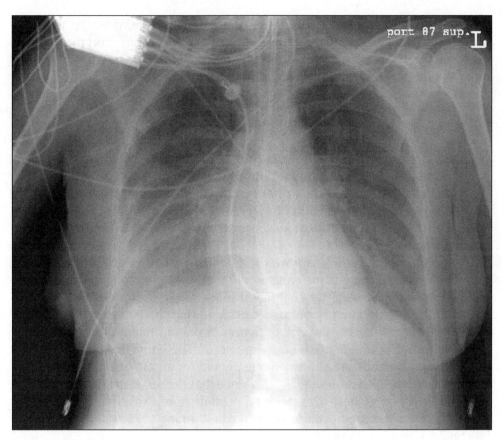

Figure 2-1 Chest radiograph published on an internet listserv.

consumer can require a health care provider with incorrect information in its files to show a correction. For example, if incorrect patient history information is included in a file, showing that one of the patient's parents had tuberculosis, the patient can demand that this error be corrected. HIPAA provides guidance on how this right is enforced.[7]

---

[7]See http://www.aldewitt.com/book%20links.htm

HIPAA privacy rights also protect confidential communications in a hospital environment. A patient retains the right to receive and send mail, and to do so privately. A hospital patient may consult with an attorney while still a patient, and has the right to participate in religious ceremonies.

11. Does a Patient Have a Right to Be Protected from Harm?

Hospital patients are, by their nature, somewhat helpless. A patient in a hospital may not be able to protect himself from assault or battery. A patient may not be able to protect his or her family members. Hospitals are under a duty to protect the patient from known harms, and harms that could reasonably be anticipated. The duty arises because of a special relationship between hospitals and their patients.

In *Young v. Huntsville Hospital,* the plaintiff was admitted to the hospital for treatment of kidney stones and while there, was sexually assaulted. She sued because the hospital was negligent in its failure to protect her from sexual assault. The Alabama Supreme Court held that the general rule was that *"absent special relationships or circumstances,* a person has no duty to protect another from criminal acts of a third person." The court noted that while it was "difficult to impose liability on one person for an intentional criminal act by a third person," that there was "evidence that the relationship between the hospital and Young here was a 'special relationship or circumstance' that would except this case from the general rule." *Young v. Huntsville Hospital,* 595 So.2d 1396 (Ala. Sup. Ct. 1992).

Hospital patients must be protected because they are weak, frail, helpless, and in a dependent condition. Hospitals must take special care to safeguard infants and children from harm by third persons, and especially, from abduction. Although there are few reported cases arising out of infant abductions, the negative publicity alone is enough to destroy a hospital. All hospital employees should be exceptionally vigilant in patient care areas and should report to security any person who does not appear to belong in the institution.

12. Can Hospitals Restrict Visitation?

Hospitals do not have the inherent right to restrict visitation of patients, subject, of course, to the security qualifiers above. An incompetent patient may need a guardian to make visitation decisions. However, it is the patient, generally, who has the right to say who may visit.

A hospital, however, may impose certain time, place, and manner limitations on visitors and patients for the good of the staff and other patients. Said another way, the patient's right to freedom of association and autonomy stops at the end of her airway. If they are an infection hazard, or if they are behavior-disordered and present a hazard to other patients, their right and ability to move about in the hospital may be limited.[8] A hospital may limit the number of visitors to protect a patient, for example, in the ICU. A hospital may limit the amount of time visitors may visit, again, to protect the patient. An institution might well place manner of visitation restrictions, requiring visitors to gown, mask, and glove before being admitted to visit a patient. And the patient may himself be limited in his movement if he presents an infection hazard or a hazard to others.

13. Can Hospitals Employ Restraints?

One of the most significant rights a patient has is personal liberty, and thus any restriction on that liberty by virtue of restraints is examined very carefully by the courts. Federal regulations restrict the use of restraints to short periods with physician orders. When restraints are used, the least restrictive environment possible is supposed to be employed. This is due to the government's concern that patients not have their liberty restrained without sound medical indications.[9]

Federal law requires a physician's order for the placement of restraints, but it does not stop there. If a physician gives an order for restraints, that order must be based on some rationale described in the medical record that clearly sets out the basis for the restraint. The physician is also required to review the decision to impose restraints every 24 hours and to remove them as soon as possible.

For example, suppose a patient is intubated and there is some fear that the sedated and confused patient will extubate himself if his hands are not restrained. The physician can write an order for hand restraints for 24 hours and can renew that until the patient is extubated. After extubation there would be no further need for the restraits.

---

[8]42 CFR § 483.10 provides that residents in nursing facilities have the right to visitation by family members and clergy on a 24 hour per day, 7 day per week basis.

[9]This policy is not all bad. Attorneys used to bring lawsuits because of a facility's failure to restrain a patient who suffered injury. "Failure to restrain" cases are now defended by reference to the federal regulations that prohibit restraints without specific reasons.

14. Do Special Rules Apply in Mental Health and Nursing Home Settings?

In many states, patients or residents in mental health or nursing facilities have special rights in health care enumerated in statutes. While it is beyond the scope of this text to list them all, any therapist providing care in the mental health or nursing home setting should take care to investigate the rights of these residents in order to ensure that they do not violate them. Violating patients' rights in these settings can result in civil penalties from the state, criminal prosecution, and, of course, significant verdicts in civil court.

15. Can Patients Be Awarded Punitive Damages for Violations of Their Health Care Rights?

No discussion of patient rights would be complete without a discussion of the one major way that courts and lawyers have of enforcing patient rights. Punitive damages are awarded to a plaintiff when there is clear and convincing evidence of evil motive or reckless indifference to the rights of a patient.

In recent years, some states have tightened up on when punitive damages can be awarded to a patient in a medical negligence case. Some states, like Missouri, require a finding by the jury that the actions of the defendant were "tantamount to intentional conduct" that caused harm. In other words, no matter how negligent a person might be in health care, unless their conduct was so dangerous and reckless as to be the equivalent of an intentional act meant to harm a patient, punitive damages would not be recoverable.

But certain statutes, particularly those aimed at nursing home care, do permit punitive damages for the violation of patient rights. These statutes are meant to ensure that patients are treated with care and respect. Unfortunately, these statutes can be turned against a provider.

Whenever an act of a therapist might be said to go against the basic rights set out in this chapter, particularly where the conduct is particularly egregious, there is a danger of punitive damages being awarded to the plaintiff. For this reason therapists must never be permitted to substitute their judgment for the judgment of the patient. If the patient refuses a therapy, that must be documented, but as long as the patient is competent, they have the absolute right to terminate or limit the care they receive. When a therapist proceeds to place a mask over the face of a restrained patient and administer medication to the patient without his consent, that therapist is committing a battery. Battery is an intentional tort. If the therapist admits that they knew

the patient had a right to refuse therapy and that the therapist simply substituted her judgment for the judgment of the patient, half of the battle is already won for punitive damages because the therapist has admitted to a
reckless disregard of the patient's rights.

This is true even though the therapist might be motivated by what she believes is the best interest of the patient. She may not want to cause harm; she
may want to prevent it. Her motivations could be completely pure. It would
not matter, however, if the patient had the right to refuse the care. There
would still be a reckless disregard at issue.

16. What About a Disagreement with a Surrogate?

Suppose Baby Jones comes into the hospital and suffers a cardiac arrest following surgery that requires her to be on mechanical ventilation. She is doing well on a mechanical ventilator, and, as a minor, does not have a written
living will. Her mother, Sue Ann, is responsible for making her health care
decisions.

Suppose there is a disagreement between the clinicians and the mother who
is the surrogate decision-maker. What is a therapist to do? The therapist
knows that the patient should remain on the ventilator and is a viable candidate to wean. The family member says "No," and tells you to disconnect the
ventilator or she will bring assault charges. Other family members indicate
she may have postpartum depression, and they are not sure she is acting in
the child's best interest. What does a principled therapist do in this situation?

Her first step is to contact hospital counsel, and to seek a court order appointing a guardian. The second step is to document all the interactions and
set forth your rationale for continuing the treatment. Documentation should
clearly indicate what you are doing and why you are doing it.

Keep in mind that in some states a parent may be guilty of child abuse by
not providing medical treatment. In situations where the issue arises out of a
health care power of attorney, remember that the durable power of attorney
may not activate until a physician declares a patient to be incompetent to act
in their own capacity. If there has not been a physician certification, and the
power of attorney requires one (see Missouri's form, Appendix D, as an example), then you can lawfully refuse the durable power of attorney's order
and act on your patient's last expressed wishes.

Also, unless a patient is adjudged mentally incompetent, or is so easily
seen as such that the issue is not seriously in doubt, the hospital must honor
the patient's wishes, not those of the holder of the durable power of attorney.

The person appointed under the durable power of attorney is an agent, and the person appointing them (the patient) is the principal. The principal always has the right to make the decision, but may give that right away. *If the wishes of the appointed agent and the principal differ, the wishes of the principal control.*

D. WHAT RIGHTS DO THERAPISTS HAVE IN ETHICAL DECISION MAKING?

Just as patients have rights in making end-of-life decisions, clinicians also have rights. A guardian or patient cannot compel a physician or clinician to take an action that the clinician believes is ethically or legally impermissible. A therapist has a right to refuse such an order.

For example, assume Sally is an 80-year-old woman who has suffered a myocardial infarction and, during code blue procedures, was intubated. She is still in mild cardiogenic shock, and requires ventilatory assistance. The family is summoned to the hospital and tells the attending physician that their mother "never wanted to be kept alive on a machine." The attending physician orders the respiratory therapist to extubate the patient and place her on a non-rebreather mask.

The therapist believes the patient is viable, can be weaned from the ventilator in a day or less, and would suffer a terminal insult if the ventilator was removed. What should the therapist do?

The therapist should address his medical concerns with the attending physician. If the physician insists, the therapist should also insist on calling in the medical director of Respiratory Care. The medical director and the attending can deal with the issues and can reach a decision about whether to extubate the patient.

In seeking help from the medical director, the therapist should try to engage the wishes of the patient. If the patient is awake and alert, her wishes, and not the wishes of her family must be followed.[10]

If the medical director and attending both agree to remove the endotracheal tube, the therapist is not without recourse. As an "interested person" he

[10]Many clinicians mistakenly believe that they must adhere to the wishes of the power of attorney even when those wishes clash with the wishes of the patient. The power of attorney has no more power than the patient (principal) gives her. A power of attorney may be terminated at any time, and no specific formalities are required to terminate it. If a patient expresses a wish different from her power of attorney, it is the patient's wish that controls. Only a court-appointed guardian may make decisions that go against the wishes of the patient, and usually only with court approval.

can seek a court order of guardianship in order to stop the extubation. This is probably not a practical solution at 2:30 in the morning, however.

A therapist does have the right, however, not to participate in health care interventions that he finds morally repugnant, religiously prohibited, or ethically improper. He has the right to refuse to carry out such an order, but he may not interfere or obstruct the physician from performing the tasks the physician orders done.

Refusing to carry out a physician's order, however, may have implications for job security. When refusing to carry out an order, a legal basis and a religious basis are often sufficient to justify that the clinician was doing what they believed to be proper. While most hospitals would not fire a therapist for refusing to take action that was morally, religiously, or ethically questionable, such terminations have occurred. Therapists should document as thoroughly as possible the reasons for their refusals in an incident report.

The bottom line: therapists should never refuse to carry out an order of a physician or a superior unless there is a real and substantive ethical issue at stake. Simple preferences, or an unwillingness to provide care to a particular class of patient do not constitute to an ethical concern.

E. KEY POINTS ON PATIENT RIGHTS

This chapter has highlighted more than a few patient rights. Most of these rights are rights every therapist knows and respects. It is important to remember these key points about patient rights:

- Patients have the right to autonomy unless they are declared incompetent or may inflict harm on others.
- Autonomy means the ability to make reasoned decisions about a person's own health care.
- Patients have the right to consent to care, to refuse to consent to care, and to later withdraw that consent.
- Clinicians may not override a patient's refusal to consent, so long as that patient is conscious and competent.
- Patients have the right to associate freely so long as doing so will not harm them or another patient.
- Patients have the right not to be restrained unless there is a sound medical rationale and the decision to restrain is reviewed every 24 hours.

- Patients have a right to have their decisions about end-of-life care respected, and to designate in advance who will make their health care decisions.
- Patients have the right to receive accurate, timely, and truthful information about their care.
- Patients have a right to expect that clinicians will protect their medical privacy and that information communicated in the privacy of the patient relationship will stay private.
- The rights patients have to privacy, autonomy, and information can be enforced in the courts.
- Patients have a right to emergency medical screening when they present in the Emergency Room.
- They cannot receive different screening on the basis of their ability to pay, or other factors than any other patient would receive.
- If a patient has a medical condition and that condition is not stabilized, the hospital cannot transport the patient to another facility unless the patient consents.
- If there is a difference of opinion between a clinician and a surrogate decision-maker (agent for health care), a clinician may have an obligation to seek appointment of a guardian if the agent is not acting in the best interests of the patient.
- If there is a difference between the agent and the patient, the patient, unless declared or adjudged incompetent, is the person with the final say.

CHAPTER 3

What Every Therapist Needs to Know About Contracts

"A verbal contract isn't worth the paper it's written on."

Samuel Goldwyn (1882—1974), Goldwyn's Law of Contracts

A. INTRODUCTION TO CONTRACTS

1. Why Are Contracts Important to Therapists?

Every therapist, at some point in her life, will sign a contract. It may be an employment contract, it might be a loan contract, or it might simply be an application for car insurance. Contracts are a routine part of business in nearly everyone's life, and they are not always obvious. For this reason, it's important to understand contract law and what a contract is and isn't.

Lawyers define a contract as "a promise that the courts, on breach of that promise, will impose a remedy on the breaching party." Like most legal definitions, it doesn't tell the average person very much. But then, that is the purpose of this chapter. Contracts are important in health care law because at one level or another all hospitals and health care entities enter into contracts. Hospitals contract for goods and services. Individuals enter into employment contracts. In the normal course of business, every hospital, health care provider, and business entity enters into some form of enforceable agreement. How those contracts are made, what those contracts contain, and how those contracts are enforced can often spell the difference between success and failure for health care business ventures. They can also affect the careers and lives of health care workers. Therefore, an understanding of basic contract law is essential for therapists.

B. WHAT IS A CONTRACT?

1. What Are the Elements of a Contract?

In order for a contract to exist there must be an offer, an acceptance, consideration, and a meeting of the minds.[1] As stated, a contract is an agreement that, upon breach, a court will impose a remedy. Contracts can be formal written instruments extending for multiple pages, or they can be handshake agreements between neighbors reached over the back fence.

There are no magic words and no magic forms that establish a contract. If all the elements exist, a contract is formed. The existence of a contract, however, does not always mean that the contract can be enforced.

One of the things that non-lawyers find galling about the law is that there is rarely a clear answer. For every situation in the law where the law lays down a rule, there are exceptions. Here, although the words necessary to form a contract have been said, Moe could say there wasn't a contract because he was only joking with Curly. In other words, Moe could simply say there never was a "meeting of the minds." Contract law, however, is rarely so simple as the made-up hypothetical examples lawyers use to discuss the principles.

A full explanation of contract law would exceed the volume reserved in this text. Because there are multiple rules dealing with oral contracts that do not apply to written contracts, this text will focus on written contracts. This is because most contracts between business entities are written as a matter of good business.

As stated earlier, in order to form a contract, there have to be four things. There must be the extension of an offer, and that offer must be accepted. In addition, there must be "consideration" for the contract. Finally, there must be a meeting of the minds—that is, both parties must agree about what they are doing. It is the actions, and not the intentions or suppositions of the parties, which determine whether or not there is a contract and the terms of the contract.[2]

In addition to an offer, the acceptance of that offer, and consideration supporting the agreement reached, an additional and always essential element of a contract is that the parties have the legal capacity to contract.[3] That means that the parties must be of legal age, must be competent mentally to enter into a contract, and must be in charge of their affairs (meaning, for ex-

---

[1]*Chisholm v. Ultima Nashua Industrial Corp.*, 834 A.2d 221 (N.H. 2003).

[2]*L.B. v. State Committee of Psychologists*, 912 S.W.2d 611, 617 (Mo.App.1995).

[3]For more information on this subject refer to 17A Am.Jur.2d Contracts § 23, at 51 (1991); Restatement (Second) of Contracts § 12(1) (1981).

ample, that they do not have a guardian or conservator who is appointed by the court to make contractual decisions for them). A contract signed by someone who is not of legal age is void, as is a contract signed by a person not mentally competent to enter into a contract.

2. What Is an Offer?

All contracts must contain mutual assent. That is, both persons must agree to the promises made in the contract. This mutual assent is usually given through an offer and acceptance. An offer is a "manifestation of willingness to enter into a bargain, made so as to justify another person in understanding that his [or her] assent to that bargain is invited and will conclude it."[4] Courts look for the existence of an offer objectively, not subjectively. That means that a court considers not whether a party actually believes they have made an offer, but rather, whether a reasonable person would believe that an offer has been extended on the basis of the statements made or the actions taken.

The test for an offer is whether it induces a reasonable belief in the recipient that he or she can, by accepting the offer, bind the other person. That means the offer has to be definite. If an offer is not definite, there is no intent to be bound. "How about I sell you some of my land," is not a definite offer. "Would you like to buy my lower forty acres for $1,500 an acre," however, is a definite offer. Once a party communicates an offer to a third person, and a reasonable person would believe that by accepting the offer, the person making it would be bound to perform, the element of "offer" has been satisfied.

3. What Is an Acceptance?

A binding contract also requires acceptance of the offer.[5] Acceptance is the second prong of mutual assent. Acceptance can be accomplished in a number of different ways. A person may either accept the offer verbally, or they may accept the offer by performing, if some performance is requested in the offer.[6] An offer that invites an acceptance by performance is deemed accepted by such performance unless there is a manifestation of intention to the contrary.[7]

---

[4]See Restatement (Second) of Contracts § 24.

[5]See 17A Am.Jur.2d Contracts § 66, at 91.

[6]It is established law that an acceptance, unless otherwise specified, may be communicated by any means sufficient to manifest assent. 1 Corbin on Contracts, 1963 Ed., s 67, p. 275; American Law Institute, Restatement of Contracts, ss 61, 64, pp. 67, 70.

[7]Id. § 100, at 117.

If Shemp offers Moe five hundred dollars to paint his house, Moe can accept the offer either by agreeing verbally to paint the house, or by actually painting the house. In either instance once the assent is given verbally, or the first brush stroke is applied to the building, there exists a contract between the two parties.

Courts generally look at the conduct of the parties in determining whether an offer has been accepted or rejected.

4. What Is Meant by Consideration?

The third element necessary and essential for a contract to exist is the element of consideration. Consideration essentially means an exchange of either something of value or a promise.

Courts have stated as a general rule that "consideration" as the term is used in legal parlance, regarding simple contracts, consists of some benefit or advantage to the promisor, or some loss or detriment to the promisee.[8] It has been held that "there is a consideration if the promisee, in return for the promise, does anything which he is not legally bound to do, or refrains from doing anything which he has a right to do, whether there is any actual loss or detriment to him or actual benefit to the promisor or not."[9]

Consideration is an important concept in a contractual relationship. Both sides have to either give or receive something for a contract to exist. A contract cannot be all one-sided.

None of the elements of a contract have to be spelled out in writing (unless required by the Statute of Frauds). As long as a court can look at the facts and determine that there is evidence that the parties intended to reach an agreement, the court can enforce that agreement.

5. What Is a Meeting of the Minds?

A meeting of the minds occurs when the parties to a contract agree on the things they want to accomplish, and on the ways they choose to accomplish them. Thus, if there is a contract to power-wash a house for $50, and the par-

---

[8]See, e.g., the following cases: *Exum v. Lynch,* 188 N.C. 392, 125 S.E. 15; *Cherokee County v. Meroney,* 173 N.C. 653, 92 S.E. 616; *Leaksville-Spray Institute v. Mebane,* 165 N.C. 644, 81 S.E. 1020; *Findly v. Ray,* 50 N.C. 125.

[9]17 C.J.S. 426. *Spencer v. Bynum,* 169 N.C. 119, 85 S.E. 216; *Basketeria Stores v. (Public) Indemnity Co.,* 204 N.C. 537, 168 S.E 822; Grubb v. (Ford) Motor Co., 209 N.C. 88, 182 S.E. 730. *Stonestreet v. (Southern) Oil Co.,* 226 N.C. 261, 37 S.E.2d 676; *Bank (of Lewiston) v. Harrington,* 205 N.C. 244, 170 S.E. 916.

ties both agree that a power-washer will be used to carry out this task, there is a meeting of the minds.

Frequently parties say there was not a meeting of the minds when there is an issue regarding enforcement of the contract. This is especially true in situations where the parties to a lawsuit settle their lawsuit and then, for whatever reason, choose to avoid a settlement agreement. When they do, they frequently claim that because there was a mutual mistake, they did not bargain for what they received.

In a recent case, clients involved in a business dispute agreed to settle their claim in exchange for a dismissal of a state court case. Specifically excluded from the settlement were all claims related to patent law. Before the settlement could be finalized a dispute arose when one party sued the other party under the patent laws, and brought a claim that the other party thought it had extinguished by its settlement. In arguing that there was no settlement agreement, the defendant essentially alleged that there had been "no meeting of the minds." Eventually the defendant dropped this claim and settled the litigation.

C. MUST CONTRACTS BE IN WRITING?

Some contracts are in writing because they must be, and some are in writing because it makes good business sense. How do you tell the difference? Contracts to buy houses, contracts to buy capital equipment, and similar contracts are written out every day both by lawyers and by business-savvy business people. A contract doesn't need magic words to be enforceable.

Sometimes, however, a contract is reached in principle, on the basis of a handshake or the word of the promisor, and that creates a binding contract just as surely as if the contract was in writing.

Two rules of law apply to contracts and the need to be in writing. The first is the Statute of Frauds, and the second is the Parol Evidence Rule.[10]

1. What Is a "Statute of Frauds"?

The Statute of Frauds is a state statute that requires that certain contracts, to guard against fraud and perjury, be in writing. The Kentucky statute of frauds says:

No action shall be brought to charge any person:

---

[10]This is pronounced pah-role, like parole from prison, not like a word that rhymes with Carol.

(1) For any representation or assurance concerning the character, conduct, credit, ability, trade, or dealings of another, made with intent that such other may obtain thereby credit, money, or goods;

•••

(6) Upon any contract for the sale of real estate, or any lease thereof for longer than one year;
(7) Upon any agreement that is not to be performed within one year from the making thereof;
(8) Upon any promise, agreement, or contract for any commission or compensation for the sale or lease of any real estate or for assisting another in the sale or lease of any real estate; or . . .

•••

In essence the statute says that certain contracts must be in writing, and must be signed by the person that the plaintiff wants to enforce the contract against. Thus a lease in Kentucky for more than one year can't be oral, and neither can a contract to sell land. Both of these must be in writing.

That does not mean, of course, that the entire contract must be a master work of draftsmanship prepared by the largest law firm in the state. Rather, it means that some writing must exist showing the essential terms of the deal. Under Kentucky law, a contract for sale of land could be very simply written:

I, John Doe, agree to sell my 50 acres of bottom land known as the Doe Run Farm, located on Highway 36, to Fred Roe, in exchange for $5,000 to be paid to me on or before July 1, 2005. On July 1, 2005, I will vacate the premises and turn over possession.

As long as both John and Fred sign the document, the contract is a binding document. No special forms or magic words need exist.

Of course, a party only gets the rights they bargain for, so a contract for sale should be drafted by an attorney, and reviewed by the attorney of the seller, in order to avoid problems later on. This is because the parties may want to provide what happens if one party fails to perform (if the buyer fails to pay, or the seller fails to vacate). The parties may want to allocate the risk of loss during the period between sale (the day the contract is signed) and closing (the day the loan is funded and possession changes). These are important contingencies because houses do burn down, and as in Florida, hurricanes do come blowing through.

2. What Is "The Parol Evidence Rule"?

The Parol Evidence Rule is a rule of law that forbids the introduction of evidence that contradicts the terms of writing on a contract. If the contract says "Joe agrees to pay $100 . . ." and Joe has signed that agreement, Joe can't offer testimony that he really meant to only pay $10.

The parol evidence rule is justified on the basis of two premises: (1) a written document is more reliable and accurate than fallible human memory, and (2) varying written terms by testimony of interested parties opens the door to perjury.[11] "It is not a rule of evidence. In a proper case for the application of the rule, even if the parol evidence be received without objection, it must be ignored."[12] "The writing itself becomes and is the single and final memorial of the understanding and intention of the parties."[13]

That doesn't mean the rule always applies. For example, if Joe wanted to testify that when he signed the document, the handwritten number had been $10 instead of $100, that might well be different since the testimony there doesn't contradict the contract so much as prove the fraud (if any) that existed.

Similarly, the rule is liberally applied by the courts in many cases, and the tendency is for courts to do "the right thing" and admit that evidence that will aid them in determining the issues.

D. HOW DO COURTS LOOK AT CONTRACTS?

While courts do not require that contracts be in writing, most contracts are written contracts. "In contractual interpretation, the primary rule is to ascertain the intent of the parties and then give effect to that intent. When there is no ambiguity in the contract, the intent of the parties is to be gathered from [the contract] alone."[14]

The reason courts look to the written contract is that they want to find out what the parties intended, and the clearest evidence—the evidence least susceptible to change—of what the parties intended is in their written document.

---

[11]*Poelker v. Jamison,* 4 S.W.3d 611, 613 (Mo.App.1999).

[12]*Commerce Trust Co. v. Watts,* 360 Mo. 971, 231 S.W.2d 817, 820 (Mo.1950).

[13]*Ibid.*

[14]*Marshall v. Pyramid Development Corp.,* 855 S.W.2d 403, 406 (Mo.App. W.D.1993).

1. Why Is Intent Important?

Why is intent so important? Because without knowing the intent, the court can't fashion an appropriate remedy. Contracts are normally written so that all the important terms are found within the document itself. In some jurisdictions a contract containing blank forms is considered unenforceable. When a court is asked to "construe" the contract, or apply the terms inside the contract to a particular fact situation, it must determine, from the language used in the document, how the parties intended to deal with the issue. But of course, contracts, being written by fallible humans, sometimes have clauses that seem to cancel one another out.

The goal, however, is always to give effect to what the parties intended when they reached their agreement. In doing that, courts look at the words used in their common and ordinary meaning, unless the parties to the agreement have defined their terms differently:

> *Contracts are to be construed according to the sense and meaning of the terms which the parties have used. Words in a written contract are to be interpreted according to their common, ordinary, and usual meaning.*[15]

In addition to the general rules set out above, courts have the power to apply special rules in special settings in order to reach the right result. If a contract fails to specify a date for delivery of a product, the courts will interpret that as requiring delivery at a reasonable time. If the parties are firm in their agreement, courts are apt to interpret their agreement to "do justice" and justify the expectations of the parties.

Sometimes, however, parties reach vague and indefinite agreements. When the parties reach an agreement, it must be definite and certain to be enforceable. Thus, for example, an agreement to agree in the future is not a contract. Courts do not require exact language, merely language that is clear and can be understood to have a definite meaning.

Sometimes agreements are complete and understandable when they are written, but later events cause the parties to be uncertain about the meaning of certain words. In these instances the courts step in with a series of special rules to guide the interpretation of contracts.

When a contract is clear, only the words of the contract can be used by the court to decide the issues. A complete and unambiguous contract in

---

[15]*West v. Ankeny,* 134 N.E.2d 185 (Oh. Ct. Comm. Pl 1956).

writing cannot be varied or contradicted by what the courts call extrinsic evidence.[16]

2. What Does Ambiguity Really Mean?

What is an ambiguous contract? It is a contract that is susceptible to two reasonable but different constructions. *Yerington v. La-z-boy Incorporated*, 124 S.W.3d 517 (Mo. App. S.D. 2004). In other words, if a contract can be read to mean two different but equally plausible things, it is ambiguous.

When a court finds an ambiguity in a contract, it will receive evidence of what the parties intended so as to clear up the ambiguity. *Wolf v. Superior Court*, 114 Cal.App.4th 1343, 8 Cal.Rptr.3d 649, (2004). In addition, another rule of contractual interpretation comes into play when a contract is ambiguous. That rule places responsibility for any ambiguity on the party who drafted the agreement, and that the ambiguity is construed against the drafter.[17] This rule, which is a rule that courts routinely use to reach the right result in contract cases, requires a person drafting a contract to be precise and specific in order to avoid being penalized later if the contract needs interpretation.

E. WHAT CONTRACTUAL REMEDIES DOES A PERSON HAVE?

When people suffer the breach of their contract they may have many remedies, or they may have only a few. As a general rule, so long as the contract provides for remedies, and those remedies do not in some way go against the settled law, then those remedies are what the injured person may use to enforce the contract.

Contracts frequently spell out what happens if one party or the other doesn't honor their obligations. Most automobile purchase contracts, or contracts for automobile loans, include a clause that requires the losing party to pay the attorney fees in the event any collection action is necessary.

Below we'll discuss the remedies that a person has when a contract is breached.

---

[16]"Extrinsic evidence" would be evidence obtained by asking the parties, under oath, what they intended when they signed or negotiated a contract. This is not permitted under most state laws. See State ex rel. *Missouri Highway and Transp. Com'n v. Maryville Land Partnership*, 62 S.W.3d 485, 489 (Mo.App. E.D.2001).

[17]See *Webb v. James*, 147 F.3d 617, 623 (7th Cir.1998).

1. Breach of Contract

Just as the parties in drafting an agreement may specify what it is they intend to accomplish, they can similarly spell out what happens in the event of breach. Not only can the contract lawfully set out what remedies are available, the parties can agree on where the lawsuit will be tried, what state's law is to be applied, and whether to submit to some form of alternate dispute resolution.

The remedies set out in contracts generally are of two forms: legal and equitable. Legal remedies usually center around the payment of money. Equitable remedies usually focus on acts that are to be taken by certain parties.

2. How Are Money Damages Calculated?

Damages are limited to what the injured party would have realized if the deal had been properly consummated. Complicating matters, parties to a contract have a duty, under the law, to "mitigate" their damages. They cannot intentionally take action that makes their damages greater (for example, a therapist could not claim breach of an employment contract with employer A, and refuse to take a new job with employer B so as to increase his damages in his suit against employer A).

In addition to economic damages, sometimes a person who breaches a contract may be liable for incidental or consequential damages.[18] Suppose a promoter pays an arena $50,000 for the right to hold a concert at the state fairgrounds, and on the eve of the concert, the entertainer cancels. The entertainer is not only responsible to pay for the lease of the arena, he may also be responsible for the loss of profits and any damage to the promoter's reputation that came about as a result of his breach.

3. What Is "Specific Performance"?

Sometimes no amount of money will compensate for the breach of a contract. This is especially true where the contracted item is something like a particular piece of property. It is also true when an executive or similar employee goes to work for a competitor and takes business contacts and trade secrets with him. One way of enforcing the contract (in addition to liquidated

---

[18]Under the Uniform Commercial Code regulating contracts for the sale of goods, incidental and consequential damages are not permitted, except in very limited circumstances.

damages clauses, discussed later) is for a court to order an injunction that forbids the employee from working for the competitor. Injunctive relief and other court orders to do or refrain from doing something are called "equitable remedies" because they do not call for a party to pay legal damages and because they are based on the principle of fairness.

When a person buys real property, that particular piece of property has value above and beyond the amount of money paid for it. There is only one property that has the attributes of that piece of property. Since the land is unique, the only thing that can make the person trying to buy the land "whole" if the seller breaches his contract is the equitable remedy of "specific performance" or simply put, a court order to complete the sale of the property.

Specific performance, however, arises in more than just real estate cases. For example, where a person agrees not to compete with a former employer, and breaches that promise, a court may, through specific performance, compel the person to honor his agreement. Sometimes that agreement takes the form of an injunction.

4. What Are Liquidated Damages?

A liquidated damages clause is a way of looking at a situation in advance and saying "it would be hard to measure the damages, so we agree that $X represents the amount of damage for a breach of this agreement." Normally these clauses are contained in personal services contracts where the value of the services might be hard to estimate.

Liquidated damages clauses are also common in contracts that require the completion of a project by a certain date (for example, for every day the building is not finished, contractor pays $100). They are likewise common in real estate and property purchases, where, for example, if a buyer cannot get financing he forfeits his earnest money as "liquidated damages for lost sales opportunities."

But courts will not enforce liquidated damages clauses where the clause is not designed to compensate for damages, but rather, to inflict a penalty on the other party for breach (or for partial breach) of the contract.[19] Courts

---

[19]In what must seem like a really bad idea to most folks, the doctrine of freedom of contract says that contracts are encouraged, and that a party should be free to breach a contract as long as he is willing to be responsible for the consequences. One basis for this rule is that where parties disagree, it is better to sever a business relationship than be in a situation where violence might erupt.

traditionally encourage freedom of contract, and so are willing to enforce a reasonable liquidated damages clause, but are unwilling to enforce penalties because they are against public policy.

When is a liquidated damages clause a penalty rather than a true damages clause? In analyzing such a case, a court would look first at whether the amount of the liquidated damages would be a reasonable approximation of the harm, and whether the amount of damages might be truly difficult to measure. Does the amount of liquidated damages reasonably approximate the amount of damage that one party would sustain if the other breached its agreement? If not, the clause is more likely a penalty than a true liquidated damages clause.

5. Can a Contract Provide for an Injunction?

Another equitable remedy available in contract actions is an injunction. An injunction is an order from the court to a party telling them to do something (take down a fence built on a neighbor's land, for example), or requiring that they stop doing something (stop parking their commercial vehicle in a particular subdivision).

Injunctions are not limited to contract cases, but are sometimes used to enforce contractual rights. In order to get an injunction, a party must show irreparable harm if the court does not grant relief. So, for example, where the issue was one of money damages, and the damages would simply get larger if the injunction were not entered, the trial court won't enter the injunction.

On the other hand, if Joe worked for Sam and knew all of Sam's trade secrets, his going to work for Sam's competitor might cause the disclosure of hundreds of trade secrets that would seriously damage Sam. In this instance a court would likely grant an injunction, provided that the contract provided for one.[20]

F. ARE WARRANTIES CONTRACTS?

Warranties (offered with the sale of new or used goods) are contracts. When General Motors promises to fix your car within the first 36 months or 100,000 miles, that is a binding promise that, subject to the exclusions contained in the warranty, is valid in all 50 states.

A warranty is a contract that gives the buyer very specific rights. Almost any time a person gets a warranty on a new piece of equipment, it is a bind-

---

[20]In some cases the Uniform Trade Secrets Act would mandate such an injunction.

ing contract, and the only remedies for repair and/or replacement are found in that warranty. For that reason, if a warranty requires you to perform maintenance at required intervals, and you fail to do so, your warranty rights may disappear.

Importantly, every warranty also has exclusions. When a new warranty is issued to you, you should read it and find out not only what is covered, but what is not covered.

New car warranties are a good example. They cover the defects in materials and workmanship, but not normal wear and tear. If your car fails at 19,000 miles because you have never changed the oil in it, that is a failure that is not covered under the warranty.

Since a warranty is a contract, and since the seller doesn't have to do anything other than what is called for in the warranty, it is always a good idea to be familiar with the rights you have under any warranties.

G. HOW SHOULD PER-DIEM STAFFING CONTRACTS BE COMPLETED?

Every hospital, from time to time, needs extra help, and most contract with a "staffing agency" to obtain that help. The hospital and the agency should define their relationship in writing so that if there is a problem later, arising out of nonperformance or negligence, the parties have remedies.

From the position of the hospital, there are two major concerns. First is patient safety. Any staffing agency must certify that the staff it supplies would be subject to hiring by the hospital if the hospital were to independently evaluate those employees. Every contract should place the burden on the staffing agency to secure background checks of each leased employee. The staffing agency should also ensure that each person's credentials are in proper order, and that proper licenses have been secured for each practitioner.

The second issue is one of tort liability. Although the individual employees who provide care through an agency are considered to be employees for the purpose of respondeat superior (because the hospital controls the way they do their jobs), the ultimate liability for the negligent acts of agency supplied staff should be made to rest with the agency supplying those employees.

There are two ways to accomplish this. One way is to ensure that there is an indemnification and hold harmless agreement in the contract that protects the hospital. When a party agrees to "indemnify" the other party in an agreement, he essentially agrees to pay any judgment rendered against that party in a court of law. When a party agrees to hold another party harmless, they are agreeing to be responsible for the costs of litigation associated with any claim. So when a hospital enters an agreement with a staffing agency it should ensure that the agency is able and willing to bear the costs of any litigation and stand good for any harm that its employees cause.

Agreements between providers and hospitals should also include an agreement to require that the hospital be named as an "additional insured" under the staffing agency's policy of insurance. Essentially the hospital wants to take advantage of any insurance contract purchased by the staffing agency and be able to require that insurance company to defend it against any claims.

In addition to the foregoing, the hospital should include certain "escape clauses" in the contract that permit it to cancel the contract if the staffing agency fails to perform, or worse, if the staffing agency becomes insolvent. One of the first expenses cut by people in financial crises is the cost of insurance, and when a provider no longer maintains insurance it should not be permitted to do business with the hospital.[21]

H. WHAT ARE THE THREE MOST IMPORTANT RULES FOR ANY CONTRACT?

Most people don't come to their lawyer before they sign a contract. Some do, and these people are richly rewarded because they are not held to terms that are onerous. At the very least, if they do agree to onerous terms, they understand them. By and large, most people come to a lawyer only when they have problems and someone tells them that their contract bars a course of action they want to take.

There are three golden rules for handling all contracts. The first rule is: Read the Contract.

1. Why Is It Important to Read the Contract?

It is a source of constant amazement to me that people will bring in a contract and when I ask "what does the contract say about that," they will answer that they do not know. If they do not know what the contract says, how could they possibly have agreed to all its terms? Yet, written in bold type right above their signature is the statement I HAVE READ THIS CONTRACT

---

[21]Physicians who fail to maintain liability insurance should also be dealt with, as their failure to maintain insurance makes it more likely that some fault will be apportioned to the hospital.

COMPLETELY AND I UNDERSTAND ALL ITS TERMS AND AGREE TO ABIDE BY IT.

When I point this out, many times people simply gasp and say "I didn't see that." I always want to ask how they could have failed to see it, since it was in boldface type directly above where they signed.

In most cases, the contract says exactly what the opposing party says, and the client is stuck living up to an agreement they do not like. Make no mistake, the first golden rule of contract law is READ THE CONTRACT! And, of course, it goes without saying that you do that **before** you sign it.

The case of **Whitney v. Alltel** is a good example of why reading the contract is important. Mr. Whitney went to the phone store and bought a cellular phone and arranged for service through Alltel. He signed an application, and they told him that the actual contract would be sent to him in the mail.

The contract they sent to him had "terms and conditions" attached and contained the following provision mandating arbitration:

Any dispute arising out of this Agreement or relating to the Services and Equipment must be settled by arbitration administered by the American Arbitration Association. Each party will bear the cost of preparing and prosecuting its case. We will reimburse you for any filing or hearing fees to the extent they exceed what your court costs would have been if your claim had been resolved in a state court having jurisdiction. The arbitrator has no power or authority to alter or modify these Terms and Conditions, including the foregoing Limitations of Liability section. All claims must be arbitrated individually, and there will be no consolidation or class treatment of any claims. This provision is subject to the United States Arbitration Act.

Alltell asserted the arbitration provision to try to avoid a class action lawsuit filed against it. At the time he got his telephone, Mr. Whitney didn't even know that there was an arbitration provision. But the terms and conditions included some additionally sneaky language. The agreement said: "BY USING ANY ALLTEL COMMUNICATIONS SERVICES OR EQUIPMENT YOU ARE AGREEING TO THESE TERMS AND CONDITIONS."

The agreement also provided that "[i]f you are a new customer and do not wish to be bound by these terms and conditions, do not begin using the services or equipment, and notify us immediately." Mr. Whitney never saw the terms and conditions because he assumed, falsely, that what he signed (an application which purported to include those terms) was the long and short of his agreement with the phone company.

The Alltel case illustrates another important concept in contract law. Be certain you know what you're agreeing to; and that dovetails into the next golden rule of contractual relations: Understand the Contract.

2. Why Is It Important to Understand the Contract?

The second golden rule of contract law is: You must understand the contract. If the cell phone contract says that it will account for time in tenths of an hour, and you agree to this, that is how time will be accounted. If you do not understand that this means that you get billed the same amount of time for a 30-second phone call as a six-minute phone call, then you have the obligation to speak up and ask the question.

Of course, most people get presented a contract at the end of the deal, when they have agreed on a price and are on great terms with the salesman. It sometimes doesn't seem wise or nice to read the contract and ask questions. It might imply you don't trust the salesman. Should you immediately assume that the salesman is not dealing fairly, even if you know them?

Absolutely! Do not ever trust someone who has an incentive to take money away from you. Instead, trust yourself. If you do not understand the contract, you absolutely, positively **must** ask questions. If the answers are not what you like, don't sign. If you ask questions and still sign the contract, no court is going to believe you didn't understand what you were signing.

3. Why Is It Important to Get an Attorney to Read and Approve Any Contract You Sign?

Because you are not an attorney, it is important for you to employ one on any contract that involves your life, your livelihood, or your commitments. If you are signing a two-year employment contract agreeing to work in the Saudi kingdom, you need to have an attorney look it over in the event there are issues that relate to how you will be paid, and your fringe benefits.

If you're signing a contract to obtain a loan, and you don't understand the information in the financing statement, or how the interest rate is calculated, don't sign it until an attorney explains it.

Unless you know everything there is to know about the contract, and understand the contract as clearly as if you'd written it, you will save money in the long run by having your attorney look over the contract first.

I. WHAT ABOUT INSURANCE CONTRACTS?

The one contract that almost everyone has, which they often fail to think of in terms of its being a contract, is a contract for insurance. Insurance is a contractual agreement between an insurance company (insurer) and the holder of the contract (insured) where the insured is required to do certain things (pay money, give truthful information to the insurer, and cooperate with the insurer). In return, the insurance company will agree to defend and indemnify the insured under certain conditions.

While it is beyond the scope of this text to fully discuss insurance, what follows is a discussion of the basics and some of the little known rules that govern the insurance company's agreements with its insured.

1. How Are Insurance Policies Written?

Insurance policies are written generally to state coverage, and then to exclude certain acts or harms from coverage. So a typical insurance contract says:

Pinched Penny Insurance will indemnify you against any claims for personal injury arising out of any <u>covered harm</u> in this policy . . . except that this policy will not provide coverage for any <u>excluded harms</u> or causes . . .

When the consumer reads the policy he finds that covered harms, in a homeowner's policy, include fire, wind, rain, tornado, ice, lightning, and similar hazards. When the consumer reads the exclusions he finds that he is not covered for flood, earthquake, hurricane, volcano, certain natural disasters, and acts of God. Thus, to determine if you have coverage, you first have to see whether the harm is covered, and then, if covered, whether it is excluded later in the contract.

2. How Do Homeowner's Policies Work?

Understanding how insurance policies work is an important tool for the consumer. A typical homeowner's policy is usually broken down into coverage of the property, and coverage for liability.

The property protection is usually further broken down into four sections:

- Dwelling (covers the house and any attached structures)
- Other Structures (covers any detached structures)

- Personal Property (This typically covers personal property, including the contents of your home and other personal items owned by you. This protection can be based on actual cash value or replacement cost.)
- Loss of Use (usually provides for living expenses if you cannot live in your home while repairs are being made)

Endorsements are available to cover additional structures, vacation homes, jewelry, camera equipment, computer equipment, and to protect against credit card fraud. You can buy either actual replacement value or cash value insurance. Replacement value insures that you will be able to replace the thing lost. So if an antique 1928 Tiffany Lamp is destroyed, replacement value insurance will fund the cost of finding and replacing the Tiffany Lamp. Actual cash value insurance, however, only provides payments based on what was paid, less any amount of depreciation. Thus, a new computer purchased two years ago would net about half the value of the computer. Actual cash value is cheaper, but replacement value insurance probably makes more sense.

Like property insurance, the liability insurance is normally broken down into two areas: liability payments and medical payments.

The Personal Liability section provides liability coverage against a claim or lawsuit resulting from bodily injury or property damage to others caused by an accident on your property or as a result of your personal activities anywhere. This coverage usually does not provide protection for use of your automobile or any use of your property arising out of business-related incidents.

Medical Payments coverage simply provides for payments to individuals who are injured on your property or through your negligence without any requirement that the insurer assume any liability. So if someone slips and falls on your front porch, medical payments coverage will make a small payment (normally up to about $5,000) for medical costs without the injured person having to prove any fault or sue.

After an insurance contract spells out what is covered, it next takes away things that are not covered through "exclusions." Exclusions in a policy are meant to deny coverage to situations where homeowners or others might abuse the process. A typical homeowner's policy does not cover damage to motor vehicles, aircraft, or boats. Nor do these policies typically cover losses due to floods, mudslides, natural disasters, and the like. Every insurance contract should be read very carefully to determine not only what is covered, but what is excluded.

Normally, intentional conduct is not covered by an insurance policy. If you go next door and break the nose of your next door neighbor in a fistfight, you are going to bear that expense personally. If you are tossing a softball around and it strikes your neighbor in the nose, fracturing it, your insurance company will most likely cover you.[22]

Similarly, if you are waiting in your doctor's office with your legs out, and someone trips over your feet and breaks their hip, you are most likely covered for this by your homeowner's policy since it insures you no matter where the accident occurs. Any time you are named as a defendant in a lawsuit that does not arise out of your business or professional activities, you should immediately contact your insurance company.

3. How Do Business Policies Work?

Comprehensive General Business Liability policies (sometimes called CGL policies) are designed to protect businesses. Like homeowner's policies, they are designed to protect against harms that come up as a result of operating a business. If your visitors or customers are injured on your premises, a CGL policy protects you.

CGL policies do not protect automobiles, nor do they protect against intentional acts. They may provide insurance for a variety of other harms, however, including consumer fraud based on false advertising. Like a homeowner's policy, a CGL policy covers buildings and structures, and provides liability coverage. These policies also have exclusions, and like any policy, should be read carefully.

4. How Do Automobile Policies Work?

Unlike homeowner's and CGL policies, automobile polices are designed to provide coverage to specific drivers for specific vehicles and for specific periods of time. Like all insurance policies, they are written so as to give broad coverage, but also scores of reasons for the insurance company to later deny liability if the policy holder turns out to be a drunken driver or fleeing felon.

The best thing you can do for yourself is read your automobile policy. You might be surprised not only at what is covered by your policy, but what is not.

One coverage you should have if you do not is uninsured and underinsured motorist coverage. These coverages protect you in the event you are in-

---

[22]Unless, of course, you purposefully throw the ball at your neighbor with the intent to break his nose.

jured as a result of some other driver's negligence when the other driver has insufficient insurance (or no insurance) to pay for your injuries.

Uninsured motorist coverage is not really "coverage" in the way you expect. In order to be paid on such claims, most motorists have to sue their insurer. But if you are hit by a hit-and-run driver who leaves the scene of the accident, such coverage can be vital in ensuring that your medical bills are covered.

5. Professional Liability Policies

Professional Liability (or professional malpractice) policies are different from almost every other form of insurance. They are priced and rated differently, and they are usually easy to get if an individual has not sustained claims for negligence. These policies provide coverage for negligent acts and come under the heading of Claims Made and Occurrence policies.

a) What Is a "Claims-Made" Policy?

A claims-made policy covers a therapist at the time that a claim is made. This form of insurance is very good for individuals who work in pediatrics or neonatal fields. In pediatric and neonatal medicine, a child may take up to 18 years to bring a claim for damages. So if you purchased a policy in 1998, and remained with the same company renewing your policy every year, the policy limits in effect at the time the claim is made control.

This is because the claims-made policy covers you for the policy amount you have **when the claim is made.** This is an advantage for you because every time you increase your policy limits, you are covered for the higher limits for every year you have carried the claims-made policy.

This increased coverage keeps pace with inflation and rising jury verdicts, and may represent a good value for some therapists.

b) What Is an "Occurrence" Policy?

An occurrence policy covers you for a specific dollar amount for each individual year. An occurrence policy might go into effect on May 1, 2004, and expire on April 30, 2005. During that year, any occurrence is covered at the policy limits purchased.

If a therapist carries an occurrence policy for $100,000/$300,000 in 2002 and a patient files a claim against that therapist in 2003, the policy limits in effect in 2002 control, even if the therapist has a larger policy in 2003.

c) Which Type of Professional Liability Insurance Policy Is Best for Me?

Confusion abounds in the medical professions about which type of professional liability policy to purchase. As previously indicated, claims-made policies do keep pace with inflation better. Occurrence policies, however, also have some advantages. If a therapist practices for only 10 or 15 years, and then pursues another field of endeavor (no longer giving patient care), that therapist probably wants an occurrence policy because once they stop practicing, they can stop buying insurance. The occurrence policy covers them for the time when they were practicing, and that coverage extends indefinitely.

Claims-made coverage, however, is better suited to a therapist who expects to enjoy a 20- or 30-year career at the bedside because he or she can purchase "tail" coverage once they stop practicing, and claims-made policies are significantly less expensive than occurrence policies. Of course, one reason those policies are less expensive is that, unlike occurrence policies, once they are not renewed or cancelled they stop working. In view of the many policy-providing companies that have gone bankrupt or been found insolvent by regulators, occurrence policies may be the better deal.

6. Do Insurance Contracts Impose Obligations on the Buyer?

Many people think that if they have an insurance policy the relationship is one way. That is, if they have a claim, their premium payment is what triggers the necessity for the insurance company to pay. That is, unfortunately, not always the case. The insurance contract will usually impose duties on the buyer to do, or not do, certain things. For example, in a recent case, a State Farm policy was found to contain this language:

3. Other duties under the physical damage coverages when there is a loss, you or the owner of the property also shall;
. . . e. Answer questions under oath, when asked by anyone we name as often as we reasonably ask and sign copies of the answers.

5. Insured's Duty to Cooperate With Us. The insured shall cooperate with us, and when asked, assist us in:
. . . b. securing and giving evidence.

a) Duty to Answer Questions

As set out previously, almost every insurance contract can require an insured to answer questions under oath in order to determine whether the company has liability. In one recent case, a car was stolen and later found burned in a distant county. The insurance company suspected fraud, and sent out an investigator. Once it became clear that the insurance company was not going to pay, the insured hired a lawyer who advised her not to talk to the insurance company further. The insurance company then arranged to have criminal charges brought against the insured.

When a jury acquitted the insured of insurance fraud, the insured then sued the insurance company for bad faith refusal to settle, for breach of contract, and for the tort of malicious prosecution. The insurance company essentially suggested there was no breach of contract because, as noted in the previous paragraph, the insured had a duty to answer questions. The court ultimately disagreed, but only because the failure to answer questions did not prejudice the company.

b) Duty to Cooperate

Every person who is insured has a duty to cooperate with the insurer. The duty to cooperate is contained in nearly every insurance policy. Although the language may vary, the duty to cooperate is designed to protect the insured's financial interest and prevent collusion between the insured and the claimant.[23] For example, a policy holder will be required to help investigate and defend a claim made by someone who purports to have been injured by the conduct of the policy holder, and may be asked to provide documents or submit to an examination under oath when they seek direct reimbursement from the insurance company (for example, on an automobile accident or homeowner's insurance claim). The duty to cooperate usually prevents an insured from settling directly with a third-party claimant. In exchange for the insured's cooperation, the insurer assumes complete control and direction of the claim.

An insured is required to notify its insurance company whenever it might require coverage for a covered harm. Normally insurance policies place these obligations on policy holders so that the insurance company can make appropriate decisions regarding how to handle the claim.

---

[23]*Clark Equipment Co. v. Arizona Property and Casualty Ins. Guar. Fund,* 189 Ariz. 433, 442, 943 P.2d 793, 802 (Ariz. Ct. App. 1997).

When an insured fails to cooperate with the insurance company, the insurance company may deny coverage. This could leave the insured on the hook for any damages later awarded by the court.

In order to curtail an insurance company's ability to claim that a minor or technical breach of the duty to cooperate clause eliminates all insurance coverage, most states require the insurance company to deny coverage only where it has suffered prejudice as a result of the insured's failure to cooperate.[24] Prejudice simply means that the insurance company has suffered some harm as a result of the failure of the insured to do as he was required to do.

One frequent problem with the duty to cooperate is that too few people know what is actually covered by their homeowner's insurance policy. For example, most homeowner's policies cover your personal property wherever it is in the world, subject to your deductible. If you are moving from Michigan to Rhode Island, and your U-Haul catches fire in Indiana, your homeowner's insurance policy covers the goods as surely as if they were resting quietly in your home. If the goods are stolen en route to their new location, the policy provides coverage.[25]

It is difficult for a policy owner to cooperate if they don't know what their policy requires. Frequently in a fire or other loss, the policy burns up along with the household goods. For this reason it is a good idea to always keep a copy of any homeowner's insurance policy in a safe deposit box.[26]

7. What Obligations Does an Insurance Company Have?

In order to understand the duties of insurance companies, it is important to understand the difference between first party and third party claims.

A first party claim is common in an automobile policy. John buys a new Taurus and on the third day backs into a tree. If John has collision and

---

[24]See, e.g., *Darcy v. Hartford Ins. Co.*, 407 Mass. 481, 488-89, 554 N.E.2d 28, 33 (1990)(citing *Clemmer v. Hartford Ins. Co.*, 22 Cal. 3d 865, 881-82, 587 P.2d 1098 (1978); *Rochon v. Preferred Accident Ins. Co.*, 118 Conn. 190, 198, 171 A. 429 (1934); *Brooks Transp. Co. v. Merchants Mut. Casualty Co.*, 36 Del. 40, 55, 171 A. 207 (1933); *American Fire & Casualty Co. v. Vliet*, 148 Fla. 568, 571, 4 So. 2d 862 (1941); *Farley v. Farmers Ins. Exch.*, 91 Idaho 37, 40, 415 P.2d 680 (1966).

[25]Certain high value items, like computers, jewelry, and negotiable instruments may not be covered unless you have specific "riders" or "endorsements" to your policy.

[26]The same is not true for life insurance policies. A person's right to enter their safe deposit box ends on death, and many banks require a court order to open the safe deposit box of a deceased person. For this reason it is always a good idea to keep life insurance policies and last wills and testaments in a safe place other than a bank vault.

comprehensive coverages on his automobile, then he can ask the insurer to fix his car. There is only one party involved (John) and any duty the insurance company owes, it owes only to John.

A third party claim is different. If John runs over Sam and breaks both his legs, Sam has the right to sue John. If Sam sues or threatens to sue, John can ask his insurance company to take over. If it assumes control of the litigation it is in "third party" mode. The insurance company has two duties. The first is to indemnify the insured against damages arising from the lawsuit. That just means pay any damages that might result from litigation.

It also has a duty to defend the insured against the claims brought by any third party.

a) What Is an Insurance Company's Duty to Defend?

Courts traditionally state that an insurer's duty to defend is greater than its duty to indemnify. In other words, while an insurance company might escape paying on a claim, it usually can't escape providing a defense to any lawsuit brought against you.

In August 2001, Robert Courtney, a Kansas City pharmacist, was arrested and charged with diluting the chemotherapy medications of thousands of Kansas City area patients. The news broke on August 15, 2001, and the first lawsuit against Courtney and his pharmacy was on file the next day.[27]

Courtney deliberately and with full knowledge that what he was doing was going to kill innocent patients, substituted sterile water for chemotherapy and pocketed millions of dollars in profit as a result. His actions were certainly intentional in that regard.

Lawyers who brought claims against Courtney, however, were careful to include claims for negligence in addition to their claims for intentional conduct, because including negligence claims triggered insurance coverage.

Since most professional liability insurance contains an exclusion for intentional acts, Courtney's insurer sent him a letter as soon as the news broke. It stated it would deny coverage on any damages claim successfully brought against him. In other words, it would refuse to pay any damages claims.[28]

---

[27]This author filed that lawsuit on behalf of a respiratory therapist who received chemotherapy from Courtney.

[28]In sending this "reservation of rights" letter the insurance company sought to minimize its liability to the plaintiffs who were suing Courtney.

But in spite of this refusal to provide indemnification, the insurer, Pharmacists Mutual Insurance of Iowa, provided a team of attorneys to help defend the more than 350 lawsuits brought against Courtney within the next two years.

The insurer provided legal defenses for all of Courtney's many lawsuits. Lawyers conducted depositions, discovery, and participated in hearings. At least one legal scholar estimated that the insurance company spent in excess of $500,000 in legal fees and travel expenses in the case.

How does an insurer decide whether to defend a case? It looks at the pleadings in the case filed by the plaintiff, and if it might be liable under its policy for any of the claims, it has a duty to defend.

Sometimes insurance companies make really dumb decisions and refuse to defend cases they should defend. When they guess wrong, they wind up on the hook not only for damages covered by the policy, but for all damages.

b) What Is the Duty to Indemnify?

Insurance companies are notorious for selling insurance to clients and then refusing, when a claim is made, to pay the damages. This is due in no small part to how insurance companies write their contracts for insurance.

In a typical insurance contract, the coverage is broadly stated ". . . we will indemnify you for any amounts you are legally obligated to pay for damage . . . relating to your negligence . . ." This broad language is then modified by later language in the policy that provides for exclusions. "We will not pay any claims where the damages are the result of the intentional acts of the insured."

Understanding how insurance companies work is particularly important. When the insurance company receives notice of a claim, it must "set a reserve." A reserve is the maximum amount of money it will be forced to pay if the plaintiff is successful. The reserve amount is then deducted from the company's books as an item of expense.

The file is then given over to an adjuster who investigates the claim and determines whether the policy provides for any exclusion that might apply. If the policy provides for such an exclusion, he sends the insured a "reservation of rights" letter that lets the insured know that the insurance company does not think it has an obligation to pay on the claim.

At some point, the insurance company will either settle the case for a sum within the policy limits, or it will pay the verdict amount, up to the policy limits. Any money left over from the reserve becomes "profit" to the insurance company.

Insurance companies make money in two ways. If they take in more premiums than they pay out damages, they make money on what is called the "spread" between the premiums and the payouts. The other way they make money is by investing the premiums in the stock or bond markets. This means that an insurer has a strong incentive to (1) deny coverage and (2) delay payment.

Denying coverage results in a profit to the insurance company. Delaying payout allows the insurance company to continue to make money on the interest it receives from its investments.

Normally insurance companies deny coverage for damages when it is clear that an exclusion prevents payment. But this is not always the case. Sometimes they deny coverage for an improper reason, like corporate profits. When that happens, the insurance company may be guilty of "bad faith."

c) What Is a "Reservation of Rights"?

When an insurance company determines it has a duty to defend, but thinks it might not have to pay any damages because the allegations state intentional acts, for example, it issues a "reservation of rights" letter to the insured. The letter essentially tells the insured that the company will defend him, but that if he gets hit with damages, he will have to pay them. The letter says "we will reserve our right to assert the intentional act [or some other] exclusion and deny indemnification should the facts so warrant." Hence the term "reservation of rights" letter.

In some states, a person given that letter may refuse to allow the insurance company to defend them and may opt to settle with the plaintiff in exchange for the plaintiff taking only what the insurance company will pay. When this happens, the insured is in a position adverse to the insurance company that is supposedly protecting its interests.

When an insurance company acts contrary to the best interests of its insured, it is said to have engaged in "bad faith."

d) What Is "Bad Faith"?

When an insurance company has a duty to indemnify, it also has a duty to protect the insured from excess liability. Thus if the insurance policy provides for liability coverage up to $400,000, and the plaintiff's injuries exceed $500,000, the insurance company has an obligation to settle the case within the policy limits. If it subjects its insured to excess liability by refusing to settle a meritorious case within the policy limits, it may be liable for any damages to its insured under the doctrine of bad faith.

This is important in terms of medical negligence cases because many health care practitioners carry policies worth only $1,000,000 and that policy may not be enough to compensate a plaintiff who suffers severe and long-term injury. Thus, if a plaintiff makes a demand for $999,999 for settlement, and the insurance company refuses to pay that demand, it may later be on the hook for any judgment rendered in excess of that amount.

In one case, while trying to save $5,000 in coverage, Shelter Insurance Company exposed itself to more than $4,000,000 in liability. Insurance companies frequently make this error.

An insured, informed of an insurance company's refusal to settle within the policy limits, has the right to demand coverage and settlement from the insurance company. The insurance company still is the only entity that can make the decision to settle, but if the insured requests settlement and the company fails to settle, the company is almost always obligated to pay.

Health care practitioners sometimes are in the opposite position. The insurance company wants to settle a claim, and the health care practitioner doesn't want to settle the claim, either because they feel strongly about it, or because they do not wish a report made to the National Practitioner Database. Some medical malpractice policies have "consent" clauses that say an insured must consent to any settlement. When this happens, there is no bad faith in the insurance company's refusal to settle because it is the insured who is at fault, not the insurance company.

Frequently, insurance companies defend under a "reservation of rights." They put up a spirited defense, and still lose. In 2003, plaintiffs suing Robert Courtney were treated to a judgment in excess of $200,000,000 for the pharmacist's dilution of chemotherapy medication for Georgia Hayes, a Kansas City cancer patient.

As mentioned, Courtney's insurer, Pharmacists Mutual Insurance Company, had told Courtney that it would refuse to indemnify him for any damages. Courtney was sent to jail for 30 years at the end of the case, and so had no incentive to push his insurance company toward settlement.

Plaintiffs used the law to their advantage by filing an "equitable garnishment" action against the insurance company. The garnishment sought to force the insurance company to pay. The legal theory is that the insurance company owed a duty to Courtney to pay, and that the plaintiffs, as the persons harmed, had a right to demand that the insurance company honor its contract.

Pharmacists Mutual took every possible legal step to avoid paying. It filed motions and declaratory judgment actions in state and federal court. In those actions, it cited the policy language of its professional liability policies that indicated that it would not be liable for intentional acts.

Courtney, however, in his "allocution" before the federal court on federal drug charges, indicated that his actions were not intentional. "I never meant to hurt anyone," he told the Court.[29] Plaintiffs used this language to argue that Courtney was negligent.

A sizeable portion of the damages awarded to Hayes were punitive in nature. Insurance policies do not cover punitive damages, so plaintiffs were seeking to recover their damages for Courtney's negligent conduct in diluting the chemotherapy.

In the meantime, the insurance company began totaling up the legal bills. If its position was sustained on appeal, it would still likely pay out millions in interest and even more to its own attorneys. After nearly three years of wrangling, in January of 2004, it reached a confidential settlement with the plaintiffs. In so doing it avoided not only a claim of bad faith, but also potential bankruptcy, since its reserves and policies were never meant to cover claims by more than 360 plaintiffs.

c) Are There Rules Governing Claims Procedures?

Almost every state has a Department Of Insurance. That department (or branch of the department) issues regulations to control how insurance companies handle claims. Another area where therapists may have frequent interactions with insurance companies is where they are a "third party beneficiary" under a contract of insurance. A hospital or home health care organization is a third party beneficiary whenever a person's insurance is required to pay for care or treatment. This is because the person who bought the insurance bought it so that their health care workers (or the workers of those they injured) would be paid if they were injured.

Dealing with insurance companies is rarely a treat. Lawyers deal with insurers on a regular basis, and often it is the most difficult and disagreeable part of the job. But in almost every state, the sales and marketing of insurance, as well as the handling of claims, is managed and supervised by the State Department of Insurance. Normally the statute that formed the department

---

[29]Courtney's claims were difficult to believe. He diluted chemotherapy for hundreds of people and his actions touched thousands of lives. Nevertheless, he claimed that he was not acting intentionally.

20 CSR 100-1.020 Misrepresentation of Policy Provisions
PURPOSE: This rule effectuates or aids in the interpretation of section 375.1007(1), RSMo.

(1) No insurer shall fail to fully disclose to first-party claimants all pertinent benefits, coverages or other provisions of an insurance policy under which a claim is presented.

(2) No insurance producer shall conceal from any first-party claimant the benefits, coverages or other provisions of any insurance policy when these benefits, coverages or other provisions are pertinent to a claim.

(3) No insurer shall deny any claim for failure to exhibit the property without proof of demand and unfounded refusal by a claimant to do so.

(4) No insurer shall deny any claim based upon the insured's failure to submit a written notice of loss within a specified time following any loss, unless this failure operates to prejudice the rights of the insurer.

(5) No insurer shall request a first-party claimant to sign a release that extends beyond the subject matter that gave rise to the claim payment.

(6) No insurer shall issue any draft in partial settlement of a claim under a specific coverage, when endorsement of the draft would totally release the insurer or its insured from liability.

Chapter 20, Code of State Regulations, Section 100, subsection 1.020

Insurers can't use dirty tricks to coerce people into settling their claims.

Figure 3-1—Missouri's rules regarding insurance claims.

also empowered it to write regulations (see Figure 3-1). In those regulations, health care workers will find wonderful tools for dealing with errant insurance companies.

J. KEY POINTS

- Contracts are agreements.
- To have a valid contract all that need be present is an offer, an acceptance, consideration, and a meeting of the minds.
- Most contracts can be oral or written.
- An oral contract is as enforceable as a written contract, unless the oral contract is forbidden by the statute of frauds.
- When a contract is written, courts won't usually allow any extrinsic evidence about what the contract means, and will decide the contract based on the writing.
- Breach of contract is a failure to perform under the contract.

- Damages are available for breach of contract.
- Equitable remedies like an injunction or specific performance of the contract are available for breach of contract.
- Liquidated damages, where parties agree in advance to a damage amount, are enforceable if they are not a penalty provision.
- Insurance contracts place obligations on both the insurer and insured.
- The insured has a duty to cooperate and answer questions.
- The insurer has a duty to indemnify the insured from damages and pay any claims he makes.
- The insurer has a duty to defend the insured from lawsuits, and that duty is greater than the duty to indemnify.
- When an insurer acts in bad faith, the insurer can be sued for bad faith.
- You must read and understand the terms of any contract before signing it.
- The best protection from a contractual error is in the form of attorney review.

K. SUMMARY

Contracts are an important part of life. Contracts are no more than agreements that courts will enforce. For every claim under a contract, there is usually a defense, and contract cases are among the more difficult of those tried by a civil court.

One of the most common contracts a person enters into is an insurance contract. Understanding how insurance carriers handle claims and enter into policy terms is important. While an insurance company may not always have a duty to pay damages, it almost always has a duty to defend its insured.

CHAPTER 4

Essential Employee Rights in Contracts and Benefits

"All may dismiss their employees at will, be they many or few, for good cause, for no cause[,] or even for cause morally wrong, without being thereby guilty of legal wrong."

Payne v. Western & Atlantic Railroad Co.,
81 Tenn. 507, 519–520, (Sep. term 1884)

A. INTRODUCTION

In most cases, when you work in health care, you are an employee. Unless you own the business, you are employed by an organization to help it accomplish its goals. The nature of that relationship will often provide you both with the most enjoyment and most frustration you are likely to encounter in your life.

Employment law is a broad topic, and this chapter deals with the topic as it pertains to the employee. Employment law, as it applies to employees, is not always clear, and not always fair. Of all the areas where lawyers get involved and often do the least amount of good, the area of employee-employer relationships stands out. Employment is not a situation where the parties usually enjoy equal bargaining power, and as a result, most agreements are very one-sided.

B. WHAT'S THE HISTORY OF EMPLOYMENT LAW?

The history of employment law begins with the time in our country when the rich were those making the decisions, and the poor were most often in a "take it or leave it" position with respect to employment. As early courts addressed the issue of employment, they looked at it from the position of Freedom of Contract.

1. What Is Freedom of Contract?

When Ford gets ready to buy tires from Goodyear, both are in equal bargaining positions. Both are represented by counsel, and both have engineers and salespersons to make sure that both parties get out of the agreement exactly what they intend. When the parties agree on a number of tires and an amount of money, that agreement is between two equals. If a disagreement erupts later, there is no claim that one party bullied the other.

The employment relationship is almost never like that, except when the employee is a business-savvy CEO being hired by a business-savvy Board of Directors. In the real world of employer-employee relations, the scales are seldom, if ever, balanced. The employee wants a job; the employer is willing to hire her on its terms, not the employee's terms. The employer sets the terms and conditions of employment, as well as the salary, and the benefits the employee will receive. The employee can negotiate almost nothing (or, at least, this is the implication given to the employee). In most cases, it is a "take it or leave it offer." Most employers believe that they can find a replacement for any employee. In many situations at the staff level, they can.

The inequality in bargaining position, however, sometimes winds up creating a relationship between employee and employer that is less than fair. Sometimes all the power is vested in the employer, and the employer or its agents abuse that power. The result is a situation that begs for lawsuits and litigation.

This chapter examines the employment relationship and the "employment at will" doctrine. It examines discrimination in employment, as well as the state and federal remedies that are available to employees. It examines issues related directly to health care, including staffing and the right to direct how tasks are accomplished. It provides guidance to employees on critical issues in the employment context.[1]

---

[1] In this regard, the chapter aims at the rank and file employee facing tough decisions, who may have to make decisions that affect her life and her family's life. The emphasis is on protecting the employee from the employer who might take advantage of the employee, or deal unfairly. Most employers are not prone to treating employees badly. But this chapter makes the assumption that the person reading it needs to know the "worst case" scenario and be advised on his or her rights as if the employer is not as close to God as the CEO's mother would like to think.

C. IS THE EMPLOYMENT RELATIONSHIP A CONTRACT?

No. Unless it is in writing, the employment relationship between an individual and a company is simply that—an employment relationship. Unless there are other facts involved, it is not a contract.

Americans, unlike the people of almost every country in the world, enjoy almost universal freedom of contract. As long as the aims of a contract are lawful, and as long as the fulfillment of the contract will not violate any public policy, Americans are free to structure their contractual relationships. Employment, however, unless you have a written contract, is what is called "quasi-contractual" under the law. That means it has lots of the same attributes of a contract, but with some serious differences.

1. How Does Employment Differ from a Regular Contract?

Essentially, if it isn't in writing, it does not exist. Contracts can be verbal or written and still be enforceable. In most instances an employment contract that is not in writing is invalid.[2] In the business world, freedom of contract means that Ford has the right to buy tires from Goodyear, or, if it desires, Bridgestone. The grocery store can choose to do business with a local farmer or pay a produce supplier. Generally, the market benefits from competition in that competition keeps prices down. With very few exceptions (like electric utilities and telephone companies), the government doesn't regulate the contracts or what buyers charge sellers.

Similarly, with very few exceptions, the government doesn't regulate the relationship between any individual and any corporate entity. The corporation is free to hire candidates for jobs on the basis of who is best qualified, so long as the company doesn't discriminate or terminate employees on the basis of certain protected statuses.[3]

Employment occurs when a willing worker goes to work for a willing employer. When an employer agrees to hire a worker for $10 per hour, and that worker accepts, the employment relationship is formed. Oddly enough, even though it conforms to the rules of contracts, employment is a matter that is only contractual (irrespective of the rules of contracting) when there

---

[2]There are some exceptions to this general rule. See below.

[3]In short, a corporation cannot discriminate on the basis of race, creed, color, national origin, pregnancy, gender, age, or disability. It must treat all persons equally in its hiring decisions, giving no preference or special treatment to any person or group of persons over any other person or group of persons. While the goal is a noble one, it is difficult to apply, as will be seen later.

is a formal written contract between persons or an intention to extend contractual terms. Otherwise it is "at will."

2. Are There Circumstances That Can Create a Contract?

There is one situation where an employment contract can result, even though there is no written agreement, and even though the employer may not actually have intended to contractually bind themselves to an employee.

The doctrine of "Promissory Estoppel" is a way of going around the requirement for a written contract. It is an "equitable" doctrine, meaning of course that it has its roots in basic fairness. It is not a "legal doctrine" in that it isn't based on contract law, but rather, on the law of Remedies. It provides that if a person makes a promise that a reasonable person would expect to be relied upon, and someone relies on that promise, that promise is enforceable.

But promissory estoppel is a very dangerous route to take. It essentially recognizes that the party seeking estoppel has no legal claim, and must base their case on fairness. Often the doctrine is not enforced by the courts, primarily because employers usually have a stable of well-paid lawyers and employees frequently do not.

3. What Is "At Will" Employment?

It's the type of employment most people have.

When a therapist is hired for $25 per hour in a hospital environment, that employment, unless specified otherwise, is not contractual but "at will." That means that there is no specific agreement to retain the employee for any particular time frame, but rather, only for so long as the employer may need the employee to work. Simply put, when you go to work for a company at an hourly wage, you have no right to expect continued employment at the end of the day. The employer can terminate your employment at that moment. This is called "at will" employment because the employment is literally at the will of the employer. If the employer decides that he no longer needs 18 employees, and wants to have only 16, there is no reason he cannot let two persons go.

4. What Is the History of Employment at Will?

The doctrine of at will employment has its origins in a strange place. Horace C. Wood, a legal "scholar" in the 19th century, wrote a legal treatise called "Master and Servant," and in section 134 stated:

With us the rule is inflexible, that a general or indefinite hiring is prima facie a hiring at will, and if the servant seeks to make it out a yearly hiring, the burden is upon him to establish it by proof. . . . It is an indefinite hiring and is determinable at the will of either party, and in this respect there is no distinction between domestic and other servants.[4]

Wood, however, might be criticized for his approach, because he cited four authorities that did not support this position. Nevertheless, the idea caught on. Unfortunately, nearly every state has adopted, at some level, the at will employment doctrine. The most common reason asserted for this doctrine is the freedom of contract rationale just described. An employee must be free to go to work for anyone at anytime, and cannot be bound to remain employed. If an employee cannot be bound, it is unfair to bind the employer to such a relationship.

5. Are All States Employment at Will?

No. Some states have different rules, but the majority of them are still governed by employment at will. Fortunately, in recent years the doctrine has come under attack and employees have made numerous gains in overcoming the doctrine via litigation.

At present, however, the doctrine is still the law in most of the 50 states. An employer can terminate the employment of a person for any reason, or for no reason, but not for an unlawful reason.

State and federal law proscribe several broad reasons why an employee may not be terminated. Obviously, if the employee is terminated because of race, creed, color, religious affiliation, gender, pregnancy, or age, this runs afoul of the Civil Rights Act of 1964 as amended. In 1990, the Americans with Disabilities Act was signed into law, and with it came additional civil rights protections for the disabled. If a person is fired for a reason that would violate these laws, they are fired for an unlawful reason.

In addition to the federal law, most states have their own anti-discrimination laws, and some of those laws are more protective than the federal law.

6. What Remedies Exist Under State Law for Termination?

Different states have different remedies, and you should always consult an employment lawyer if you are unfairly terminated.

---

[4]Horace G. Wood, *A Treatise on the Law of Master and Servant* § 134, At 272 (2d Ed. 1877).

One problem that often exists for employees is knowing exactly why an employer terminated them (otherwise, how do you know it wasn't fair?). The information given to the employee in the termination interview seldom, if ever, makes it into the written record. Employers have been known to invent tardiness, absenteeism, and other rationales for termination even though the real reason was something quite other than documented.

7. What Is a Service Letter?

Missouri and several other states have service letter statutes. A service letter is a letter an employee requests that allows them to learn the true nature of their discharge. In Missouri it can be found at § 290.140, RSMo. (2003), and it requires a manager or supervisor to provide a written letter "setting forth the nature and character of service rendered by such employee to such corporation and the duration thereof, and truly stating for what cause, if any, such employee was discharged or voluntarily quit such service."

The service letter fills an important void in the area of employment law. It essentially requires the employer to set out in writing the reason that the employer will give to those calling for references for the termination. If the employer says the employee was terminated because of a "contraction of work opportunities" (a layoff) and then later says in a reference that the employer was terminated for "bad work performance," the employee has a right to sue based on defamation, since the employer has already set out the "true cause" of the termination in writing in the service letter.

This can frequently be a source of problems for supervisors and managers who may not be privy to the actual reasons listed in an employee's discharge paperwork. Many employers now give terminated employees information about their termination and, in effect, provide a voluntary service letter that sets out the reason for their discharge.

Secondarily, those employers also often refuse to provide any reference of any kind to prospective employers. They will confirm the dates of employment, and, if asked, state whether the employee is eligible for rehire, but they will generally not provide a reference that speaks to the employee's job performance.

Sometimes Human Resources persons work around their counterparts in the other organization and call the department director or shift supervisor directly, and sometimes at home, in order to find out what they perceive to be the "real reason" that an employee was terminated, or to get a reference they could not get from the employer's human resources department.

If the shift supervisor reveals information that is not in the service letter, or worse, says defamatory things about the employee in the reference, they may subject themselves and their employer to liability. This is the reason why most employers no longer provide any real references for their former employees.

Recently, however, there has been a new wrinkle in this area called "Compelled Self-Publication" that suggests that when a former employer won't give out references, the former employee is compelled to self-publicize the reasons the employer gave, even though they may disagree violently with those reasons. It is for this reason that many employers are now either providing a voluntary service letter, or, in the alternative, verifying only the basics of employment at the organization.

D. WHAT CONSTITUTES AN EMPLOYMENT CONTRACT?

In order to have an employment contract, the essentials of a contract must exist. There must be an offer, an acceptance, consideration, and a meeting of the minds, and all of this must be recorded in writing.

Because the world of "at will" employment has been shrinking, and because the courts have imposed additional remedies on employers in recent years, there has been an increasing trend in employment to use employment contracts for supervisory-type positions, and even for some line positions in instances where an employee may gain access to trade secrets.

Employment contracts are written documents that spell out the terms and conditions of employment, as well as all benefits. They specify what rights an employee has in her employment, and frequently that means no rights whatsoever. They provide for remedies for the employer if the employee should breach the agreement (usually termination), and they may also provide for a period of non-competition in some circumstances. Worse, some contracts may require that binding arbitration or some other form of alternate dispute resolution be applied. Employment contracts that specify the hours and wages and appear to give an employee enforceable rights may seem like a good thing; frequently they are not.

1. Why Would a Therapist Need a Contract?

The only reason a therapist needs a contract is to protect herself from unlawful or unfair termination or employment practices. Generally speaking, if you fear an employer is going to engage in this kind of conduct, why take the job in the first place?

The first, and perhaps most important, issue in the area of employment contracts is deciding whether or not one is necessary. If an employer offers an employment contract, generally it is to secure for itself some right it cannot get in the normal course of business. Frequently, the major reason an employer wants a contract is to prevent the employee from taking information and knowledge gained from it, and going to work for himself or for the competition. The employer may want to prevent disclosure of sensitive information through a "non-disclosure" agreement.

Another reason is to codify the reasons why an employee may be terminated. Generally this is stated very broadly and with sweepingly general statements like "any act that brings discredit upon the organization." An employee signing such a contract is wise to clarify any broad language in a contract.[5]

2. What Are "Non-Disclosure" and "Non-Compete" Clauses?

These onerous clauses in employment contracts impose restrictions on what a person may disclose and what work a person may secure after voluntary or involuntary termination.

By far the most onerous of all clauses in an employment contract is the clause regarding competition. The employer usually has reasons for asking for such a clause. An employee may be privy to management meetings in which the strategy of the hospital or other sensitive information is shared.

The employer may count on the personal force of the employee to generate business, for example, by working directly with doctors and other referral sources to send business to the hospital. The last thing the employer may want is to have those personal relationships developed through the good offices of the hospital pirated by a competitor.

In the world of home care, sales, and other similar enterprises, an employee's list of contacts and his agreements with individual buyers may be a large part of the success of the business. If the employee takes that list with him, it might inure to the harm of the business. Employers expect to own the fruits of their employees' labor, while employees traditionally think of their

---

[5]Unfortunately, clarifying it verbally with your new boss is not good enough. You need to get the clarification in writing. Most contracts have a clause that says there are no side agreements, and that everything the parties agree to is included in the contract. If you do not get clarification in writing before you sign the contract, you may be bound by whatever construction the employer places on the language at some later point in time.

contact information as personal property. In order to prevent this, most employers, when they hire by contract, impose both non-disclosure and non-competition clauses in the contract.

a) What Does a Non-Disclosure Agreement Require?

A non-disclosure agreement requires the person signing it to keep secret the information that the company tells her is secret. Like many agreements for employment, the contract and clause often do not spell out what is confidential and what is proprietary information. This allows the employer, later, to argue that the list of contacts, forms, letters, documents, policies, procedures, and similar information obtained and used by the employee during the course of employment is confidential and/or proprietary information. It is a blank check for the employer.

3. If My Employer Insists on Such an Agreement, What Should I Do?

Run.

Okay, maybe not run, but at the very least, get your guard up. An employer who wants an agreement including a confidentiality clause wants something from you, and you have to be sure that you aren't signing away valuable rights. This is particularly true when you live and work in the same town, and have for the last ten years. You do not want to give up valuable investments in your home if you lose your job.

An employee should be careful to read and understand such an agreement; and, let's be honest, these agreements are written in such a way as to make that difficult. Trained lawyers often have difficulty agreeing on what a term or clause means in one of these contracts. I have personally spent more than 20 hours on the phone and in drafting, trying to clarify what a 14-sentence agreement meant.

Let's examine these agreements. The agreement provides for injunctive relief, even if it does not provide for payment of legal expenses. As a result, an employer might well fire an employee to prevent vesting of benefits and then attempt to enforce its rights to keep that employee from competing with it by suing for an injunction after an employee has already started work for a competing employer.

Some employers try to limit this problem by requiring employees, upon starting employment, to sign an agreement that includes a restriction on bringing confidential information from former employees to the new employer.

In addition to insulating itself from damages from any former employer, most companies have policies that require the return of documents. In the age of HIPAA, which requires that patient information be maintained in a safe and secure format, and not be disclosed to third parties, most hospitals now have policies on separation. Those policies require that anything that might conceivably be considered a patient record or to contain patient information be returned to the hospital on separation, and that failure to do so will be prosecuted as the theft of proprietary information.

4. How Are Agreements Enforced?

Employment agreements are frequently enforced by injunction (a court order requiring that the individual cease employment for the competitor) or through what is called a "liquidated damages" clause. The purpose of the clause, under contract law, is to approximate the amount of damages an employer might sustain, to preclude actual proof of damages. In setting the amount of liquidated damages employers must be careful, because a liquidated damages amount that is extreme may be considered to be a penalty by certain courts, and not enforced.

Keep in mind that confidentiality and non-disclosure agreements are a species of agreement where the devil is always in the details. An employee asked to sign such an agreement should ask for an exclusive list of proprietary and confidential information so that he or she can either comply with the agreement, or, in the alternative, refuse to sign the agreement. If an entity cannot answer this question, it probably means they have not thought about the answer. If that's the case, it is the most dangerous situation for all concerned. The employer doesn't know what it considers proprietary, and the employee, therefore, can't know either. If the question can't be answered, the employee should submit a non-exclusive list of things that are excluded from the confidentiality agreement like:

(1) personal rolodexes or similar date and contact managers
(2) contacts made through professional societies
(3) information developed by them while in the capacity of an employee but not on the direction of the company (for example, a novel written by the employee).

In this way, the employee can be reasonably sure that these items will be exempted from the confidentiality clause. Again, this must be done before the agreement is signed, and specifically referenced within the agreement.

Another frequent trick is the "ADR" clause in the employment contract. The "ADR" clause (which stands for alternate dispute resolution) will usually include mandatory arbitration of employment claims, and may even require you to give up the right to join in class action litigation.

As a general rule, it is never a good idea to sign an arbitration clause because doing so mandates arbitration, and arbitration is rarely in the employee's best interests.

5. What Happens If You Violate an Agreement?

Failure to carefully read an agreement can be disastrous, because corporations and their cultures change. Just ask Richard A. Albert, a former salesman for Kforce, Inc., a publicly traded staffing agency.

Albert was employed subject to two employment agreements. Both agreements included confidentiality and non-compete clauses that were designed to protect Kforce's proprietary information, as well as language that precluded Albert from soliciting any of Kforce's current customers if he were to leave. This was important because Albert was Kforce's top producer, managing accounts worth millions of dollars to the company.

As frequently happens in business, the company that Albert went to work for changed and became a company he no longer cared to be associated with. Although he was approached by a competitor in November, 2003, and accepted a position with the company at that time, he did not resign from Kforce until after January, 2004. He went to work for the competitor immediately, however, and began to approach his current customers at Kforce with the idea that they should switch to the competitor.

Once Albert's resignation was effective, Kforce learned of his work for the competitor and filed a lawsuit to enforce the confidentiality and the non-competition agreements.

At trial, Albert admitted that he breached his agreements with Kforce, but told the judge he wasn't to blame. After all, he reasoned, the corporate culture had changed. He was effectively forced out of his position.

When it became clear that Kforce would prevail, the parties settled their matter with Albert paying his former employers $20,000 in liquidated damages and agreeing to an injunction.

The lesson to be learned from Albert's case is that courts are apt to enforce agreements that individuals intentionally breach, and the results can't be good for the employee.

a) What Is a Covenant Not to Compete?

A covenant not to compete is merely a promise that an employee will not engage in work that competes with the activities of the current employer. To be effective, a covenant not to compete must be offered before employment begins, or it must receive a separate consideration. For example, if the employer, previously not concerned with competition in the home care business, learns of a competing enterprise opening across town, he cannot gather his employees and force them on pain of termination to sign a non-competition agreement unless he gives them something, or refrains from doing something (see Chapter 3).

6. Are Covenants Not to Compete Limited in Any Way?

A covenant not to compete must satisfy several requirements to be valid. It must be for a reasonable time, and have a reasonable geographic limitation.

A covenant not to compete must be for a reasonable time. Courts tend to enforce agreements between 18 and 24 months, but not to enforce those that go for longer periods of time because they tend to be viewed as unlawful restraints on trade. The covenant not to compete must also be reasonable in view of the geographic limitation.

If a salesperson has a territory consisting of Iowa and Missouri, a restriction forbidding competitive employment in the continental United States would be overbroad from a geographic perspective. It also would be more than would be necessary to protect the trade secrets or true competitive aspects of the company seeking to enforce it. However, if that employee were the national sales manager, a court might well enforce such a clause against the employee who went to work for the nearest competitor.

7. What Distinguishes Valid Non-Compete Clauses?

A non-compete agreement must be something that legitimately protects a company's financial and economic interests, not merely a punishment for changing jobs. If the employee doesn't have proprietary information, if they do not have trade secrets, if they did not work with sensitive functions, and if they merely handled paperwork, a covenant not to compete might not be enforced.

An agreement cannot be against public policy either.[6] An agreement is against public policy if what it accomplishes by contract is forbidden by some other means. Consider the case of Ronald Elwell, a former GM employee. Elwell testified as a design engineer for several years in cases brought against General Motors. Elwell and GM had a falling out, and they each sued the other. In a settlement of their lawsuits, the parties agreed to the entry of an injunction that prevented Elwell from testifying on behalf of plaintiff. Elwell and GM agreed to this injunction in exchange for General Motors paying to Elwell a certain sum of money.

By taking the money, Elwell agreed he could not be compelled to testify against GM. GM and Elwell exempted situations where Elwell was called as other than a paid witness. Meanwhile the Bakers, who had a wrongful death case pending in Missouri, wanted to depose Elwell on the design of the fuel system. The district court in Missouri permitted this, and the Eighth United States Circuit Appeals Court overruled the district court. The Supreme Court stepped in to decide who was right.

The constitutional issue was "full faith and credit." GM wanted Missouri to give "full faith and credit" to the injunction issued against Elwell in Michigan. Full faith and credit does not allow one state to prevent its citizens from testifying in another state, however, and thus Michigan could not reach into Missouri and control litigation there. The case is *Baker by Thomas v. General Motors Corp.*, 522 US 222 (1998). See Appendix C-4.

In essence, an employer may not accomplish by contract what it may not otherwise legally accomplish. General Motors could not legally prohibit Elwell from testifying about what he knew. Thus, it could not, under pretense of contract and injunction, prohibit him from testifying in plaintiff's personal injury cases. An employer cannot muzzle an employee or require him not to obey a subpoena; doing so is against public policy.

8. What Are Choice of Law Provisions?

A "choice of law" provision decides which state's law governs a contract. Often, Company A, a Delaware company, hires John Doe who lives in Arizona. When issues arise under the employment contract, the employer may find itself litigating in Arizona, under Arizona law, instead of its more friendly territory of Delaware. For that reason, another frequent target of

[6]For this reason confidentiality agreements that have been sued on in order to keep incriminating documents out of the hands of federal prosecutors routinely are not enforced by the courts.

employment contracts is called the "choice of law" provision, which establishes which state's law applies.

A choice of law clause is most often the by-product of whatever firm is doing the company's legal work. For example, if the firm's lawyers are Illinois lawyers, they most likely stick an Illinois clause into their contracts because they are experts on Illinois law. This is true even if the company is located in Wisconsin. If a person agrees to a choice of law, they'll probably be stuck with it later if the contract must be construed. It is always a good idea to get an attorney to review any choice of law clause in an employment contract.

9. What Is Choice of Forum?

Think of it as a choice of venue. A choice of forum clause restricts the case to being heard in a particular court or jurisdiction. This is because another favorite trick of lawyers drafting employment contracts is to require that all cases arising under the contract be litigated at the home office of the company or institution, where the company often has the most political clout.

Like the choice of law clause, a forum selection clause will most likely be enforced so long as doing so doesn't violate the public policy of the state where litigation is brought. Some states do not allow parties to choose a forum other than that set out by the statutes or rules of the jurisdiction, and refuse to enforce these clauses on public policy grounds. For this reason, it is a good idea to have an attorney examine the contract for employment before you sign it, to ensure that any problems with the choice of forum can be addressed.

10. What About Teachers? Is Tenure and Quasi-Contract Different?

Yes. Teachers enjoy a statutory contract if they are tenured, and essentially have "at will" employment if they are not tenured. Whether a respiratory care educator at a public or private school is tenured is usually a question of either contract or state education law.

Educators often have issues in contracts that deal with whether tenure will be granted or withheld. In most states and county systems, tenure is a right given to teachers who are contracted with the system. The tenure right essentially prevents the firing of the teacher or instructor for any reason other than cause, and the causes are stated in a statute or regulation. Any clause in a contract that obviates tenure rights should be stricken, as it may be against the law and public policy to deny a tenure-track employee tenure status for any reason other than those set out in the tenure statutes and regulations.

If tenure is discussed in an employment contract for a teacher of respiratory care, the therapist-educator should immediately seek legal assistance. Since statutory rights are at issue, it is vital to have those issues fully explored prior to signing any contract for employment.

11. Should I Agree to Alternate Dispute Resolution?

In most cases, no. Alternate dispute resolution frequently works against the employee. Nonetheless, more and more employers, particularly those with employees in multiple judicial districts, are selecting binding arbitration as a way of heading off litigation over employment contracts. Binding arbitration clauses are used to forestall litigation because they require that any dispute arising out of the employment relationship to be submitted to a binding arbitration proceeding rather than being heard in a court of law.

Importantly, a federal statute called the Federal Arbitration Act, passed in 1925, has recently been used to compel arbitration where the matter involves interstate commerce. Thus, if a hospital hires an employee from a distant state and insists on an arbitration clause in the contract, in most cases it falls within the Federal Arbitration Act. While many state courts are reluctant to enforce arbitration agreements, the Federal Arbitration Act mandates that enforcement if the matter involves interstate commerce.

Some states do not allow a party to agree to give up the right to sue in a court of law, but more and more states are upholding arbitration agreements as valid.

In arbitration, the employer picks an arbitrator, and the employee picks an arbitrator, and the two arbitrators pick a third person as a neutral to hear the case. Evidence is not presented under the rules of evidence, and many things that could not be admitted in a court of law are admitted in an arbitration proceeding. The arbitrators decide who is right and who is wrong, and frequently there is no appeal from the decision of the arbitrator. In essence, the parties agree up front to not go to court if they reach disagreement. While the process saves time, it usually works to the disadvantage of the employee because some employment attorneys will not handle arbitration cases, leaving the employee to try to navigate his way through that maze alone.

Unless an attorney advises otherwise, you should never sign an agreement with a binding arbitration clause. Doing so gives up valuable protections under the law, and exposes you to having your case heard by someone other than a jury of 12 citizens.

E. WHAT RIGHTS ARE PROTECTED BY LABOR RELATIONS LAWS?

Labor laws protect the rights of employees to organize and engage in activity for mutual protection. They apply to almost all non-supervisory employees, not just those in unions. In other words, even though a union does not exist at a hospital, the National Labor Relations Act protects employees who band together for mutual protection.

The history of labor relations in this country is tortured. Workers at the turn of the 20th century did not enjoy very many rights. Many worked 12- to 15-hour days and received precious little pay for their work. They worked in dismal conditions without proper sanitation. The factories of the 1920s were, in many ways, no different from the slave plantations of the 1860s, except that the divisions were economic instead of racial. From these deprivations was born the American labor movement, and the rich history of the AFL-CIO is still with us today.

Most health care workers enjoy a quality of work environment and standard of living that makes union membership unnecessary and unwarranted. While some hospitals have unionized, most have not. While this author is generally not in favor of unions, he is willing to recognize that conditions at some employers cannot be made better without them.

Until the 1930s, however, unions did not have much political clout. When they finally achieved a measure of respect, they were able to get the National Labor Relations Act (NLRA) passed and signed into law. That act, normally thought to apply only to organizations that are unionized, in fact applies to every organization that meets the tests under the act. As a general rule, so long as an employer meets the tests of the requisite number of employees and so long as they do business that affects interstate commerce, they are required to conform to the law.

1. How Is the Right to Organize Protected?

The first and most hard fought right that unions won with the NLRA was the right to organize. That meant that employers could not forbid employees from conversing with other employees and attempting to organize the workers into a union organization. Although the employer has a right to restrict access to the hospital to certain individuals, and to insist that workers do not engage in activity on company time, they are literally powerless to resist the efforts of employees to organize.

An employee cannot be terminated, demoted, or otherwise suffer a job action (nor can they be interrogated by management) as a result of being part of a union organizing action. Thus, employees cannot be threatened with discharge, or given bad assignments simply because they are working to bring a union into a facility.

If an employer attempts to restrict the right of workers to organize (for example, by selectively enforcing rules against organizers that are not enforced against other employees) they are committing an unfair labor practice.

2. Is the Right to Group Action Protected?

Employees have the right to act on each other's behalf for mutual aid and protection. This is provided under Section 157 of the NLRA:

> *§ 157. Right of employees as to organization, collective bargaining, etc.*
>
> *Employees shall have the right to self-organization, to form, join, or assist labor organizations, to bargain collectively through representatives of their own choosing, and to engage in other concerted activities for the purpose of collective bargaining or other mutual aid or protection, and shall also have the right to refrain from any or all of such activities except to the extent that such right may be affected by an agreement requiring membership in a labor organization as a condition of employment as authorized in section 158(a)(3) of this title.*

3. What Is Concerted Activity?

Although the term "concerted activity" is not defined in the act, according to the courts "it clearly enough embraces the activities of employees who have joined together in order to achieve common goals."[7] In other words, if employees are concerned that they are being asked to work without sufficient staff, and one employee raises this concern to management as the representative of the others, that is protected concerted activity. That employee can't be singled out.

The phrase "to engage in concerted activities" does not refer only to the situation in which two or more employees are working together at the same

---

[7]*NLRB v. City Disposal Systems, Inc.*, 465 U.S. 822, 829, 104 S.Ct. 1505, 1510, 79 L.Ed.2d 839 (1984).

time and the same place toward a common goal.[8] That is a rather narrow construction that the courts have routinely rejected. Instead, courts recognize that an individual employee may be engaged in concerted activity when he acts alone in several other situations: that in which the lone employee intends to induce group activity, and that in which the employee acts as a representative of at least one other employee.[9] Thus, an employee who addresses peers and supervisors in a meeting and who urges therapists not to work extra shifts until management hired additional staff might well be engaging in protected concerted activity, even though he is advocating something that only a few workers are likely to agree with.

Generally, to qualify as "concerted activity" under the National Labor Relations Act, 29 USC § 151, et seq., courts require that the conduct "appear at the very least that it was engaged in with the object of initiating or inducing or preparing for group action or that it had some relation to group action in the interests of the employees."[10] Any conduct that appears oriented toward group action qualifies. So writing a memo, talking to other employees, and setting meetings with supervisors all qualify.

A conversation, for example, may constitute a concerted activity although it involves only two people, but to qualify as such, it must appear that it was engaged in with the object of initiating or inducing or preparing for group action or that it had some relation to group action in the interest of the employees.[11] If the conversation centered around name calling—"That evening shift supervisor is a dork"—the communication is probably not protected or concerted. However, if the conversation centered around changing working conditions—"That evening shift supervisor is treating certified people differently than registered people, and someone should let management know"— it most likely is a protected concerted activity.

When an employee approaches the management and says that, on behalf of all the therapists in the department, he would like to see the on-call policy changed, he cannot be reprimanded or disciplined for acting on behalf of his fellow employees. He has an absolute right to engage in activity for mutual aid and protection.

Unfortunately, very few managers know this, and they tend to deal harshly with that employee who asserts his right to act on behalf of others.

---

[8]*Ibid.* at 831.

[9]See *ibid.*, citing e.g., *Aro Inc v. NLRB*, 596 F.2d 713, 717 (6th Cir. 1979).

[10]*NLRB v. Buddies Supermarkets, Inc.*, 481 F.2d 714, 718 (5th Cir. 1973).

[11]See *Mushroom Trans. Co. v. NLRB*, 330 F.2d 683, 685 (3rd Cir. 1964).

In fact, many managers will treat a person more harshly if they say "I'm not the only one that feels this way."

When an employee is demoted or disciplined for activity within the scope of mutual aid and protection, they have a right to file a complaint with the National Labor Relations Board, and to have the NLRB act on that complaint.

4. How Does the NLRB Work?

If you are an employee, it works pretty well. If you are the employer, the supposition is that you are wrong. If that seems like a harsh judgment, it is simply because I've defended small companies in front of the NLRB, and the presumption is always that the company is in the wrong. That's how the NLRB approaches things.

The National Labor Relations Board functions as prosecutor, judge, jury, reviewing court, and executioner in an action brought by an employee. It is an exceptionally favorable forum for the employee, and an exceptionally unfavorable forum for the employer. The NLRB is a powerful ally for the employee.[12]

Complaints related to enforcement of rights can be made to the NLRB. A list of regional offices is found at Appendix E.

5. Must Hospitals Give Notice of Closings?

The last thing anyone wants is to have a hospital close or go out of business. But it does happen, and when it does, generally the hospital must provide notice of the closing to all employees 60 days in advance, provided the hospital is of a sufficient size.

With certain exceptions, every employee who works for a company with more than 100 employees is covered by the Worker Adjustment and Retraining Act, 29 USC § 2101. The Act, passed during the Clinton Administration, provides for 60 days' notice to any employee in an organization of any impending plant closing or layoff.

The Worker Adjustment and Retraining Act provides not only for a private right of action against the employer if it violates the act, but also provides for attorneys' fees and civil penalties against the employer.

---

[12]Unfortunately for the rank and file, it is often the truly incompetent and lazy employees who are most successful in NLRB actions.

If the layoff or closing is caused by natural disaster, flood, or strike, the act does not apply. In addition, if the closing results from circumstances that could not have been predicted, the act does not require notice. For example, a manufacturer in New York City, whose access to the facility was blocked after the terrorist attacks in September 2001, would not have been required to issue notice under the act.

F. ARE THERE EMPLOYMENT RIGHTS UNIQUE TO HEALTH CARE?

Yes, and there are responsibilities too. Health care employees have some specific rights that vary from state to state. These rights are usually found in licensing statutes and in certain other federal statutes protecting health care workers.

1. What Issues Affect Staffing?

Hospitals, nursing homes, and other health care institutions have an obligation to their patients to provide a safe level of staffing. This obligation is enforced through inspection (JCAHO) and Medicare regulations. Employees should be aware of this fact.

A safe level of staffing is that level at which there are sufficient workers to deliver patient care. Most states do not specify specific staffing ratios or limits on staffing, but rather, expect that hospitals and nursing homes will have sufficient staff to meet the needs of their patients.

Medicare, as a condition of participation, requires that care be delivered in accordance with generally accepted professional standards in the community. As a result, when a hospital does not have sufficient staff to meet the needs of the patients, and patient needs go unmet, that creates a fraud situation for the hospital or nursing home. It is billing Medicare for services that are supposed to meet professional standards when they in fact do not meet those standards.

Clinicians have few options when they find themselves in this position. Although they may choose to report the health care facility to state and local licensure boards, frequently these boards take no immediate action, and the only result tends to be the imposition of punishment on the whistleblower.

If the facility has a Corporate Compliance Officer (CCO), this is the individual to whom it would be appropriate to complain, and most CCOs allow anonymous complaints. A compliance officer is normally charged with reporting this information up the chain of command, and if enough reports are made, frequently changes follow.

If a CCO is not available, the next best reporting agency would be the State Board of Health (the entity licensing hospitals in your state) and the Joint Commission for the Accreditation of Healthcare Organizations (JCAHO). Anonymous reports to these entities should produce investigations, and possibly change.

The last approach may well be to retain a private attorney for the purpose of bringing a whistleblower lawsuit. An in-depth explanation of this subject follows.

2. What Issues Affect Workload?

The major issue is your duty to the patients. A therapist has an independent duty to every patient he or she treats. That independent duty requires that the therapist exercise that degree of skill, learning, and expertise necessary to protect the patient from harm and treat them for their medical conditions. When a therapist is assigned a workload that is so excessive that no other therapist could reasonably be expected to handle the workload, it would be impossible to deliver appropriate care.

Sadly, the difference between staffing and workload is a critical one. While a hospital is required to staff properly, it is not required to apportion workload properly. As such, there is little if any regulation of therapist workload, absent union work rules.[13]

When a therapist is continually assigned workloads in excess of what a reasonable person can accomplish, the appropriate response is quite simply to vote with your feet. If a hospital does not permit you to practice within the bounds of the law, then you should change employers.

There are several good reasons to do so, one of which is patient abandonment.

3. What Is Patient Abandonment?

When you are assigned to a patient, and you do not fulfill the assignment to the best of your ability, that is abandonment. If a therapist has an independent duty to a patient, that duty extends to every patient that he is

---

[13]Therapists do not normally set the amount of care they give; that is a function of medical orders. However, certain unions do impose work rules through bargaining that restrict the number of treatments or patient interactions a therapist may be expected to provide in a certain work period.

assigned to, even if that assignment is unreasonable. If the workload is such that he cannot reach a patient, even in the exercise of all due diligence, then the employee may be considered to be abandoning his patient during the shift, and that could be an issue for a licensure board at some point.

Worse, if because of short staffing you make a choice to not see patients because you don't have time, and you do not take reasonable measures to see to it that the patients are seen by someone, that can be abandonment.

Finally, if you receive an assignment, and that assignment is unreasonable and unworkable, and knowing that there are insufficient staff you walk off the job, that is also abandonment of the patient.

But there are other, closer calls. For example, suppose the night shift therapist calls in and says "I'm going to be 10 minutes late." You have something to do at home, and you accept his word that he'll be there in 10 minutes, and you leave the hospital to the two remaining therapists on the night shift. The therapist doesn't arrive until 25 minutes later, and in the interim there are two codes. Patient treatments get missed. Are you liable for patient abandonment?

Quite probably you are. You did not have relief present before you left, and you accepted the word of another therapist and gambled that a third person would not be needed. That is a gamble that impacted the patients, and you and your employer are most likely liable for any harm caused to a patient by the shortage of staff.

What about the situation where the patient is an infant who requires transport to a Neonatal ICU, and the manager or supervisor is unreachable. As the supervisor, can you send the only other therapist out of the hospital with the infant, knowing that there is more work than you can do alone?

Again, it is a close call that could be argued either way, but the doctrine of triage would tend to protect you here. Here, the situation is not of your creation, but is due to external forces. You owe a duty to the infant to properly transport her to the distant facility, and you also owe duties to patients already at the institution. Sending the therapist and continuing to call on the supervisor or manager for back up is a reasonable alternative, and one more closely aligned with triage than with bad attitude.

4. What Is the Difference Between Triage and Abandonment?

Triage is caring for the sickest patients first, and spending time on more stable patients only after the critical needs are met. It is a universally accepted method of rationing health care in an emergency situation. The key word, however, is emergency.

While triage is a necessary and proper part of patient care when emergency situations occur, triage should not be a regular occurrence. If a therapist is routinely given more work than she can handle, she should consider leaving employment to protect her license against a claim of abandonment. If that is not an option, working hard within the system to protect her license is. Reports should be made to the Respiratory Care Board, to the Joint Commission, and if the practice continues, to the Office of Inspector General at Health and Human Services.

5. Should Therapists Be the Patient's Advocate?

Absolutely! Therapists also have the right and duty to speak out on behalf of their patients. Thus, whenever a patient does not receive a treatment, an incident report should be created and submitted to Risk Management. A paper trail of incident reports (a completely honest approach to the failure to deliver an ordered medication) creates an incentive in Risk Management to push for additional staffing and reduced workload for the therapists.

In recognizing their independent duty to the patient, the therapist may speak as the patient's advocate in the hospital. If insufficient therapists are providing insignificant care, then duty to the patient requires that therapists speak out. Remember, acting for mutual aid or protection (in this case, the protection of your license and the license of your peers) is protected concerted activity under the National Labor Relations Act.

G. WHAT IS WORKER'S COMPENSATION?

Worker's Compensation, sometimes called "Workmen's Compensation" in more sexist venues, is a means of providing for medical care and compensation for work-related injuries. Every employee in every state has the right to seek coverage under Worker's Compensation when they are injured at work.

1. What Is a Work-Related Injury?

A work-related injury is one suffered in the course, scope, and performance of your job duties. An accident in your personal car on the way to work is not a worker's compensation injury. Likewise tripping in the company parking lot may or may not be a work-related injury depending on state law. If you leave work on your way to the company Christmas party with the case of champagne in the trunk, and stop to buy plastic cups, and you fall carrying the cups to the car, that probably is a work-related injury.

In short, worker's compensation covers situations where an employee is injured doing his or her job, and it provides for medical treatment, partial disability payments, and permanent total disability payments.

2. What Rights Exist in Worker's Compensation?

Employees have the right to medical care, compensation for injuries, and partial continuing wages during periods of recuperation.

One of the most important rights of every health care worker is the right to a safe working environment. In most cases hospitals are safe. Most hospitals provide security, and employees are reasonably safe from assault, battery, rape, and robbery while performing their jobs or working on hospital property. Employees are also given work rules and supervisors to ensure that they are safe on the job. The recent use of "universal precautions" to prevent the spread of certain blood and body-fluid-borne ailments (Hepatitis, HIV, etc.) is but one example.

In spite of that, work injuries happen. When they do, few employees know their legal rights, and many wind up suffering chronic or even debilitating injuries for which they are never compensated. Worker's compensation is designed to help workers survive work injuries and be compensated more modestly than if they were permitted to sue their employer. It is also designed to provide quick and immediate treatment for work injuries and to provide proper restorative care.

3. Is Medical Treatment Covered?

Yes, when the injury is work related. When a work injury occurs in a hospital, usually the Employee Health Nurse or Emergency Room physician is the first person to see the employee. In that regard, work injuries in a hospital occur in the best possible place, where immediate medical care is available.

But it is important to remember that any injury that is work related is compensable and treatable under Worker's Compensation. Thus, when a therapist, as part of his job responsibilities, is riding in an ambulance that is involved in an accident, and he's injured as a result, that is a compensable work injury.[14] Similarly if they are working outside the hospital, perhaps attending

---

[14]It may also be a case where the therapist can sue some other third party. Just because the therapist has a remedy against the hospital for his work injuries does not preclude him from suing the person who ran the red light and broadsided the ambulance.

a seminar on company time, any injury that occurs is a work injury in most states.

This is important because the right to seek medical care for these injuries is one of the most important rights an injured worker has.

4. Must I Report My Injury?

Usually, yes. An employee who is injured must report the injury to their supervisor and to the company within a specific period of time, which varies from state to state. In most states, the period is 72 hours or less. Failure to report the injury does not necessarily cut off rights to treatment or partial disability payments, but it may affect the employee's ability to prove his or her case.

One thing every employee should know is to whom they report a work injury.

5. Who Chooses the Physician for Me?

Your physician is selected by the employer in most states. In most states the right to medical care is unquestioned; however, an injured employee's right to treatment is tempered by the right of the employer to select a physician. Sometimes the employer may select the same physician as the employee, or allow the employee to continue to see his own physician. In other instances, they may insist on sending the employee to some other physician. Of course, the employee can see his own physician, but that just means that the employee, not the employer, will be liable for the medical payments to that physician.

6. Do I Have a Right to Partial Disability Payments?

Depending on the nature and severity of your injury, yes. When an employee is seriously injured, such that they lose time from work, they may suffer what is termed a partial disability as a result. In nearly every state, the Worker's Compensation program has a "partial disability" program that is designed to compensate the employee for time missed from work.

While rights vary from state to state, partial disability payments are generally lump sum payments made after the disability is terminated.

7. What Is Permanent Disability?

Permanent disability payments are made for work injuries that result in permanent injury. For example, an injury to an employee's back is apt to be a permanent partial disability. The employee may have lifting restrictions and may have to be careful about how she works for many years to come. Her future employability may be affected. The employer is required to compensate her for her losses. Usually the injury is evaluated as a percentage of the whole body and employees receive an award based on the severity of their injury.

In almost every case, an attorney specializing in worker's compensation is required to advance a case for compensation for most work injuries. Fees for these cases are limited by statute in most states, with the national average being somewhere between 20% and 25% of the award. The employer is always represented by seasoned attorneys whose job is to minimize the payout to the employee. The employee who tries to negotiate with these attorneys will almost always come out behind a seasoned attorney with experience in worker's compensation cases. It is one of the areas where people who get an attorney generally get what they pay for.

8. Can an Employer Fire Me for Using Worker's Compensation?

No. It is unlawful in every state to terminate a worker for using worker's compensation benefits. It is not unlawful, however, to terminate someone for fraud on the worker's compensation insurance plan.

Sadly, it is also not improper for the employer to terminate you for tardiness even though the real reason is your use of worker's compensation benefits. When an employer engages in such conduct, it may be difficult to prove the "real reason" for the discharge and the employee may have no effective remedy.

H. SHOULD EMPLOYEES HAVE CONTRACTS?

From management's perspective, it is almost never a good idea to enter into a written contract with employees. Under the law of most states, when an employee is hired, that employee is hired "at will" meaning that they can be hired or fired for any reason or no reason, but not for an unlawful reason. The "at will" employment doctrine allows a hospital or business to release a non-performing employee without too much fear that the employee will later file a successful lawsuit against them.[15]

From an employee's perspective, sometimes it is a good thing to get a contract. Contracted employees have as many additional rights as their employ-

---

[15]The majority of wrongful termination lawsuits are dismissed before trial.

ment contract gives them. If the contract specifies a yearly salary, that has been held in some instances to be a contract to retain the employee for at least one year. Unless the employee has special skills, or is engaged to perform specific work that makes a contract desirable, line employees should never be hired under contract.

1. Do You Need a Contract?

A contract is most likely necessary when an employee is hired into an executive position, or into a position where they will come into contact with proprietary information and trade secrets. When an employee is exposed to such information, the business is investing money not only in his salary, but in his integrity. These employees should be hired under contract. The contract should be drafted by a specialist in employment law, and should be reviewed by counsel before being offered to the potential employee.

2. What Is an Independent Contractor?

Every now and then it is necessary to hire independent contractors to perform certain independent tasks. An independent contractor is an individual who is hired because of his or her special knowledge or expertise. They are responsible for the end result, and the person hiring them does not have the authority or ability to impose conditions on how they do their job.

In recent years, some employers and employees have hired staff therapists and per diem employees as independent contractors. The employee has the benefit of not having payroll taxes deducted from his or her check[16] and the employer has the benefit of not having to pay taxes and other benefits on that employee's salary.

The IRS has recently cracked down on this tactic, and explains the distinctions between contractors and employees as follows:

Independent Contractors vs. Employees

Before you can determine how to treat payments you make for services, you must first know the business relationship that exists between you and the person performing the services. The person performing the services may be

---

[16]They remain liable, however, for federal income taxes on the amounts they are paid.

- *An independent contractor*
- *A common-law employee (Employee)*
- *A statutory employee*
- *A statutory non-employee*

In determining whether the person providing the service is an employee or an independent contractor, all information that provides evidence of the degree of control and independence must be considered.

It is critical that you, the employer, correctly determine whether the individuals providing services are employees or independent contractors. Generally, you must withhold income taxes, withhold and pay Social Security and Medicare taxes, and pay unemployment tax on wages paid to an employee. You do not generally have to withhold or pay any taxes on payments to independent contractors.

Caution: If you incorrectly classify an employee as an independent contractor, you can be held liable for employment taxes for that worker, plus a penalty.

Who is an Independent Contractor?
A general rule is that you, the payer, have the **right to control or direct only the result of the work** *done by an independent contractor, and* **not the means and methods of accomplishing the result.**

Example: Vera Elm, an electrician, submitted a job estimate to a housing complex for electrical work at $16 per hour for 400 hours. She is to receive $1,280 every 2 weeks for the next 10 weeks. This is not considered payment by the hour. Even if she works more or less than 400 hours to complete the work, Vera Elm will receive $6,400. She also performs additional electrical installations under contracts with other companies, which she obtained through advertisements. Vera is an **independent contractor.**

Who is a Common-Law Employee (Employee)?
Under common-law rules, anyone who performs services for you is your employee if you can control what will be done and how it will be done. This is so even when you give the employee freedom of action. What matters is that you have the right to control the details of how the services are performed.

To determine whether an individual is an employee or independent contractor under the common law, the relationship of the worker and the business must be examined. All evidence of control and independence must be considered. In an employee-independent contractor determination, all information that provides evidence of the degree of control and degree of independence must be considered.

Facts that provide evidence of the degree of control and independence fall into three categories: behavioral control, financial control, and the type of relationship of the parties. Refer to Publication 15-A, <u>Employer's Supplemental Tax Guide</u> for additional information.

Who is an Employee?
A general rule is that anyone who performs services for you is your employee **if you can control what will be done and how it will be done.**

Example: Donna Lee is a salesperson employed on a full-time basis by Bob Blue, an auto dealer. She works six days a week, and is on duty in Bob's showroom on certain assigned days and times. She appraises trade-ins, but her appraisals are subject to the sales manager's approval. Lists of prospective customers belong to the dealer. She has to develop leads and report results to the sales manager. Because of her experience, she requires only minimal assistance in closing and financing sales and in other phases of her work. She is paid a commission and is eligible for prizes and bonuses offered by Bob. Bob also pays the cost of health insurance and group-term life insurance for Donna. Donna is an employee of Bob Blue.

Sometimes it is necessary and advisable to hire an independent contractor. For example, when a department wants to conduct training under HIPAA so that all its employees know and understand the new privacy rules, it might well contract with an attorney or with a seminar company to come in and train its employees.

Here, the hospital should insist in its contract what subjects the contractor covers in its lectures, but should not specify the way that training will be conducted (other than, perhaps, to specify that it be done on all three shifts and training series held on multiple days at multiple times).

The hospital should not, however, hire a part time or per diem employee to perform routine patient care services for it under this kind of arrangement. This is important because when a therapist performs patient care services, he does so subject to the rules and regulations imposed on the department by the hospital and the medical staff. The therapist does not decide independently how to treat patients, what medications to give, and how best to accomplish the goal of preventing atlectasis. Instead he relies on policies, procedures, and protocols, developed by the hospital.

While the hospital physician is probably an independent contractor (because the hospital does not have the right to control the manner in which he cares for his patient), the therapist is not such a contractor, and treating him like one will result in penalties from the IRS.

There is another issue with respect to independent contractors that should be discussed briefly here. A contractor who is truly "independent" and who, while performing services, injures a patient, does not subject the hospital to liability under respondeat superior in most instances.[17] So, in some instances, there are advantages to having an independent contractor relationship. As a general rule, how a relationship is structured for a person performing services for a hospital or business should be discussed with counsel prior to entering into any contract or agreement.

I. KEY POINTS

- Freedom of Contract means that employers are free to contract with employees.
- One side-effect is that employment is not a contract, instead, it is an "at-will" status.
- At will means you can be fired for:
  - Any reason; or
  - No Reason; but
  - Not for an unlawful reason.
- A Service Letter allows an employee to know the "true reason" his employment was terminated.
- An employment contract must generally be written.
- Where an employee moves from one location to another, or suffers some detriment from acting on a promise by an employer of continuing employment, there may be a case of "promissory estoppel."

---

[17]If the hospital holds the independent contractor out as its employee, for example, by giving him a lab coat that says "St. Mary's Hospital ER Physician" such that a reasonable person might think he was an employee of the hospital, the independent contractor rule may give way to the doctrine of "ostensible agent." When entering into any independent contractor relationship, contracts should be reviewed by counsel and should require the contractor to indemnify and hold harmless the hospital for any acts of negligence committed by the independent contractor.

- You need an employment contract if you want to protect yourself from unlawful termination, but
- An employer normally gets more rights in an employment contract than does an employee.
- These rights can include:
  - Non-compete agreements
  - Non-disclosure or confidentiality agreements
  - Return of Documents provisions
  - Notification of Employers provisions; and
  - Ban on Solicitation of Employees provisions.
- Covenants not to compete must be for a valid time and valid geographic area.
- A covenant not to compete must not be against public policy.
- The National Labor Relations Act governs every employee in an organization with 50 or more employees, and not just those in unions.
  - Employees have the right to organize.
  - Employees have the right to act for mutual aid and protection.
  - Employees have the right to organize and act for mutual aid even though they are not in a union.
- Hospitals must usually give notice of closing when a layoff or shutdown is imminent.
- There are certain rights unique to health care.
- Patient care persons must not abandon patients, no matter how bad staffing is.
- Worker's Compensation gives a worker the right to medical treatment.
- The employer has the right to choose the employee's doctor for Worker's Compensation treatment.
- The Employee has a right to permanent, and partial disability payments.
- Employers may not retaliate for an employee's use of Worker's Compensation insurance.

CHAPTER 5

Essential Employee Rights Granted by Federal and State Law

Unquestionably, there is progress. The average American now pays twice as much in taxes as he formerly got in wages.

H. L. Mencken
1880–1956, American Editor, Author, Critic, Humorist

A. WHAT ARE MY WAGE AND HOUR RIGHTS?

On June 25, 1938, Congress passed the Fair Labor Standards Act, which set minimum guidelines for compensation of employees. Since the passage of this legislation, more than $1 billion has been computed in back wage liability, against employers, by agents of the federal government. Most of this money was unknowingly not paid to employees because employers were unaware of the interpretation or application of the federal and state regulations.

1. What Is the Fair Labor Standards Act (FLSA)?

It is a federal law applicable to almost every employer. The Fair Labor Standards Act (FLSA) provides minimum wage, equal pay, overtime pay, record-keeping, and child labor standards. These requirements apply to:

- employees engaged in interstate commerce,
- employees involved in the production of goods for interstate commerce,
- employees in certain enterprises that are engaged in interstate commerce.

There are, however, some exemptions from these requirements. Some employees in certain establishments and in certain occupations are not covered. For the most part, respiratory therapists and employees in hospital and health care work are covered by the FLSA.

The Act is administered by the Wage and Hour Division of the United States Department of Labor. The equal pay provisions of the FLSA are administered by the Equal Employment Opportunity Commission. This presents some problems for employees who have to know which agency to go to for enforcement assistance.

2. What Is Covered by Federal Wage and Hour Law?

The FLSA covers the hours a person may lawfully work, and the amount of money that person must be paid is covered by wage and hour laws. In addition to the FLSA, certain state regulations under state laws apply in those situations where the federal laws do not apply (e.g., only two or three employees). See Appendix F.

Federal Regulations—The FLSA applies to any employee who is not specifically exempt and is individually engaged either in interstate commerce activities or in the production of (including handling and working on) goods for interstate commerce, or is employed in an enterprise that is covered under the act.

An establishment is covered if its annual gross sales exceed $500,000. Almost every hospital is going to meet this threshold. For those that don't, however, the employees are still covered under the individual coverage rule. Individual coverage simply means that if an employee, as part of her work in the workweek, is involved in engaging in interstate commerce or in the production of (including the handling of or working on) goods for interstate commerce, or in activities essential to interstate commerce, she falls under the FLSA. So, for example, if a hospital brings in ventilator circuits manufactured in another state or that have components from other states, a therapist works with or works on goods produced for interstate commerce. Clerks and housekeeping employees whose work is closely related and directly essential to any interstate operations are also covered, as are employees regularly engaged in interstate communication by telephone, telegraph, or the mail. Therapists routinely assist in transports, and many of those transports extend across state lines. Therapists also make telephone calls to physicians and obtain patient information through the mail. Therapists would be considered workers involved in interstate commerce.

3. What Are Minimum Wage and Overtime Pay Rights?

This information has recently changed, and may be changing again depending on Congressional action. New regulations took effect in 2004, and the full impact of those regulations is still unknown. What follows is a discussion of the pre-2004 rules, which may be reinstated.

As of September 1, 1997, covered non-exempt employees are entitled to a minimum wage of not less than $5.15 an hour and to overtime pay at a rate of not less than one and one-half times their regular rates of pay for hours worked in excess of 40 hours in a workweek.

Where meals, lodging, or other facilities are customarily provided for the benefit of the employee, the reasonable cost or fair value is considered wages under section 3(m) of the act except to the extent that such costs are excluded by the terms of a bona fide collective bargaining agreement. (See Regulations, 29 CFR Part 531.)

If the facilities furnished by the employer are primarily for the employer's benefit instead of the worker's, their cost may not be included in computing wages. For example, if the hospital furnishes scrubs for its employees who work in critical care, this is for the benefit of the hospital in securing infection control, and is not a basis for deduction from wages.

4. How Do Employers Compute Overtime Pay?

Employers calculate pay according to state or federal law. All non-exempt employees (generally those who are working in a non-supervisory/non-salaried position) must be paid at not less than one and one-half times their regular rates of pay for all hours worked over 40 in a workweek. Nothing requires that a therapist be paid each week, or even every two weeks. The employer may make the wage or salary payment at other regular intervals, such as every two weeks, every half month, or once a month. The act does require that both the minimum wage and any overtime pay be computed only on the hours actually worked each work week; the employer can't average hours over two or more workweeks to "smooth out" overtime.

A workweek is a regular recurring period of 168 hours in the form of seven consecutive 24-hour periods. The workweek need not be the same as the calendar week. It may begin on any day of the week and at any hour of the day. Once established, however, an employee's workweek may not be changed unless the change is intended to be permanent. So the workweek may begin on a Thursday and end on a Wednesday, so long as that rule is always followed.

The regular rate of pay can always be more than the applicable minimum wage (and for therapists, almost always will be) but it cannot be less. The regular rate includes all remuneration for employment except certain payments excluded by the law itself.

Payments that are not part of the regular rate include payment for business expenses; discretionary bonuses; gifts and payments in the nature of gifts on special occasions; payments pursuant to certain profit-sharing, welfare, or thrift and saving plans; and payments for occasional periods when no work is performed due to vacation, holiday, or illness.

Other payments such as production bonuses, attendance bonuses, commissions, piece rate earnings, and other payments for work performed must be added to the employee's hourly or weekly earnings and then divided by the hours worked during the workweek to determine the regular rate. All time worked in excess of the statutory workweek applicable to the employees must be paid for at the premium rate required by the act.

5. What Counts as Hours Worked?

Many activities count toward hours worked. An employee subject to the act in any workweek must be paid in accordance with its provisions for all hours worked. In general, "hours worked" includes all time the employee is required to be on duty or on the employer's premises or at a prescribed workplace, and all time the employee is permitted to work for the employer.[1]

Meal Periods present a unique challenge. Meal Periods during the scheduled workday are not work time if the employee is completely relieved from duty for the purpose of eating regular meals. Ordinarily 30 minutes or more is long enough for a bona fide meal period. In order for an employer to deduct a meal period from time paid, the employee must receive 30 minutes or more of an uninterrupted meal period.

It is the "uninterrupted" issue that creates problems for therapists. Where an employee's otherwise bona fide meal periods are uninterrupted except for rare and infrequent emergency calls, the meal period can be excluded from compensable working time except on those occasions when the period is actually interrupted.

On the other hand, if the meal periods are frequently interrupted by calls to treat patients in the ICU and ER, the employee is not to be considered relieved of all duties and the meal periods must be counted as hours worked. So a therapist with the ICU beeper, with the ER beeper, or with a requirement to return in an emergency to his or her work area, who does so on a more than infrequent basis (e.g., more than once a pay period) must be compensated for the meal time as work time, and no deduction is permissible.

---

[1]*Federal Regulation, Part 785.*

6. What About On-Call Time?

Therapists who are not required to remain at the hospital, and are free to engage in their own pursuits, subject only to the understanding that they carry a beeper or cell phone, or make other arrangements to be reached, are not working while on call for the purpose of the act.

When such employees are called into the hospital the actual time worked is counted as hours worked and must be paid. If calls are so frequent or the "on-call" conditions so restrictive that the employees are not free to use the intervening periods for their own benefit, then such time would be counted as hours worked. For example, if a hospital required the on-call therapist to be present at the hospital, but allowed her to sleep until called, the conditions might be considered too restrictive and the on-call time would be paid time.

7. Are There Exemptions to the FLSA?

a) Who Are Salaried Persons?

Executive, administrative, or professional exemption: An exemption from both the minimum wage and overtime pay requirements is provided in section 13(a)(1) of the act for any employee employed in a bona fide executive, administrative, or professional capacity, as these terms are defined and delimited in Regulations.[2] An employee must meet all of the criteria of an exemption test in order to be considered exempt from the minimum wage and overtime requirements.

b) Must Employers Put Up a Poster?

Each covered establishment must display a Wage and Hour poster where the employees may readily see it. This poster, which briefly outlines the act's basic requirements, may be obtained free from the nearest office of the Wage and Hour Division. Employers should also post the Employee Polygraph Protection Act poster and the Family Leave Medical Act poster, if applicable.

c) Are Breaks (Lunch—Meal—Rest) a Requirement?

Federal regulations do not require that breaks be provided for any employees. Some states, like Maine and California, do require break periods. But technically, nothing in the federal law requires an employer to provide a meal break.

---

[2]29 CFR Part 541.

d) Who Can Enforce These Rights?

Authorized representatives of the Wage and Hour Division may investigate and gather data regarding wages, hours, and other conditions and practices of employment. The act provides these methods of recovering unpaid minimum and/or overtime wages: (1) the Administrator may supervise the payment of back wages; (2) in certain circumstances the Secretary of Labor may bring suit for back pay and an equal amount as liquidated damages; (3) an employee may sue for back wages and an additional sum as liquidated damages plus attorney's fees and court costs; and (4) the Secretary of Labor may also obtain a court injunction restraining violations of the law, including the unlawful withholding of proper minimum wage and overtime pay.

e) Is Enforcement by Employees Allowed?

It is a violation of the law to discharge an employee for filing a complaint or participating in a proceeding under the Fair Labor Standards Act or minimum wage laws. Willful violations may be prosecuted criminally and the violator fined up to $10,000. A second conviction for such a violation may result in imprisonment.

A two-year statute of limitations applies to the recovery of back wages except in the case of willful violations, in which case a three-year statute of limitations would be applicable.

f) Can Employers Be Forced to Pay Civil Money Penalties Imposed by the Department of Labor?

The United States Department of Labor can assess civil money penalties of up to $10,000 per minor against employers who violate the Fair Labor Standard Act's child labor provisions, or willfully or repeatedly violate the law's minimum wage or overtime pay requirements.

Employers who willfully or repeatedly violate the minimum wage or overtime pay requirements are subject to civil money penalties of up to $1,000 per violation.

g) What Are the Rules Regarding Garnishment of Wages for a Single Debt?

The Federal Wage Garnishment Law (Title III of the Consumer Credit Protection Act) limits the amount of an employee's earnings that may be garnished and protects an employee from being fired if pay is garnished for one debt. Title III is administered by the Wage and Hour Division of the Department of Labor's Employment Standards Administration. The law protects everyone receiving personal earnings, i.e., wages, salaries, commissions, bonuses, or income including earnings from a pension or retirement program. The law prohibits an employer from firing an employee whose earnings are subject to garnishment for any one debt, regardless of the number of levies made or proceedings brought to collect the debt. The law does not prohibit discharge if the employee's earnings have been garnished for a second or subsequent debt.

Specific restrictions apply to court orders for child support or alimony. The garnishment law allows up to 50 percent of a worker's disposable earnings to be garnished if the worker is supporting another spouse or child, and up to 60 percent for a worker who is not. An additional 5 percent may be garnished for support payments more than 12 weeks in arrears. These garnishments are not subject to the limitation noted above.

B. WHAT ARE MY RIGHTS UNDER THE FAMILY AND MEDICAL LEAVE ACT?

The U. S. Department of Labor's Employment Standards Administration, Wage and Hour Division, administers and enforces the Family and Medical Leave Act (FMLA) for all private, state, and local government employees, and some federal employees. Most federal and certain congressional employees are also covered by the law and are subject to the jurisdiction of the U.S. Office of Personnel Management or the Congress.

FMLA became effective on August 5, 1993. The FMLA entitles eligible employees to take up to 12 weeks of unpaid job-protected leave in a 12-month period for specified family and medical reasons. The employer may elect to use the calendar year, a fixed 12-month leave, or fiscal year, or a 12-month period prior to or after the commencement of leave as the 12-month period.

The law contains provisions on employer coverage; employee eligibility for the law's benefits; entitlement to leave, maintenance of health benefits during leave, and job restoration after leave; notice and certification of the need for FMLA leave; and protection for employees who request or take FMLA leave. The law also requires employers to keep certain records.

1. To Whom Does the FMLA Apply?

The FMLA applies to:

- public agencies, including state, local, and federal employers, local education agencies (schools), and

- private sector employers who employed 50 or more employees in 20 or more workweeks in the current or preceding calendar year and who are engaged in commerce or in any industry or activity affecting commerce—including joint employers and successors of covered employers.

2. Who Has FMLA Eligibility?

To be eligible for FMLA benefits, an employee must:

(1) work for a covered employer;
(2) have worked for the employer for a total of 12 months;
(3) have worked at least 1,250 hours over the previous 12 months; and
(4) work at a location in the United States or in any territory or possession of the United States where at least 50 employees are employed by the employer within 75 miles.

3. What Are My FMLA Rights?

A covered employer must grant an eligible employee up to a total of 12 workweeks of unpaid leave during any 12-month period for one or more of the following reasons:

- for the birth and care of the newborn child of the employee;
- for placement with the employee of a son or daughter for adoption or foster care;
- to care for an immediate family member (spouse, child, or parent) with a serious health condition; or
- to take medical leave when the employee is unable to work because of a serious health condition.

Spouses employed by the same employer are jointly entitled to a combined total of 12 workweeks of family leave for the birth and care of the newborn child, for placement of a child for adoption or foster care, and to care for a parent who has a serious health condition.

Leave for birth and care, or placement for adoption or foster care must conclude within 12 months of the birth or placement.

Under some circumstances, employees may take FMLA leave intermittently—which means taking leave in blocks of time, or by reducing their normal weekly or daily work schedule.

- If FMLA leave is for birth and care or placement for adoption or foster care, use of intermittent leave is subject to the employer's approval.

- FMLA leave may be taken intermittently whenever medically necessary to care for a seriously ill family member, or because the employee is seriously ill and unable to work.

Also, subject to certain conditions, employees or employers may choose to use accrued paid leave (such as sick or vacation leave) to cover some or all of the FMLA leave.

The employer is responsible for designating whether an employee's use of paid leave counts as FMLA leave, based on information from the employee.

a) Are Any Specific Terms Defined Under FMLA?

Yes. The following terms are defined:

"Serious health condition" means an illness, injury, impairment, or physical or mental condition that involves either:

- any period of incapacity or treatment connected with inpatient care (i.e., an overnight stay) in a hospital, hospice, or residential medical care facility, and any period of incapacity or subsequent treatment in connection with such inpatient care; or
- continuing treatment by a health care provider, which includes any period of incapacity (i.e. inability to work, attend school, or perform other regular daily activities) due to: (1) A health condition (including treatment therefor, or recovery therefrom) lasting more than three consecutive days, and any subsequent treatment or period of incapacity relating to the same condition, which also includes:
- treatment two or more times by or under the supervision of a health care provider; or
- one treatment by a health care provider with a continuing regimen of treatment; or
  (1) pregnancy or prenatal care. A visit to the health care provider is not necessary for each absence; or
  (2) a chronic serious health condition that continues over an extended period of time, requires periodic visits to a health care provider, and may involve occasional episodes of incapacity (e.g., asthma, diabetes). A visit to a health care provider is not necessary for each absence; or
  (3) a permanent or long-term condition for which treatment may not be effective (e.g., Alzheimer's, a severe stroke, terminal cancer). Only supervision by a health care provider is required, rather than active treatment; or

(4) any absences to receive multiple treatments for restoration surgery or for a condition that would likely result in a period of incapacity of more than three days if not treated (e.g., chemotherapy or radiation treatments for cancer).

"Health care provider" means:

- doctors of medicine or osteopathy authorized to practice medicine or surgery by the state in which the doctors practice; or
- podiatrists, dentists, clinical psychologists, optometrists, and chiropractors (limited to manual manipulation of the spine to correct a subluxation as demonstrated by X-ray to exist) authorized to practice, and performing within the scope of their practice, under state law; or
- Christian Science practitioners listed with the First Church of Christ, Scientist in Boston, Massachusetts; or
- any health care provider recognized by the employer or the employer's group health plan benefits manager.

4. What About Maintenance of Health Benefits While on Family Leave?

A covered employer is required to maintain group health insurance coverage for an employee on FMLA leave whenever such insurance was provided before the leave was taken and on the same terms as if the employee had continued to work. If applicable, arrangements will need to be made for employees to pay their share of health insurance premiums while on leave.

In some instances, the employer may recover premiums it paid to maintain health coverage for an employee who fails to return to work from FMLA leave.

5. Must an Employer Grant Job Restoration?

Usually, yes. Upon return from FMLA leave, an employee must be restored to the employee's original job, or to an equivalent job with equivalent pay, benefits, and other terms and conditions of employment.

In addition, an employee's use of FMLA leave cannot result in the loss of any employment benefit that the employee earned or was entitled to before using FMLA leave, nor be counted against the employee under a "no fault" attendance policy.

Under specified and limited circumstances where restoration to employment will cause substantial and grievous economic injury to its operations, an employer may refuse to reinstate certain highly paid "key" employees after their use of FMLA leave during which health coverage was maintained. In order to do so, the employer must:

- notify the employee of his/her status as a "key" employee in response to the employee's notice of intent to take FMLA leave;
- notify the employee as soon as the employer decides it will deny job restoration, and explain the reasons for this decision;
- offer the employee a reasonable opportunity to return to work from FMLA leave after giving this notice; and
- make a final determination whether reinstatement will be denied at the end of the leave period if the employee then requests restoration.

A "key" employee is a salaried "eligible" employee who is among the highest paid ten percent of employees within 75 miles of the work site.

6. Do Employees Have Any Notice and Certification Responsibilities?

The FMLA contains a trap for the unwary employee. Employees seeking to use FMLA leave are required to provide a 30-day advance notice of their need to take FMLA leave when the need is foreseeable and such notice is practicable. Employers may also require employees to provide:

- medical certification supporting the need for leave due to a serious health condition affecting the employee or an immediate family member;
- second or third medical opinions (at the employer's expense) and periodic recertification; and
- periodic reports during FMLA leave regarding the employee's status and intent to return to work.

When intermittent leave is needed to care for an immediate family member or the employee's own illness, and is for planned medical treatment, the employee must try to schedule treatment so as not to unduly disrupt the employer's operation.

Covered employers must post a notice approved by the Secretary of Labor explaining rights and responsibilities under FMLA. An employer that willfully violates this posting requirement may be subject to a fine of up to $100 for each separate offense.

Also, covered employers must inform employees of their rights and responsibilities under FMLA, including giving specific written information on what is required of the employee and what might happen in certain circumstances, such as if the employee fails to return to work after FMLA leave.

7. What Is an Unlawful Act Under the FMLA?

It is unlawful for any employer to interfere with, restrain, or deny the exercise of any right provided by the FMLA. It is also unlawful for an employer to discharge or discriminate against an individual for opposing any practice, or because of involvement in any proceeding related to FMLA.

8. Who Has Enforcement Power?

The Wage and Hour Division investigates complaints. If violations cannot be satisfactorily resolved, the United States Department of Labor may bring action in court to compel compliance. Individuals may also bring private civil actions against an employer for violations.

9. What Are the Other Provisions of the FMLA?

Special rules apply to employees of local education agencies. Generally, these rules provide for FMLA leave to be taken in blocks of time when intermittent leave is needed or the leave is required near the end of a school term.

Salaried executive, administrative, and professional employees of covered employers who meet the Fair Labor Standards Act (FLSA) criteria for exemption from minimum wage and overtime under Regulations, 29 CFR Part 541, do not lose their FLSA-exempt status by using any unpaid FMLA leave. This special exception to the "salary basis" requirements for FLSA's exemption extends only to "eligible" employees' use of leave required by FMLA.

The FMLA does not affect any other federal or state law that prohibits discrimination, nor does it supersede any state or local law that provides greater family or medical leave protection. It also does not affect an employer's obligation to provide greater leave rights under a collective bargaining agreement or employment benefit plan. The FMLA also encourages employers to provide more generous leave rights.

C. IS EQUAL PAY FOR EQUAL WORK GUARANTEED?

Yes, but that doesn't mean you always get it.

The right of all employees to be free from discrimination in their compensation is protected under several federal laws, including the following, enforced by the United States Equal Employment Opportunity Commission (EEOC): the Equal Pay Act of 1963, Title VII of the Civil Rights Act of 1964, the Age Discrimination in Employment Act of 1967, and Title I of the Americans with Disabilities Act of 1990.

The Equal Pay Act (EPA) requires that men and women be given equal pay for equal work in the same establishment. The jobs need not be identical, but they must be substantially equal. It is job content, not job titles, that determines whether jobs are substantially equal. Thus, even though one therapist is an RRT, and another a CRTT, for purposes of equal pay analysis, if their jobs require the same skills, efforts and responsibilities, under the terms of the EPA, they are substantially equal.

1. Are There "Male Jobs" and "Female Jobs?"

Generally speaking, there shouldn't be.

Wage classification systems that designate certain jobs as "male jobs" and other jobs as "female jobs" frequently specify markedly lower rates for the "female jobs." Such practices indicate a pay practice of discrimination based on sex. It is an unlawful employment practice under Title VII of the Civil Rights Act of 1964 to classify a job as "male" or "female" unless sex is a bona fide occupational qualification for the job. In other words, only if the job can only be done by a male is it appropriate to assign the job a male classification, and similarly, only if the job can only be done by females may it be assigned a female classification. Classifications for the convenience of the employer in hiring individuals are unlawful.

The EPA prohibits discrimination on the basis of sex in the payment of wages to employees for work on jobs that are equal under the standards that the act provides. For example, where an employee of one sex is hired or assigned to a particular job to replace an employee of the opposite sex but receives a lower rate of pay than the person replaced, a prima facie violation of the EPA exists. When a prima facie violation of the EPA exists, it is incumbent on the employer to show that the wage differential is justified under one or more of the act's four affirmative defenses.

These violations occur frequently in health care, and some of them may be justified under the affirmative defenses. But employees should know that the EEOC will investigate, and may charge the employer with violations where such obvious violations of the Act occur.

If a person of one sex succeeds a person of the opposite sex on a job at a higher rate of pay than the predecessor, and there is no reason for the higher rate other than difference in gender, a violation as to the predecessor is established and that person is entitled to recover the difference between his or her pay and the higher rate paid the successor employee. This can be a significant matter where there is a gender difference and a long-term employee is replaced by an employee of a different gender with a significant increase in remuneration.

> *Suppose John has been the Pulmonary Function Technician for ten years, and has made $18.00 per hour for the last six years. After a series of poor evaluations, John reads the handwriting on the wall and takes a job at a home care company. He is replaced by Matilda, a registered therapist with no PFT experience, who is paid $22.00 per hour to do the same job.*

This is a violation of the Equal Pay Act, and John may report the former employer to the EEOC. It is possible that John will receive back pay from his employer because of a violation of the Equal Pay Act.

Under the EPA, it is immaterial that a member of the higher paid sex ceased to be employed prior to the period covered by the applicable statute of limitations period for filing a timely suit under the EPA. The employer's continued failure to pay the member of the lower paid sex the wage rate paid to the higher paid predecessor constitutes a prima facie continuing violation. This means that every day that a person is not properly paid, there is a new "injury" and therefore, the statute of limitations is not a defense. Also, it is no defense that the unequal payments began before the statute of limitations period. For this reason, the EEOC may be very effective in getting back pay for discriminated employees.

The EEOC has issued regulations regarding the standards for determining the rate of pay under the EPA. The rate of pay must be equal for persons performing equal work on jobs requiring equal skill, effort, and responsibility, and performed under similar working conditions. When factors such as seniority, education, or experience are used to determine the rate of pay, then those standards must be applied on a sex- or gender-neutral basis. Thus, a male therapist with 10 years seniority should be paid the same as a female therapist with 10 years of seniority, and should be entitled to the same priority for job transfers, vacation, and other benefits. Failure to provide for such equal treatment can result in sanctions from the EEOC.

As noted earlier, job content is controlling for purposes of the Equal Pay Act. Application of the equal pay standard is not dependent on job classifications or titles. It depends instead on actual job requirements and performance. For example, the fact that jobs performed by male and female employees may have the same total point value under an evaluation system in use by the employer does not in itself mean that the jobs concerned are equal according to the terms of the statute. Conversely, although the point values allocated to jobs may add up to unequal totals, it does not necessarily follow that the work being performed in such jobs is unequal when the statutory tests of the equal pay standard are applied. Job titles are frequently of such a general nature as to provide very little guidance in determining the application of the equal pay standard. For example, the job title "therapist" may be applied to employees who perform a variety of duties so dissimilar as to place many of them beyond the scope of comparison under the act.

Similarly, jobs included under the title "technician" may include an employee of one sex who spends all or most of his or her working hours in the ICU, whereas another employee, of the opposite sex, may also be described as a "technician" but be engaged entirely in giving routine treatments. In the case of jobs identified by the general title "therapist," the facts may show that equal skill, effort, and responsibility are required in the jobs of male and female employees notwithstanding that they are engaged in different kinds of care. In all such situations, the application of the equal pay standard will have to be determined by applying the terms of the act to the specific facts involved.

Pay differentials are permitted when they are based on seniority, merit, quantity or quality of production, or a factor other than sex. These are known as "affirmative defenses" and it is the employer's burden to prove that these apply.

In correcting a pay differential, no employee's pay may be reduced. Instead, the pay of the lower paid employee(s) must be increased.

2. How Do Title VII, ADEA, and ADA Affect Compensation Discrimination?

They make it unlawful and actionable in court.

Title VII, the ADEA, and the ADA prohibit compensation discrimination on the basis of race, color, religion, sex, national origin, age, or disability. Unlike the EPA, there is no requirement under Title VII, the ADEA, or the ADA that the claimant's job be substantially equal to that of a higher paid person outside the claimant's protected class, nor do these statutes require the claimant to work in the same establishment as a comparator.

Compensation discrimination under Title VII, the ADEA, or the ADA can occur in a variety of forms. For example:

An employer pays an employee with a disability less than similarly situated employees without disabilities and the employer's explanation (if any) does not satisfactorily account for the differential.

A discriminatory compensation system has been discontinued but still has lingering discriminatory effects on present salaries. For example, if an employer has a compensation policy or practice that pays Hispanics lower salaries than other employees, the employer must not only adopt a new non-discriminatory compensation policy, it also must affirmatively eradicate salary disparities that began prior to the adoption of the new policy and make the victims whole.

An employer sets the compensation for jobs held predominantly by, for example, women or African-Americans below that suggested by the employer's job evaluation study, while the pay for jobs held predominantly by men or whites is consistent with the level suggested by the job evaluation study.

An employer maintains a neutral compensation policy or practice that has an adverse impact on employees in a protected class and cannot be justified as job-related and consistent with business necessity. For example, if an employer provides extra compensation to employees who are the "head of household," i.e., married with dependents and the primary financial contributor to the household, the practice may have an unlawful disparate impact on women.

It is also unlawful to retaliate against an individual for opposing employment practices that discriminate based on compensation or for filing a discrimination charge, testifying, or participating in any way in an investigation, proceeding, or litigation under Title VII, ADEA, ADA, or the Equal Pay Act.

D. ARE LIFE AND HEALTH INSURANCE BENEFITS BY EMPLOYERS REGULATED?

Yes.

Generally, there are two major issues with regard to insurance that arise in the employment context. The first is the issue of health and life insurance benefits. The second is the issue of malpractice liability insurance. This section deals specifically with these insurance issues.

1. What Are the Life Insurance and Health Insurance Issues?

An employee is not entitled to life insurance or health insurance under any set of state or federal laws. An employee gets life insurance or health insurance solely on the basis of the employer's good will. Other than the mandates of the Equal Pay Act discussed above, it is not improper for the management or senior executives of an institution to enjoy a greatly enhanced benefit package over the rank and file employees in an organization. For this reason, officers and directors of hospitals frequently enjoy cost-free health care benefits and life insurance paid for by their employer. They may also enjoy car and housing allowances that are not provided to employees generally. Certain executives, like the CEO, the Chief Operating Officer, and the Chief Financial Officer, may enjoy additional perks like country club memberships. So long as these benefits are not applied disparately among those of that level, there is no violation of federal or state laws. An organization may choose to compensate different jobs with different levels of compensation, and the employee benefit plan is likewise free to be used as a tool to recruit or retain certain levels of employees.

a) What Is ERISA (and should I care?)

Health insurance benefits are governed by a federal law called ERISA—the Employee Retirement Income Security Act. The Employee Retirement Income Security Act of 1974 (ERISA) is a federal law that sets minimum standards for most voluntarily established pension and health plans in private industry to provide protection for individuals in these plans.

ERISA requires plans to provide participants with plan information, including important information about plan features and funding; sets minimum standards for participation, vesting, benefit accrual and funding; provides fiduciary responsibilities for those who manage and control plan assets; requires plans to establish a grievance and appeals process for participants to get benefits from their plans; gives participants the right to sue for benefits and breaches of fiduciary duty; and, if a defined benefit plan is terminated, guarantees payment of certain benefits through a federally chartered corporation, known as the Pension Benefit Guaranty Corporation (PBGC).

In general, ERISA does not cover retirement plans established or maintained by governmental entities, churches for their employees, or plans that are maintained solely to comply with applicable workers compensation, unemployment, or disability laws. ERISA also does not cover plans maintained outside the United States primarily for the benefit of nonresident aliens or unfunded excess benefit plans.

b) How Does HIPAA Affect My Insurance Rights?

By making your coverage portable—you can take it from place to place.

In addition to creating headaches for hospitals in the area of medical records security, the Health Insurance Portability and Accountability Act (HIPAA) also created certain rights for employees regarding their health benefits coverages.

HIPAA, signed into law on August 21, 1996, offers protections for millions of American workers that improve portability and continuity of health insurance coverage.

HIPAA protects workers and their families by:

- Limiting exclusions for preexisting medical conditions (known as preexisting conditions)
- Providing credit against maximum preexisting condition exclusion periods for prior health coverage and a process for providing certificates showing periods of prior coverage to a new group health plan or health insurance issuer
- Providing new rights that allow individuals to enroll for health coverage when they lose other health coverage, get married or add a new dependent

HIPAA is effective for all plans and issuers with respect to the certification requirements of HIPAA beginning June 1, 1997. However, the other HIPAA provisions are generally effective for plan years beginning after June 30, 1997.

2. What Effect Does HIPAA Have on the Preexisting Condition Exclusions?

In most cases it helps ease or remove them.

The law defines a preexisting condition as one for which medical advice, diagnosis, care, or treatment was recommended or received during the six-month period prior to an individual's enrollment date (which is the earlier of the first day of health coverage or the first day of any waiting period for coverage).

Group health plans and issuers may not exclude an individual's preexisting medical condition from coverage for more than 12 months (18 months for late enrollees) after an individual's enrollment date.

Under HIPAA, a new employer's plan must give individuals credit for the length of time they had prior continuous health coverage, without a break in coverage of 63 days or more, thereby reducing or eliminating the 12-month exclusion period (18 months for late enrollees).

3. What Effect Does HIPAA Have on Creditable Coverage?

It includes prior coverage under another group health plan, an individual health insurance policy, COBRA, Medicaid, Medicare, CHAMPUS, the Indian Health Service, a state health benefits risk pool, FEHBP, the Peace Corps Act, or a public health plan.

4. What Are Certificates of Creditable Coverage?

Certificates of creditable coverage must be provided automatically and free of charge by the plan or issuer when an individual loses coverage under the plan, becomes entitled to elect COBRA continuation coverage or exhausts COBRA continuation coverage. A certificate must also be provided free of charge upon request while you have health coverage or any time within 24 months after your coverage ends.

Certificates of creditable coverage should contain information about the length of time you or your dependents had coverage as well as the length of any waiting period for coverage that applied to you or your dependents.

If a certificate is not received, or the information on the certificate is wrong, you should contact your prior plan or issuer. You have a right to show prior creditable coverage with other evidence—like pay stubs, explanation of benefits, letters from a doctor—if you cannot get a certificate.

5. Are There Special Enrollment Rights?

Yes. These are provided for individuals who lose their coverage in certain situations, including on separation, divorce, death, termination of employment, and reduction in hours. Special enrollment rights also are provided if employer contributions toward the other coverage terminates. They are provided for employees, their spouses, and new dependents upon marriage, birth, adoption or placement for adoption.

6. Are There Discrimination Prohibitions?

Yes. They ensure that individuals are not excluded from coverage, or charged more for coverage offered by a plan or issuer, based on health status-related factors.

a) What Is the Consolidated Omnibus Budget Reconciliation Act (COBRA)?

It is a law that requires your employer to tell you how to continue your health insurance after voluntary or involuntary termination from employment.

Throughout a career, workers will face multiple life events, job changes, or even job losses. A law enacted in 1986 helps workers and their families keep their group health coverage during times of voluntary or involuntary job loss, reduction in the hours worked, transition between jobs, and in certain other cases.

The law—the Consolidated Omnibus Budget Reconciliation Act (COBRA)—gives workers who lose their health benefits the right to choose to continue group health benefits provided by the plan under certain circumstances.

COBRA generally requires that group health plans sponsored by employers with 20 or more employees in the prior year offer employees and their families the opportunity for a temporary extension of health coverage (called continuation coverage) in certain instances where coverage under the plan would otherwise end.

The law generally covers group health plans maintained by employers with 20 or more employees in the prior year. It applies to plans in the private sector and those sponsored by state and local governments. Provisions of COBRA covering state and local government plans are administered by the Department of Health and Human Services.

Several events that can cause workers and their family members to lose group health coverage may result in the right to COBRA coverage. These include:

- Voluntary or involuntary termination of the covered employee's employment for reasons other than gross misconduct
- Reduced hours of work for the covered employee
- Covered employee becoming entitled to Medicare
- Divorce or legal separation of a covered employee
- Death of a covered employee
- Loss of status as a dependent child under plan rules

Under COBRA, the employee or family member may qualify to keep their group health plan benefits for a set period of time, depending on the reason for losing the health coverage. The following represents some basic information on periods of continuation coverage:

Qualified Beneficiary	Qualifying Event	Period of Coverage
Employee Spouse Dependent child	Termination Reduced hours	18 months *
Spouse Dependent child	Entitled to Medicare Divorce or legal separation Death of covered employee	36 months
Dependent child	Loss of dependent child status	36 months

*This 18-month period may be extended for all qualified beneficiaries if certain conditions are met in cases where a qualified beneficiary is determined to be disabled for purposes of COBRA.

However, COBRA also provides that your continuation coverage may be cut short in certain cases.

7. Must an Employer Tell You About COBRA Rights?

An initial notice must be furnished to covered employees and spouses, at the time coverage under the plan commences, informing them of their rights under COBRA and describing provisions of the law. COBRA information also is required to be contained in the plan's summary plan description (SPD).

When the plan administrator is notified that a qualifying event has happened, it must in turn notify each qualified beneficiary of the right to choose continuation coverage.

COBRA allows at least 60 days from the date the election notice is provided to inform the plan administrator that the qualified beneficiary wants to elect continuation coverage.

Under COBRA, the covered employee or a family member has the responsibility to inform the plan administrator of a divorce, legal separation, disability, or a child losing dependent status under the plan.

Employers have a responsibility to notify the plan administrator of the employee's death, termination of employment or reduction in hours, or Medicare entitlement.

If covered individuals change their marital status, or their spouses have changed addresses, they should notify the plan administrator.

8. Who Has the Responsibility to Make Premium Payments?

Most likely, you do. Qualified individuals may be required to pay the entire premium for coverage up to 102% of the cost to the plan. Premiums may be higher for persons exercising the disability provisions of COBRA. Failure to make timely payments may result in loss of coverage.

Premiums may be increased by the plan; however, premiums generally must be set in advance of each 12-month premium cycle.

Individuals subject to COBRA coverage may be responsible for paying all costs related to deductibles, and may be subject to catastrophic and other benefit limits.

E. WHAT ARE WHISTLEBLOWER STATUTES?

These are statutes that are designed to assist an employee in reporting wrongdoing. A whistleblower is an individual who, when confronted by an institutional wrong, rises up to report and address that wrong. Sometimes a whistleblower is internal. A therapist who reports theft of drugs from the ICU is an internal whistleblower.

Sometimes organizations do not want to know when their employees are doing things wrong. Sometimes the organization actually encourages the wrong so as to continue to profit from it. In that situation, the employee must be aware that there are state and federal statutes that protect their right to blow the whistle.

1. Does EMTALA Have a Whistleblower Provision?

Yes. As set out in Chapter 2, Patient Rights, the Emergency Medical Treatment and Active Labor Act contains a provision that protects clinicians from retaliation if they report violations of the EMTALA statute.

Under EMTALA, an employee of the hospital may not be disciplined for reporting violations of the statute. However, the statute does not give the employee a private right of action against the hospital. It merely states that the hospital should not discipline or reproach the employee for reporting the violation.

So what happens if the hospital does terminate an employee who blows the whistle? Unless the employee hires an attorney and pursues a wrongful discharge claim, usually very little. Even the impact of the statute on the law of wrongful termination is unclear.

2. What Is the Federal False Claims Act?

Among the most powerful whistleblower laws in existence, the Federal False Claims Act, 31 USC § 3729 et seq., is a statute that empowers private citizens to act as private attorneys general to go after those who commit fraud against the government. If the idea of deputizing every citizen for the purpose of preventing fraud seems to invoke images of Big Brother, consider the context in which the False Claims Act arose.

3. What Is the History of the FCA?

In 1863, the most bitter war in the history of the United States raged on, and as President Lincoln discovered, there is someone in every war whose goal is to make money from the carnage.[3] At that time, the Army Quartermaster had the authority to buy from private bidders. Military leaders often issued their personal assurances of payment to civilians in order to secure horses, wagons, or food.[4]

Unscrupulous vendors cheated the Army, giving them rancid beef or faulty weapons. As the battles wore on, President Lincoln found that the treasury was being bled dry, and much of the money being paid was for false claims or fraudulently-billed items. Lincoln sought help from Congress in the form of the False Claims Act (the "FCA" or the "Act").[5]

The Act deputized individual citizens. Citizens could sue to recover money paid by the government on a false or fraudulent claim. The Act let the government get double damages, and, in addition, it let the government get a civil penalty for each false claim submitted. As an incentive, a portion of the

---

[3]Martin Dyckman, Tallahassee Turf Fight Series, ST. PETERSBURG TIMES, Aug. 24, 1993, at 9A.

[4]For an interesting review of the history of the False Claims Act, see Phillips & Cohen (visited July 1996) http://www.phillipsandcohen.com. At that web site is a partial transcript of General Ulysses S. Grant's 1861 testimony in front of Congress regarding defective arms in use by the Union Army.

[5]See *United States ex rel. Stinson v. Prudential Life & Accident Ins. Co.*, 944 F.2d 1149, 1153 (3rd Cir. 1991); see also S. REP. NO. 99-345, at 8-10 (1986), reprinted in 1986 U.S.C.C.A.N. 5226, 5273-75.

recovery was allocated to the person bringing the action, also known as a qui tam plaintiff, or relator.

4. How Has the FCA Been Used?

After becoming law in 1863, the Act was used rather sporadically. There are few reported FCA cases from the 1800s and early 1900s. However, in the late 1970s, environmentalists and public interest attorneys began to focus on the spiraling costs of defense contractors, and these litigants filed numerous actions in federal courts.

In 1986, Congress amended the False Claims Act to make it easier for a qui tam plaintiff to bring an action.[6] The result has been a record number of new cases filed in the last few years. Under the Act, as currently codified, a relator can share between 15 and 25 percent of the government's recovery. The recovery is for three times the amount of the damages sustained by reason of the fraud, and includes a civil penalty between $5,500 and $11,000 for each false claim.[7]

The legislative history of the FCA shows it was meant to ferret out fraudulent and false billings submitted to the government. Congress's objective in establishing the FCA was "to protect the funds and property of the Government from fraudulent claims, regardless of the particular form, or function, of the government instrumentality upon which such claims were made." The purpose of treble damages provided for by the FCA was "to make sure that [the] government [was] made completely whole." By building into the Act a damage-trebling provision, and by including a civil penalty for each and every false claim submitted, Congress intended to give private citizens an opportunity to right wrongs that only they might know about. Moreover, by making it possible for a relator to share in the award (in an amount between 15 and 30 percent of the total judgment), Congress intended to provide a suitable incentive to motivate those with knowledge of fraud to come forward. At the same time, by including a provision limiting the reward where public disclosure of the fraud had taken place, Congress intended to prevent latecomers with "nothing to add" from claiming a part of the proceeds.

---

[6]See *United States ex rel. Hagood v. Sonoma County Water Agency,* 929 F.2d 1416, 1420 (9th Cir. 1991).

[7]31 U.S.C. § 3730 (1994).; 31 U.S.C. § 3729 (1994). The impact of the civil penalty on false claims recoveries is impressive. If a health care provider were, for example, to over bill only one dollar for one thousand laboratory tests, the civil penalty could exceed ten million dollars.

While the Act provides that a private citizen may bring an action, the government is the real party that benefits, and it gets the most discretion about how the case is handled. The government doesn't have to wait for a citizen to sue; it may initiate the prosecution of a false claims action on its own. Where the government initiates a criminal investigation that exposes evidence of false or fraudulent claims, the government may also bring an action under the FCA.

If the purpose of the Act is to increase recoveries into the treasury, it has been fabulously successful. Since Congress reinforced the False Claims Act in 1986, citizens have recovered more than one billion dollars for the federal government, amounting to more than one-third of all fraud recoveries. The news media has generally ignored these recoveries. The number of qui tam cases filed increases every year, and more frequently, physicians, laboratories, and other health care providers are being targeted with FCA violations.

What sets the FCA apart from other statutes is the possibility that a citizen will benefit personally from reporting the fraud. Most citizens go into that process with some starry-eyed notion of getting fabulously wealthy off their employer's wrongdoing. Frequently that is not the result because False Claims Act cases are not easy to prosecute and depend in large measure on cooperation from the federal government. When they are successful, however, the rewards can be significant.

In 1996 six therapists at Portercare Hospital became concerned that they were being asked to commit acts that were unlawful. They were being asked to overcharge Medicare, sometimes by a factor of 200%. Encouraged to put down blatant lies on their time records, some of the therapists reacted by contacting the federal government.

No one at the Colorado Department of Health would listen, and no one at the Office of Inspector General for Health and Human Services was very interested. Frustrated, the therapists shrugged their shoulders and began to press internally for an investigation.

Finally, a vice president agreed that an audit should be conducted to assure the therapists that the conduct of the hospital was legitimate. That audit began with two accountants, and by the end of the first week included lawyers and consultants. After a month of interviews with the auditors the hospital announced that it was closing the program that employed the therapists. No reason was given. No one mentioned fraud, and when the therapists asked about fraud, there was dead silence. Frustrated, the therapists hired private counsel who put together a False Claims Act case.

The case was filed and the federal government began to investigate. At first the case dragged on for nearly 18 months as investigators continually substantiated the allegations of the therapists. Before long, the federal government had a case worth more than $18,000,000 against the hospital.

Since a False Claims Act case is filed under seal, the hospital did not know what was going on until the federal government intervened. When the hospital admitted liability, they also stated they didn't have any money to pay the damages. The federal government settled for $1.5 million, and the therapists and their attorneys received awards disproportionately small to the risk they had taken.

If a therapist knows about fraud on the federal or state Medicare or Medicaid programs, or any other program that is paid for out of federal dollars, there is always a possibility that there is a good False Claims Act case. Counsel should be contacted immediately.

5. Are There State False Claims Acts?

Yes, in some states. In addition to the Federal False Claims Act, several states have enacted their own whistleblower acts. Texas, California, and several others have statutes modeled on the federal statute and designed to prevent fraud against the state government. If you live in one of these states and know of fraud on the government, it is a good idea to seek counsel familiar with these statutes.

6. Are There Other Whistleblower Statutes?

Yes, but you may have to look carefully to find them. In addition to the statutes mentioned above, the federal banking laws are routinely the subject of abuse. Borrowers defraud banks, home sellers mis-state the true value of homes in order to get government guarantees. There are lots of ways that federal banks lose money to fraud.

If you know of someone who has defrauded a federally chartered banking institution (e.g., banks, savings and loans, credit unions, etc.), then these statutes may provide an excellent way to redress that wrong. Like the FCA, these statutes provide for a reward for turning in those who steal from the government. Unlike the FCA, the rewards are not as handsome, but as a benefit they include sharing in a reward when perpetrators are brought to the criminal justice system and put out of business.

If you know of fraud on a nationally chartered bank, you should most likely consult with an attorney.

F. WHAT HAPPENS IN UNLAWFUL TERMINATION LITIGATION?

An employee takes an employer to court for a termination that the employee believes is unlawful. But employees should always understand: this is a risky and sometimes costly venture that always favors the employer over the employee.[8]

The last thing a loyal employee wants to do is think about what happens when they are wrongfully fired. Most employees work hard in their jobs doing the best job they can for their employers day after day. Most of these employees never have issues with wrongful termination. But the issues do arise, and when they do most are confronted by the employment at will doctrine and the fact that an employer cannot be made to play fair in most circumstances.

1. Must an Employee Fit Within an Exception to Employment at Will?

Usually, yes. Unless there is a written contract, there must be an exception. There are limited exceptions to the Employment at Will doctrine, and those exceptions are generally found either in statutes or in the public policy of the state.

2. What is the Public Policy Exception?

It is a way of stopping employers from committing unlawful or improper acts or firing employees who refuse to do so.

An employee should not, as a general rule, have to face the decision between keeping his job and breaking the criminal law. Unfortunately, that is often what happens to employees. When it does, and the employee chooses honesty over employment, the public policy exception to the employment at will doctrine comes into play.

Most states have now recognized the public policy exception, but some states have made the exception so narrow as to be of no practical use to employees. Texas is one such state. Generally, under Texas Law, an employee must be asked to do an unlawful act, must refuse, and must be fired for this reason before an action for unlawful termination exists.

---

[8]If an employee is discharged and wishes to contest that firing, the best and most productive way to do it is through the National Labor Relations Board system. Civil courts are much more hostile to the employee than the NLRB is.

3. Are There Statutory Exceptions?

Sometimes a state or federal statute will provide an exception to the employment at will doctrine. Generally these are very narrow and are limited to those situations where the employee's conduct is clearly proscribed by a statute, or the exception for retaliation is clearly spelled out in the statute.

The best way to find out whether a statutory or similar protection exists is to see an attorney. Much of the law in the area of employment is judge-made. There may be statutes that provide guidance, but even those statutes have to be interpreted and construed. For this reason, if you suspect you have been wrongfully terminated, the only answer is to immediately seek legal representation. Statutes of limitation, which limit your right to sue, are very short in employment law cases.

G. HOW DO FEDERAL ANTI-DISCRIMINATION STATUTES WORK?

Federal anti-discrimination laws make it unlawful to discriminate on the basis of a protected status. They provide for complaints to be filed with the Equal Employment Opportunity Commission (EEOC), and for the EEOC to investigate and attempt to help the employee redress the grievance with the employer. If the employer does not respond to the "conciliation" attempt by the EEOC, the EEOC may either investigate further and charge discrimination, bringing a federal lawsuit on behalf of the employee (something that happens once is a thousand or more cases) or the employee may get a "right to sue" letter and proceed to sue the employer with a private attorney.

1. What Kinds of Discrimination Are Affected?

There are numerous federal anti-discrimination statutes. Age, sex, national origin, race, religion, pregnancy, and disability are but a few of them. In each instance the federal law is very clear in what it requires employers to do to comply. Less clear is how employees make claims under the acts. At the outset, it should be noted that if you or someone you know believes they have a claim under the federal anti-discrimination statutes, they should immediately consult the State Office of Equal Employment Opportunity (sometimes called the State Human Rights Commission) or the Equal Employment Opportunity Commission for guidance about how to proceed.

2. What Is Age Discrimination?

Discrimination in employment against a person age 40 or more.

The Age Discrimination in Employment Act of 1967 (ADEA) protects individuals who are 40 years of age or older from employment discrimination based on age. The ADEA's protections apply to both employees and job applicants. Under the ADEA, it is unlawful to discriminate against a person because of his/her age with respect to any term, condition, or privilege of employment, including hiring, firing, promotion, layoff, compensation, benefits, job assignments, and training.

It is also unlawful to retaliate against an individual for opposing employment practices that discriminate based on age or for filing an age discrimination charge, testifying, or participating in any way in an investigation, proceeding, or litigation under the ADEA.

The ADEA applies to employers with 20 or more employees, including state and local governments. It also applies to employment agencies and labor organizations, as well as to the federal government.

3. What Is Pregnancy Discrimination?

It is discrimination against a woman on the basis of her pregnancy, planned pregnancy, or the ability to become pregnant.[9] The Pregnancy Discrimination Act is an amendment to Title VII of the Civil Rights Act of 1964. Discrimination on the basis of pregnancy, childbirth, or related medical conditions constitutes unlawful sex discrimination under Title VII, which covers employers with 15 or more employees, including state and local governments. Title VII also applies to employment agencies and to labor organizations, as well as to the federal government. Women who are pregnant or affected by related conditions must be treated in the same manner as other applicants or employees with similar abilities or limitations.

It is also unlawful to retaliate against an individual for taking any action to oppose employment practices that discriminate based on pregnancy or for filing a discrimination charge, testifying, or participating in any way in an investigation, proceeding, or litigation under Title VII.

---

[9]Employers frequently ask women (but never ask men) if they intend to have a family. Women who answer yes are often not hired because the employer views them as likely to get pregnant and likely to use health benefits they will have to pay for. Such discrimination is unlawful.

4. What About Gender-Based or Sex-Based Discrimination?

Discrimination against a person on the basis of sex or gender is unlawful.

Title VII of the Civil Rights Act of 1964 protects individuals against employment discrimination on the basis of sex as well as race, color, national origin, and religion. Title VII applies to employers with 15 or more employees, including state and local governments. It also applies to employment agencies and to labor organizations, as well as to the federal government.

It is unlawful to discriminate against any employee or applicant for employment because of his/her sex in regard to hiring, termination, promotion, compensation, job training, or any other term, condition, or privilege of employment. Title VII also prohibits employment decisions based on stereotypes and assumptions about abilities, traits, or the performance of individuals on the basis of sex. Title VII prohibits both intentional discrimination and neutral job policies that disproportionately exclude individuals on the basis of sex and that are not job related.

Title VII's prohibitions against sex-based discrimination also cover:

- Sexual Harassment: This includes practices ranging from direct requests for sexual favors to workplace conditions that create a hostile environment for persons of either gender, including same-sex harassment.
- Pregnancy Based Discrimination: Title VII was amended by the Pregnancy Discrimination Act, which prohibits discrimination on the basis of pregnancy, childbirth, and related medical conditions.

Just as with pregnancy discrimination, it is unlawful to retaliate against an individual for bringing an action or cooperating with the government in an investigation under Title VII.

5. What Is Sexual Harassment?

Sexual harassment is a form of sex discrimination that violates Title VII of the Civil Rights Act of 1964. Title VII applies to employers with 15 or more employees, including state and local governments. It also applies to employment agencies and to labor organizations, as well as to the federal government.

Unwelcome sexual advances, requests for sexual favors, and other verbal or physical conduct of a sexual nature constitute sexual harassment when this conduct explicitly or implicitly affects an individual's employment, unreasonably interferes with an individual's work performance, or creates an intimidating, hostile, or offensive work environment.

Sexual harassment can occur in a variety of circumstances, including but not limited to the following:

- The victim, as well as the harasser, may be a woman or a man. The victim does not have to be of the opposite sex.
- The harasser can be the victim's supervisor, an agent of the employer, a supervisor in another area, a co-worker, or a non-employee.
- The victim does not have to be the person harassed but could be anyone affected by the offensive conduct.
- Unlawful sexual harassment may occur without economic injury to or discharge of the victim.
- The harasser's conduct must be unwelcome.

It is helpful for the victim to inform the harasser directly that the conduct is unwelcome and must stop. The victim should use any employer complaint mechanism or grievance system available. This is important because one frequent defense in these cases is that the employee failed to exhaust remedies available through the employer.

When investigating allegations of sexual harassment, EEOC looks at the whole record: the circumstances, such as the nature of the sexual advances, and the context in which the alleged incidents occurred. A determination on the allegations is made from the facts on a case-by-case basis.

Prevention is the best tool to eliminate sexual harassment in the workplace. Hospitals and health care employers should take steps to prevent sexual harassment from occurring. They should communicate to employees that sexual harassment will not be tolerated. They should also provide sexual harassment training to their administrative, managerial, and supervisory employees. This training should focus on both identifying behavior that qualifies as discriminatory, and on taking appropriate disciplinary action against individuals who engage in the behavior. Health care institutions should also establish an effective complaint or grievance process and encourage the use of anonymous reporting. When discriminatory or abusive behavior is documented, swift and decisive action should be taken against the offender, and all claims should be investigated.

6. Must Sexual Discrimination Be Across Genders?

No. As long as the basis for the discriminatory treatment is sex or gender, it doesn't matter who engages in it. Thus a white male may discriminate against another white male on the basis of sex, and does so if he treats that person differently because the employee is a man. Similarly, a woman may discriminate against a woman on the basis of sex or gender. Man-on-man and woman-on-woman discrimination cases often arise where there is a question about sexual preference, and people act on biases.

7. What Is Disability Discrimination?

It is discrimination aimed at persons with mental or physical handicaps.

Title I of the Americans with Disabilities Act of 1990 prohibits private employers, state and local governments, employment agencies, and labor unions from discriminating against qualified individuals with disabilities in job application procedures, hiring, firing, advancement, compensation, job training, and other terms, conditions, and privileges of employment. The ADA covers employers with 15 or more employees, including state and local governments. It also applies to employment agencies and to labor organizations. The ADA's nondiscrimination standards also apply to federal sector employees under section 501 of the Rehabilitation Act.

An individual with a disability is a person who:

- Has a physical or mental impairment that substantially limits one or more major life activities;
- Has a record of such an impairment; or
- Is regarded as having such an impairment.

A qualified employee or applicant with a disability is an individual who, with or without reasonable accommodation, can perform the essential functions of the job in question. Reasonable accommodation may include, but is not limited to:

- Making existing facilities used by employees readily accessible to and usable by persons with disabilities.
- Job restructuring, modifying work schedules, reassignment to a vacant position;
- Acquiring or modifying equipment or devices, adjusting or modifying examinations, training materials, or policies, and providing qualified readers or interpreters.

An employer is required to make a reasonable accommodation to the known disability of a qualified applicant or employee if it would not impose an "undue hardship" on the operation of the employer's business. Undue hardship is defined as an action requiring significant difficulty or expense when considered in light of factors such as an employer's size, financial resources, and the nature and structure of its operation.

An employer is not required to lower quality or production standards to make an accommodation; nor is an employer obligated to provide personal use items such as glasses or hearing aids.

Title I of the ADA also covers:

Medical Examinations and Inquiries	Employers may not ask job applicants about the existence, nature, or severity of a disability. Applicants may be asked about their ability to perform specific job functions. A job offer may be conditioned on the results of a medical examination, but only if the examination is required for all entering employees in similar jobs. Medical examinations of employees must be job related and consistent with the employer's business needs.
Drug and Alcohol Abuse	Employees and applicants currently engaging in the illegal use of drugs are not covered by the ADA when an employer acts on the basis of such use. Tests for illegal drugs are not subject to the ADA's restrictions on medical examinations. Employers may hold illegal drug users and alcoholics to the same performance standards as other employees.

Just as anti-retaliation measures are built into the other civil rights statutes, so too are they present in the ADA. It is also unlawful to retaliate against an individual for bringing litigation under the ADA.

8. Is It Lawful to Discriminate on the Basis of National Origin?

Never. Whether an employee or job applicant's ancestry is Mexican, Ukrainian, Filipino, Arab, American Indian, or any other nationality, he or she is entitled to the same employment opportunities as anyone else. EEOC enforces the federal prohibition against national origin discrimination in employment under Title VII of the Civil Rights Act of 1964, which covers employers with fifteen (15) or more employees.

"With American society growing increasingly diverse, protection against national origin discrimination is vital to the right of workers to compete for jobs on a level playing field," said EEOC Chair Cari M. Dominguez, announcing the issuance of recent guidance on national origin discrimination. "Immigrants have long been an asset to the American workforce. In today's increasingly global economy, this is true more than ever. Recent world events, including the events of September 11, 2001, only add to the need for employers to be vigilant in ensuring a workplace free from discrimination."

National origin discrimination means treating someone less favorably because he or she comes from a particular place, because of his or her ethnicity or accent, or because it is believed that he or she has a particular ethnic background. National origin discrimination also means treating someone less favorably at work because of marriage or other association with someone of a particular nationality.

9. Are Foreign Nationals Covered?

Yes, some of the time. Title VII and the other antidiscrimination laws prohibit discrimination against individuals employed in the United States, regardless of citizenship. However, relief may be limited if an individual does not have work authorization. In other words, if a worker is an unlawful immigrant, they may not be able to take full advantage of their rights under the statute.

10. How Is Racial Discrimination Different?

Title VII of the Civil Rights Act of 1964 protects individuals against employment discrimination on the basis of race and color, as well as national origin, sex, and religion. Title VII applies to employers with 15 or more employees, including state and local governments. It also applies to employment agencies and to labor organizations, as well as to the federal government.

It is unlawful to discriminate against any employee or applicant for employment because of his/her race or color in regard to hiring, termination, promotion, compensation, job training, or any other term, condition, or privilege of employment. Title VII also prohibits employment decisions based on stereotypes and assumptions about abilities, traits, or the performance of individuals of certain racial groups. Title VII prohibits both intentional discrimination and neutral job policies that disproportionately exclude minorities and that are not job related.

Equal employment opportunity cannot be denied because of marriage to or association with an individual of a different race; membership in or association with ethnic-based organizations or groups; or attendance or participation in schools or places of worship generally associated with certain minority groups.

Title VII violations include:

Race-Related Characteristics and Conditions	Discrimination on the basis of an immutable characteristic associated with race, such as skin color, hair texture, or certain facial features violates Title VII, even though not all members of the race share the same characteristic. Title VII also prohibits discrimination on the basis of a condition that predominantly affects one race unless the practice is job related and consistent with business necessity. For example, since sickle cell anemia predominantly occurs in African-Americans, a policy that excludes individuals with sickle cell anemia must be job related and consistent with business necessity. Similarly, a "no-beard" employment policy may discriminate against African-American men who have a predisposition to pseudofolliculitis barbae (severe shaving bumps) unless the policy is job related and consistent with business necessity.
Harassment	Harassment on the basis of race and/or color violates Title VII. Ethnic slurs, racial "jokes," offensive or derogatory comments, or other verbal or physical conduct based on an individual's race/color constitutes unlawful harassment if the conduct creates an intimidating, hostile, or offensive working environment or interferes with the individual's work performance.
Segregation and Classification	Title VII is violated where employees who belong to a protected group are segregated by physically isolating them from other employees or from

Continued

Segregation and Classification, continued

customer contact. In addition, employers may not assign employees according to race or color. For example, Title VII prohibits assigning primarily African-Americans to predominantly African-American establishments or geographic areas. It is also illegal to exclude members of one group from particular positions or to group or categorize employees or jobs so that certain jobs are generally held by members of a certain protected group. Coding applications/resumes to designate an applicant's race, by either an employer or employment agency, constitutes evidence of discrimination where people of a certain race or color are excluded from employment or from certain positions.

Pre-Employment Inquiries

Requesting pre-employment information that discloses or tends to disclose an applicant's race strongly suggests that race will be used unlawfully as a basis for hiring. Therefore, if members of minority groups are excluded from employment, the request for such pre-employment information would likely constitute evidence of discrimination.

If an employer legitimately needs information about its employees' or applicants' race for affirmative action purposes and/or to track applicant flow, it may obtain racial information and simultaneously guard against discriminatory selection by using "tear-off sheets" for the identification of an applicant's race. After the applicant completes the application and the tear-off portion, the employer separates the tear-off sheet from the application and does not use it in the selection process.

11. What Is Religious Discrimination?

It is interference with a person's ability to exercise his or her freedom of religion or discrimination against him or her for doing so.

Title VII of the Civil Rights Act of 1964 prohibits employers from discriminating against individuals because of their religion in hiring, firing, and other terms and conditions of employment. Title VII covers employers with 15 or more employees, including state and local governments. It also applies to employment agencies and to labor organizations, as well as to the federal government.

12. How Does an Employee File a Charge of Discrimination?

Normally, the best way is to find the EEOC office, or the local human rights organization, and contact them for the forms and procedure. You may also want to see a lawyer to get advice about what to include in your complaint. Whatever else you do, act quickly. The statute of limitations is very short.

a) Who Can File?

Any individual who believes that his or her employment rights have been violated may file a charge of discrimination with EEOC. In addition, an individual, organization, or agency may file a charge on behalf of another person in order to protect the aggrieved person's identity. Thus a union may file on behalf of a member, or a non-union fraternal organization may file on behalf of a member. A co-worker may file on behalf of a co-worker under a strict reading of the act.

b) Filing the Charge

A charge may be filed by mail or in person at the nearest EEOC office.

Individuals who need an accommodation in order to file a charge (e.g., sign language interpreter, print materials in an accessible format) should inform the EEOC field office so that appropriate arrangements can be made.

Federal employees or applicants for employment should see Federal Sector Equal Employment Opportunity Complaint Processing.

c) Information Required to File a Charge

What information is needed to file the charge? This is the information requested by the appropriate forms:

- The complaining party's name, address, and telephone number;
- The name, address, and telephone number of the respondent employer,

employment agency, or union that is alleged to have discriminated, and number of employees (or union members), if known;
- A short description of the alleged violation (the event that caused the complaining party to believe that his or her rights were violated); and
- The date(s) of the alleged violation(s).
- Federal employees or applicants for employment should see Federal Sector Equal Employment Opportunity Complaint Processing.

d) Time Limits for Filing

All laws enforced by EEOC, except the Equal Pay Act, require filing a charge with EEOC before a private lawsuit may be filed in court. There are strict time limits within which charges must be filed:

A charge must be filed with EEOC within 180 days from the date of the alleged violation, in order to protect the charging party's rights.

This 180-day filing deadline is extended to 300 days if the charge also is covered by a state or local anti-discrimination law. For ADEA charges, only state laws extend the filing limit to 300 days.

These time limits do not apply to claims under the Equal Pay Act, because under that Act persons do not have to first file a charge with EEOC in order to have the right to go to court. However, since many EPA claims also raise Title VII sex discrimination issues, it may be advisable to file charges under both laws within the time limits indicated.

To protect your legal rights, it is always best to contact either an employment lawyer or the EEOC promptly when discrimination is suspected.

Federal employees or applicants for employment should see Federal Sector Equal Employment Opportunity Complaint Processing.

e) Agencies That Handle Charges Covered by State or Local Law

Many states and localities have anti-discrimination laws and agencies responsible for enforcing those laws. EEOC refers to these agencies as "Fair Employment Practices Agencies (FEPAs)." Through the use of "work sharing agreements," EEOC and the FEPAs avoid duplication of effort while at the same time ensuring that a charging party's rights are protected under both federal and state law.

- If a charge is filed with a FEPA and is also covered by federal law, the FEPA "dual files" the charge with EEOC to protect federal rights. The charge usually will be retained by the FEPA for handling.

- If a charge is filed with EEOC and also is covered by state or local law, EEOC "dual files" the charge with the state or local FEPA, but ordinarily retains the charge for handling.

The EEOC's mailing address is:

1801 L Street, N.W.
Washington, D.C. 20507
Phone: (202) 663-4900
TTY: (202) 663-4494

The toll free number connecting you to the nearest EEOC Field Office is:

Phone: (800) 669-4000
TTY: (800) 669-6820

f) What Happens When a Charge Is Filed?

The employer is notified that the charge has been filed. From this point there are a number of ways a charge may be handled.

A charge may be assigned for priority investigation if the initial facts appear to support a violation of law. When the evidence is less strong, the charge may be assigned for follow-up investigation to determine whether it is likely that a violation has occurred.

EEOC can seek to settle a charge at any stage of the investigation if the charging party and the employer express an interest in doing so. If settlement efforts are not successful, the investigation continues.

In investigating a charge, EEOC may make written requests for information, interview people, review documents, and, as needed, visit the facility where the alleged discrimination occurred. When the investigation is complete, EEOC will discuss the evidence with the charging party or employer, as appropriate.

The charge may be selected for EEOC's mediation program if both the charging party and the employer express an interest in this option. Mediation is offered as an alternative to a lengthy investigation. Participation in the mediation program is confidential, voluntary, and requires consent from both charging party and employer. If mediation is unsuccessful, the charge is returned for investigation.

A charge may be dismissed at any point if, in the agency's best judgment, further investigation will not establish a violation of the law. A charge may be dismissed at the time it is filed, if an initial in-depth interview does not produce evidence to support the claim. When a charge is dismissed, a notice is issued in accordance with the law, which gives the charging party 90 days in which to file a lawsuit on his or her own behalf.

g) How Does EEOC Resolve Discrimination Charges?

It first gives both sides a chance to reach an accommodation, if possible.

If the evidence obtained in an investigation does not establish that discrimination occurred, this will be explained to the charging party. A required notice is then issued, closing the case and giving the charging party 90 days in which to file a lawsuit on his or her own behalf.

If the evidence establishes that discrimination has occurred, the employer and the charging party will be informed of this in a letter of determination that explains the finding. EEOC will then attempt conciliation with the employer to develop a remedy for the discrimination.

If the case is successfully conciliated, or if a case has earlier been successfully mediated or settled, neither EEOC nor the charging party may go to court unless the conciliation, mediation, or settlement agreement is not honored.

If EEOC is unable to successfully conciliate the case, the agency will decide whether to bring suit in federal court. If EEOC decides not to sue, it will issue a notice closing the case and giving the charging party 90 days in which to file a lawsuit on his or her own behalf. In Title VII and ADA cases against state or local governments, the Department of Justice takes these actions.

h) When Can an Individual File an Employment Discrimination Lawsuit in Court?

A charging party may file a lawsuit within 90 days after receiving a notice of a "right to sue" from EEOC, as stated above. Under Title VII and the ADA, a charging party also can request a notice of "right to sue" from EEOC 180 days after the charge was first filed with the Commission, and may then bring suit within 90 days after receiving this notice. Under the ADEA, a suit may be filed at any time 60 days after filing a charge with EEOC, but not later than 90 days after EEOC gives notice that it has completed action on the charge.

Under the EPA, a lawsuit must be filed within two years (three years for willful violations) of the discriminatory act, which in most cases is payment of a discriminatory lower wage.

If the EEOC is unable to help, that is clearly not the end of the issue. Thousands of cases are litigated every year by private attorneys under the 90-

day rule stated above. An attorney should be involved at the earliest possible stage of the litigation to assist and guide the employee in making a complaint through the EEOC.

i) *What Remedies Are Available When Discrimination Is Found?*

The "relief" or remedies available for employment discrimination, whether caused by intentional acts or by practices that have a discriminatory effect, may include:

- back pay,
- hiring,
- promotion,
- reinstatement,
- front pay,
- reasonable accommodation, or
- other actions that will make an individual "whole" (in the condition s/he would have been but for the discrimination).

Remedies also may include payment of:

- attorneys' fees,
- expert witness fees, and
- court costs.

Under most EEOC-enforced laws, compensatory and punitive damages also may be available where intentional discrimination is found. Damages may be available to compensate for actual monetary losses, for future monetary losses, and for mental anguish and inconvenience. Punitive damages also may be available if an employer acted with malice or reckless indifference. Punitive damages are not available against the federal, state, or local governments.

In cases concerning reasonable accommodation under the ADA, compensatory or punitive damages may not be awarded to the charging party if an employer can demonstrate that "good faith" efforts were made to provide reasonable accommodation.

An employer may be required to post notices to all employees addressing the violations of a specific charge and advising them of their rights under the laws EEOC enforces and their right to be free from retaliation. Such notices must be accessible, as needed, to persons with visual or other disabilities that affect reading.

The employer also may be required to take corrective or preventive actions to cure the source of the identified discrimination and minimize the chance of its recurrence, as well as discontinue the specific discriminatory practices involved in the case.

H. KEY POINTS

- States all have minimum wage laws, some of which are more generous than federal law.
- Employees have the right to wages and, when they are not exempt, to overtime.
- Overtime rules have changed and most professionals cannot get overtime.
- Salaried workers are exempt from overtime.
- There are recordkeeping requirements for employers.
- Employers must post all workers' wage and hour rights.
- Some states have rules regarding breaks.
- HIPAA and COBRA both give employees rights to continue health insurance and obtain new health insurance.
- Employees can enforce their rights under federal and state wage and hour laws.
- The Equal Pay Act, Age Discrimination in Employment Act, Pregnancy Discrimination Act, Americans with Disabilities Act, and Civil Rights Act mandate that employers not engage in discrimination on the basis of:
    - Age
    - Race
    - Sex
    - National Origin
    - Skin Color
    - Religion
    - Gender
    - Pregnancy
    - Disability
- The EEOC and Department of Justice investigate violations of these acts.
- Employees can enforce their rights to a workplace free of discrimination even if the EEOC does not.

CHAPTER 6

Essentials of Employment Law for Managers

The magic formula that successful businesses have discovered is to treat customers like guests and employees like people.

Thomas J. Peters
American Management Consultant, Author, Trainer

INTRODUCTION

This chapter is written for employers, and for supervisors and managers. It expands and builds upon the information presented in Chapter Four regarding employment law. When you look at the area of employment law from the perspective of a manager, it may seem as if the law unduly favors the employee, and in some areas, like discrimination, it does. But generally if organizations and managers comply with a few basic rules, they can operate a fine organization without running afoul of the law.

The key principle I share with clients is that your organization should be prepared to defend, on the front page of the local newspaper, any employment action you take against your employees. If you can defend what you're doing or attempting to do honestly, then you should take the action you want to take. If you can't do that, or if you have to rationalize the behavior, then you should think twice.

B. HOW DOES FREEDOM OF CONTRACT—EMPLOYMENT AT WILL AFFECT MANAGERS?

As fully set out in Chapter Four, employers have great latitude on hiring because most courts support the notion that individuals should not have a right to continued employment under most circumstances. But that doesn't mean employers have carte blanche to treat employees poorly. In fact, an organization that does not try to recruit and retain the best help and does not try to work with marginal employees to improve their performance is the aberrancy in America.

Still, there are many employers who just don't understand the technical rules of law that govern the workplace, and as a result, they do dumb things. These dumb things become employment law issues and create lawsuits against managers, supervisors, and organizations.

In the Waggoner case, presented in Chapter Four, the hotel had a bad employee. They had the absolute right to terminate her for bad performance. If they had done so properly, there never would have been a case of unfair labor practices. But the hotel manager made a critical mistake. Although it was not the reason the employee was terminated, she mentioned to the employee the fact that the hotel had learned of her purported plans to lead a walkout. With that admission to the employee, she placed her employer squarely in the sights of the National Labor Relations Board.

The manager felt that leading a walkout was a bona fide reason to fire the employee. Most similarly situated managers would have felt the very same way. That is dangerous thinking for a member of management. The purpose of this chapter is to remove ideas you may have as to the common sense ways you go about hiring and firing employees, and replace them with appropriate ways to prevent workplace litigation.

The first principle of employer-employee relations is that employers have freedom to hire and fire so long as they adhere to the basic rules of employment law. This is freedom of contract. Employers are free to hire and retain a worker for as long as they choose. They are not required to pay anything more than the minimum wage, so long as they do not violate the Equal Pay Act or discriminate by paying workers different wages based on race, sex, or religion.

The first place these principles get tested in the employer-employee relationship, however, is in hiring (or more commonly, the refusal to hire) individuals.

1. What Are the Rules on Hiring?

Employers have the right:

- To hire anyone they want for the job, so long as they do not commit unlawful acts while hiring.

- To use both objective and subjective criteria to determine who is better suited to a job, so long as the subjective criterion is not a mask for discriminatory processes.
- To set the objective standards for a position, so long as those objective standards are applied objectively to all candidates.
- To make a decision about candidates who are otherwise equal in objective measures on the basis of subjective standards, so long as those subjective standards are not a mask for discriminatory processes.
- To advertise for the employee they want, so long as that advertisement does not indicate an intention to discriminate.
- To screen employees on objective criteria, so long as those objective criteria are directly related to the performance of the job.
- To specify that a position is a "male only" or "female only" position, so long as there is a genuine bona fide occupational qualification for the worker to be of a specific sex.

2. What Are Employers Prohibited to Do?

Employers, however, simply cannot:

- Advertise a job as being male or female without the gender of the worker being a bona fide occupational qualification.
- Fail to follow internal policies or procedures when hiring or promoting.
- Treat employees differently on the basis of:
  - race,
  - sex,
  - national origin,
  - age,
  - disability,
  - pregnancy,
  - color, or
  - gender.
- Ask questions that reflect any improper motivation for an employment decision.

One of the very first things employment attorneys look for is a telltale sign in the employment interview that indicates improper motivations for hiring. For example, you should not ask the questions in the table below for the reasons expressed:

Question	Problem
So, are you married?	If she (or he) tells you, that's fine. But otherwise you shouldn't care. It might mean you pay married women differently than married men, or it may violate sex discrimination laws.
You know, we've really hit it off here today. I don't see a wedding ring on your finger. Are you seeing anyone?	This screams what lawyers call "quid pro quo" sexual harassment. An employee might well say "I went out with her because I was afraid she wouldn't hire me if I didn't." Relationships with employed subordinates are strictly improper and should never be permitted, and therefore, neither should a manager ask questions like this.
Are you planning on having children?	The Pregnancy Discrimination Act forbids different treatment based on pregnancy or the ability to get pregnant. The impression is that if you're asking this question, you care about the person becoming pregnant and having children, and are apt to hire someone who isn't going to get pregnant.
Did I understand it right that you're married to an African-American man?	First, it's irrelevant. Second, it violates the Civil Rights Act as Discrimination on the basis of color.
Well, with a name like Woslowski, you must be Polish. . . .	Suggests national origin discrimination.
Are you in good health?	Employers may not make health inquiries until after a job is offered under the Americans with Disabilities Act.

Question	Problem
Seventh Day Adventist? Does that mean you'll be wanting every Saturday off?	Religious discrimination.
Let me just ask you, since you're almost 42, do you think you can do as much therapy on the floors or in the ICU as a 20-year-old therapist?	Age Discrimination in Employment Act.
As an African-American male, I bet the cops really hassled you growing up. Did you ever get arrested for anything?	Why would you assume that because someone is African-American they would be more likely to be arrested? Questions like this scream discriminatory practice. This is a question you do not want to ask.

The list above is not meant to be exhaustive, but illustrative.

In general, employers have the right to pick and choose their employees so long as in so doing they do not violate the state or federal antidiscrimination statutes. One way to run afoul of those statutes is to engage in questioning during the interview that tends to suggest you're making an improper inquiry on the basis of protected status.

The purpose of those antidiscrimination statutes is to protect workers from being judged unfairly on attributes that do not, in any way, affect their worth as employees. An Hispanic worker is no better nurse than someone of Asian ethnicity, and all things being equal, the decision to hire should not be made on the basis of national origin when that does not affect the performance of the job.

For obvious reasons, managers cannot simply ask the questions they want to ask, and cover those questions with some blanket statement about not being discriminatory. "Miss Jones, I see that you want this job as a secretary, and you tell me you're newly married. Now, I don't want you to think that this would affect our hiring decision, but tell me, do you and your husband plan to have children?"

If the question doesn't matter, or figure into the hiring decision, then why are you asking it? If you refuse to hire Miss Jones and instead hire a 32-year-old woman who has no children, Miss Jones may well have a claim under the Pregnancy Discrimination Act because the court will discount your statement that the question did not figure into the hiring decision based on the person you hired.

C. ARE ALL FORMS OF DISCRIMINATION UNLAWFUL?

Unfortunately some forms of bigotry are still permitted. Although a person's sexual preference plays little role in their ability to give respiratory care treatments, there are still individuals who will not hire a person on this basis. At this writing, the decision not to hire on the basis of sexual preference is not protected under federal law, and it is still lawful to discriminate against gays and lesbians. While some states have more powerful antidiscrimination laws applicable to sexual preference, at present most states do not regulate this area.

D. WHAT IS AN EXAMPLE OF IMPROPER HIRING?

The hiring process starts with the process of making it known that a vacancy exists in your organization. How a position is described in any advertisement or position announcement becomes the baseline for determining, at some later point in time, if the organization complied with the law. While normally this process begins and ends in the Human Resources Department in a large organization, for smaller businesses, it often begins on the desk of the owner.

One way to run afoul of the law is to advertise the position as requiring a male or female when the job doesn't require it. For example, a delivery person for a home care company could be either a man or a woman; there would be no reason either could not handle the job. Advertising a job as "man wanted for delivery company" is an example of how a seemingly innocent advertisement can get a company sued. A person challenging the advertisement by saying the company was discriminating on the basis of sex would have proof in the copy of the newspaper.

Of course, a person's intent when hiring is hard to discern, except, of course, from the questions they ask and the qualifications they require in their advertisements. It is important to keep good notes of job interviews. If a prospective employee volunteers that she is married, that's okay, but should not go into your notes. It is also important not to follow up on a statement like that. You shouldn't care to whom the person is married.

You should keep a list of the questions you ask and the responses you received. If you reject an applicant after an interview your notes should reflect a reason why you refused to hire. The reason should be based on appropriate criteria. It is okay to write "therapist told me he didn't like critical care work, and position requires critical care background." It is not okay to write "we don't need another [Italian/Polish/Mexican/Black/Female] therapist around here."

You should always send a letter to interviewees thanking them for their time and declining to hire them. It is not a good idea to state, in the letter, why you didn't hire them, as often there are any number of creative rationales that can be invented to show that this reason is pretextual. A good decline letter is one paragraph. It states:

> *We appreciated your coming in for an interview. Regrettably, we have decided to hire another applicant. We wish you the best in your future endeavors.*

The hiring process requires that you adhere to certain rules. If your hospital does a credit check of applicants, that should be disclosed on the application, and permission should be sought for that check. You should tell applicants that background checks will be required, and that references will be checked prior to hiring.

Some good guidelines to use in hiring include:

- Advertisements must have non-sexist speech.
- Selection and screening criteria should be based on objective criteria that relate directly to the job.
- Interviews should be used to document attitudes and biases that may indicate a bad employee.
- Subjective findings should be documented.
- When a candidate says something that excludes him, it should be written on his resume or application as the reason for his non-selection.
- Records should be kept on non-selection for at least 18 months (because the statute of limitations is less than one year).
- The same rules that apply to sex apply with respect to race, religion, national origin, skin color, pregnancy, and age.

1. Are There Rules Governing Promotion and Transfer?

While the rules on promoting individuals are the same as the rules for hiring, the way most employers run afoul of the law is by having favorite employees to whom they steer certain opportunities.

Margaret is quitting her position in the Pulmonary Lab in order to raise her children. Lisa is a staff therapist who has worked hard to advance, having recently taken and passed the Pulmonary Function Technologist Exam from the NBRC. Lisa has filled in from time to time in the PF lab when Margaret's children were sick. Dan, the department manager, can think of no one he would like better in that job than Lisa.

Fred, on the other hand, has been a bit of a pain. He recently led the effort to get new scrubs for RT personnel paid for by the hospital because the hospital paid for nursing scrubs in clean areas. He has filed six job grievances through the hospital HR department, and five of the six have been ruled against him. He has worked at the hospital for two years, and for the four years before that he was a pulmonary function technician in another state. Fred not only has more experience with pulmonary functions, he has been a CPFT much longer. Fred is 40 years old, and Hispanic. Lisa is 23, and Caucasian.

Dan approaches Lisa and tells her that the position is opening. He says, "I can't post the position or Fred will want it, and I don't want to even consider him." He asks Lisa if she wants the PF position. She agrees.

Dan has:

1. Committed an unfair labor practice because his refusal to consider Fred for the position in the PF lab could be tied to his "protected concerted activity" of getting scrubs purchased for the department;
2. Violated the Civil Rights Act, because Fred, an Hispanic male, was denied the opportunity to bid on a job that went to a white female; and
3. Violated the Age Discrimination in Employment Act.

Positions must be offered to all those individuals who are qualified. The hospital policy (assuming one exists) must be followed. A manager cannot take shortcuts. All qualified individuals have to be interviewed and given an equal chance to compete for the position.

Dan's failure to even consider Fred in the above example would be fatal to any defense in a discrimination or unfair labor practice case. His statements to Lisa to the effect that he didn't want to give Fred a chance to compete would make it very hard to defend the hospital from a charge of purposeful discrimination.

That does not mean that Dan could not have had the person he wanted for the PF lab. If the objective requirements for the position included current experience in pulmonary function, or experience with the current brand of pulmonary function equipment, those factors might have weighed against Fred.

Similarly, if in the interview Dan determined that Fred did not relate well, or could not communicate well with patients because he was impatient and brusque (but not because he was Hispanic), then on the basis of those factors Fred could have been denied the position. Fred might still have challenged the decision. An unfair labor practice claim might still have been filed, as might an EEOC action. However, the defense of those actions would be much easier with at least the appearance of fairness in the process.

2. What Are the Rules on Firing and Demotion?

Frequently employees do not work out. When they do not, one common reason is an inability to get along with their peer group. Sometimes, employees will demand that a worker be let go because they are not pulling their own weight, or for reasons that they feel breed conflict.

Of all the potential land mines that a manager can step on in the area of employment, firing employees is the largest. There are literally hundreds of ways to violate the various federal and state laws, and precious few ways to comply with all of them.

At the outset, it should be noted that the rule of law is still that an employee may be fired for any reason, or no reason, but not for an unlawful reason. From a practical point of view, however, an employee should only be fired for a good reason related to business purposes.

If this sounds contradictory, consider the import of a decision to fire an employee for no reason. If the employee is told there is no reason for his termination, he has a strong incentive to invent one. Most employees don't need an incentive, but when told there is no reason for their termination, quickly reach the conclusion that it is because of some protected status.

And, of course, every single employee a manager has is a member of a protected class. That is because every single employee is either male or female, and is therefore a member of a class protected from sex discrimination.

While conventional wisdom suggests that sex discrimination only applies in the context of a woman denied a job by a man, the fact is that courts do not make that a requirement. A man can be sexually harassed by another man. A woman can be sexually harassed and discriminated against by another woman.[1] Similarly, it is unlawful to discriminate on the basis of national

---

[1] In fact, this is frequently the most invidious discrimination. There are numerous cases of women discriminating against other women when the object of the discrimination is also a rival for the affection of some other person.

origin. In many parts of the country where a person's family comes from is an important consideration (even though it should not be). Because every employee in your organization can claim at least one, and usually several bases for discrimination, it is never a good idea to terminate an employee for no reason. Rather, they should be terminated only for a very good reason that has something to do with job performance.

At one Catholic hospital, a manager was heard to grouse that the only way an employee ever got terminated was "to be caught on video tape ax-murdering a nun." While I suspect this was a bit of hyperbole, the fact is that many HR departments will only approve a job action against an employee if the job action can be substantiated under the hospital's rules.

Importantly, almost all employers have what is called a "probationary period" where an employee can be discharged without cause, for any reason or no reason, without incurring liability for things like unemployment insurance. Any new employee's first month on the job should be the hardest possible. They should be given the most challenging assignments and their ability and attitude evaluated closely. A manager should not assume that "no news is good news." In fact, quite frequently the situation is just the opposite. The employee is so bad that everyone else is sure that someone's said something.

An excellent resource for managers is peer review of new employees. Every new employee should be subject to peer review. Each individual in the department with more than one year's experience should rate the new employee in terms of knowledge, experience, and ability, and should sign that evaluation and submit it without allowing the new employee to know the results. One or two isolated bad marks should be discounted. If everyone thinks the employee doesn't know the job, the manager should pay attention and terminate the employee.

Keep in mind that although a warm body may be preferable to a vacancy in many cases, that's only until the first lawsuit is filed. And a wrongful termination lawsuit is cheaper to defend than a wrongful death lawsuit.

3. Should I Be Concerned About the NLRB?

Yes! For example, in one instance, an employee with known union affiliations, who had been active in leading a union organizing attempt, was accused of having contributed to the death of a neonate by not being able to assemble an ambu bag during a code. The manager sought to terminate him on the basis of the behavior. The HR department concluded that other employees had made similar errors (e.g., a nurse had given the wrong medication, resulting in patient death), and the hospital had not terminated the employee. The employee who had failed to fix the ambu bag received only a written warning for his conduct.

The hospital had acted carefully because the National Labor Relations Board was involved. The employee filed an unfair labor practice charge. The NLRB investigated and ruled against the employee.[2] Part of the reason it did is that the hospital convinced the NLRB that it applied only the discipline necessary to address the behavior, and did not consider the union actions of the employee in reaching the decision. The memorandum of the manager recommending termination, and the memorandum of the HR Vice President explaining that this was against the discipline policy, factored heavily into the decision.

Across the country thousands of employees are terminated every day. Only about one half of one percent of these employees ever bring a legal action for the termination. But for those who do, the costs are significant. Thus, the termination process normally begins with a violation of a work rule or standard of conduct.

The most important factor to consider in making the decision to terminate is whether the standard of conduct and work rules are being fairly applied. In other words, "is the employee being terminated for violation of a rule that no one else would be terminated for?" If the answer is yes, then the termination should not go forward.

4. How Important Are Investigation Procedures?

One factor central to the concept of fairness is that when a work rule violation occurs, unless it is physically witnessed by the manager responsible for the termination, an investigation into the conduct is necessary. As a general rule, the investigation should not be conducted by the person who is the ultimate decision maker with respect to termination. It should be done by someone who is as neutral as possible, and should be reported to a person who can make a determination about termination fairly.

If the department director does the investigation, he should defer the decision about termination to the next higher level in the chain of command to avoid the impression that he is judge, jury, and executioner. If a supervisor does the investigation, he should report his findings and recommendations to the department director.

---

[2]This is, frankly, rare. The NLRB normally reviews things in the light most favorable to the employee.

The employee should receive a copy of the supervisor's report, and should have an opportunity to present mitigating evidence or challenge the facts.

No supervisor should ever rely on hearsay statements or statements from people who "don't want to be named." If an employee does not want his or her name to appear in the report, their information should not be considered. If an employee saw something, and reported something to management, they should be as accountable for what they report as the individual sought to be held accountable for a work rule violation.

One thing that must always be considered in doing any investigation, even if it is the worst employee in the department, is that sometimes people do not tell the truth. It is completely possible for 13 people to be wrong about something.

Often, bad conduct takes on its own life. An employee sees another employee taking a pill. Later, he or she sees the employee stumble in the hall. The two events are unconnected, but the rumor that circulates later is that the employee was seen taking drugs and stumbling in the halls. The "drug" is aspirin, and the stumbling is from errant clumsiness. The employee hasn't done anything wrong.

As Pure Prairie League once observed, "the tales grow taller on down the line." By the time the department director hears the tale, third hand, from a shift supervisor on the following shift, the employee was "popping pills" and "stumbling around like a drunken sailor."

If the department director initiates an investigation, the first thing he will most likely do is call the employee in for a drug urine test. If the drug test is negative, or cannot be explained by prescription medications, then all the probable cause necessary for termination is available.

If the director waits, and misses the opportunity to do drug testing, then the potential "smoking gun" is likely to be missed. The department director will now have to rely on observations by other persons. The person who made the original observation, because he knows it to be blown out of proportion and motivated by his own desire not to have to work with the employee, refuses to make a written statement.

At this point, the investigation is over.

Ultimately, the decision should be made only after a full day's reflection in order to avoid the appearance of a rush to judgment, or in fact, the appearance that the judgment was reached prior to the offense being committed. All decisions, those that involve hiring, firing, discipline, and promotions, should be rigorously documented.

5. How Important Is Documentation?

No one ever went into a trial, got up on the stand, and said, "Gosh, I wish I hadn't kept such good notes." In fact, almost always, the expression is just the opposite. "I wish I had kept better notes."

Documentation, made contemporaneously with the event being documented, is the single best record a person can have to defend themselves at any subsequent legal proceeding.

At a minimum, good documentation of a personnel decision includes:

1. A memorandum regarding how the matter was called to the attention of the decision-maker.
2. A report from a supervisory employee assigned to investigate.
3. Copies of statements from employees who witnessed events, and who have told what they saw to the supervisor.
4. An analysis of any harm caused to any patient as a result.
5. A memorandum to the employee setting out the evidence, establishing the basis for personnel action, and permitting the employee to submit any evidence of material he wants to submit.
6. The employee's evidence; and
7. A memorandum regarding the personnel decision being made, and how the evidence figured into it.
8. A final memorandum to the employee setting out the decision.[3]

There is a very real danger to the organization, however, in setting out in detail any disciplinary action that is taken in response to a patient care incident that results in patient harm. If a wrongful death or patient malpractice suit is brought as a result of the conduct and the information appears in the employee file, it will be discoverable by the plaintiff's attorney.

For this reason, the employee should be provided with a memorandum setting out the basis for termination, but that memorandum should not contain any identifying patient information. The personnel information should be recorded only in the briefest and most succinct of manners (e.g., "terminated for cause").

The file of the investigation, and all the statements made should be referred to the Quality Control Committee for presentation to the committee

---

[3]No memorandum given to the employee should contain information from any patient care record. This would violate HIPAA.

and recommendations by the committee. The information submitted to the committee should be stored separately in the Quality Assurance department, and not in the HR or Respiratory Care department to prevent its discovery or later misappropriation.

In some states, no matter how carefully the record of a termination is hidden, it may be discoverable. Some states do not permit an investigation and termination file to be shielded if the facts are otherwise discoverable.

6. What Is a Hostile Work Environment?

Just as it is wrong to fire an employee for an unlawful reason, it is just as wrong to create a hostile work environment for them. While Hostile Work Environment as a cause of action has been principally limited to sexual harassment suits, there is some authority for expanding this ground of termination to other forms of discriminatory treatment. If the department's only male team member is continually locked in the men's room by the women in the department, that is evidence of hostile work environment. If the department's only Asian team member is constantly subjected to offensive and stereotypical ethnic jokes—that too can create a hostile work environment. Managers should remember that the test is an objective one. Courts do not impose a remedy for the hurt feelings of one person, but rather, they impose a remedy if the conduct would be such as to create a hostile work environment in the minds of a reasonable person.

7. What Is Constructive Termination?

Going hand-in-hand with the doctrine of Hostile Work Environment is the doctrine of Constructive Termination. Constructive termination is where an employer creates a situation so untenable that an employee is faced with a Hobson's choice.

For example, Judy is an employee who works 3 to 11. She works this shift because her husband works 7 to 3, and they live a block away from the hospital. Judy's children have a parent available at all times.

Judy's new supervisor doesn't like her. She moved her out of the ICU, where Judy loved to work, and assigned her to the Long Term Care unit. Judy complained, but kept working. Now she has decided to transfer her to days. Judy has explained this is not the shift she signed up for, and that it does not work out for her. The manager says, "Take it or leave it."

This is constructive termination. Judy has been terminated, even though she ultimately is the one who resigns, because her employer created a situation where she was forced to resign.

Just as it is unwise to engage in this kind of behavior, it can be the basis for a claim of discrimination just as surely as can a termination, demotion, or refusal to hire.

E. CAN THE EMPLOYER SET CONDITIONS OF EMPLOYMENT?

Just as the employer has the right to obtain the employees he or she wants, within the limits of the federal and state antidiscrimination statutes, so too does the employer have the right to set the conditions of employment. In other words, he has the right to say how much an employee will be paid, what shifts they will work, how many people they will work with, what benefits they will receive, and what other perks they may enjoy as a result of their employment. In doing that, the organization and its managers must follow federal and state antidiscrimination laws.

1. What Controls Wages?

An employer is guided in setting wages by three factors: state law, federal law, and the local market. As set forth in Chapter Four, he must pay the employee a rate equal to or higher than the state and federal minimum wage. If the state minimum wage is higher than the federal minimum wage, he has to pay that rate, unless state law exempts the employer for some reason.

The employer is required to comply with the record-keeping requirements of the Federal Labor Standards Act. Similarly, the employer must comply with state record-keeping requirements.

The real factor affecting wages, however, is the local market. Whatever the local market pays for therapists is what is most likely to affect the wages a therapist receives. Usually only unskilled labor positions are affected by minimum wage.

It is the employer's desire to keep wages as low as possible, and it is in the employee's interest to keep the wages going up. Generally, when an employer cannot recruit and retain employees, it routinely raises its wage scale.

So long as the employer complies with federal and state laws on the amount of minimum wages paid, and maintains proper records, wages will seldom be a problem for the employer.

2. Are Hours Regulated?

Yes, in some states employees can only work so many hours in a row. Employers have the right to set the hours an employee will work. Some hospitals use 10- and 12-hour shifts. Others use eight-hour shifts. Still others use a combination of shifts and flexible time. Generally speaking, no federal law really speaks to the amount of time an employer may require a worker to spend on the job. Federal laws do require that if an employee is made to work 24-hour shifts, that sleeping time is not deducted from the hours paid.

Some states, like Florida and Illinois, have maximum numbers of hours that an employee can work in a week or in a day. See Appendix G for a list of states and various meal and hours requirements.

3. How Are Employee Benefits Regulated?

As noted in Chapter Four, while an employer does not have to offer health care benefits to all employees, when health care benefits are offered, they are subject to ERISA, HIPAA, and COBRA federal statutory requirements.

Employers are required to comply with these mandates. Failure to comply can result in civil money penalties, and sometimes, criminal sanctions.

4. Are Workloads and Staffing Regulated?

Although federal and state wage and hour laws govern meal breaks, wages, and hours of work, there are no federal standards setting out what safe staffing levels are in a hospital, nursing home, or other health care facility. The only source of regulation of the adequacy of staff is, in fact, the medical negligence standards to which hospitals are held.

Hospitals are free to staff at a level that makes the most economic sense, but factored into the economic equation is the cost of medical negligence lawsuits. These lawsuits cause a huge disruption in the provision of care, create stress for workers, and ultimately work against the mission of the health care entity, which is usually to provide compassionate and cost-effective care.

For this reason, while employers have the right to cut the corner on staffing, sending people home when workloads are low, they also have the responsibility to ensure that sufficient staff are available in an emergency. In an age of cost-cutting, this is not an insignificant task.

A word of caution is in order here. The quickest way to create a malpractice problem is to create a situation where your staff is short of help on an evening or night shift. If there are not sufficient people to do the job, then the managers and supervisors must find them, or work themselves.

This has the power to create great problems for managers who want to spend time with their families. But supervisors and managers have the absolute obligation to their staff and to their patients to secure adequate numbers of persons to provide care.

Some states and certain unions allow employees to fill out "staffing protest" forms, which document low staffing. If your hospital has this policy in place, or if staff routinely document poor staffing, you may be setting yourself up for a lawsuit.

F. DOES THE EMPLOYER HAVE THE RIGHT TO CONTROL THE WORKPLACE?

Yes. In addition to the other rights an employer has, the employer has the right to control the workplace and set workplace rules. For example, even though state statute might give the employee the right to wear a concealed weapon, the employer can mandate that as part of the agreement for employment, the employee will not wear such a weapon while at work. The employer can't control the employee's behavior off site, but on site the employer has a great deal of control.

Similarly, the right to control the workplace gives the employer the right to make safety rules. In organizations where certain types of patients are treated, such as patients with tuberculosis, the employer can mandate the wearing of positive pressure respirators. These respirators cannot achieve a tight seal without the wearer being clean shaven. When the employer mandates that an employee work in a particular area, he has the right to mandate that they be clean shaven.[4]

G. WHAT IS THE TARASOFF DOCTRINE?

When an employer knows that a patient, visitor, family member, or other individual on hospital property has a grievance against, or has made a threat to an identifiable person, there may be a duty to warn that individual, even if that information was communicated in the context of a request for medical help.

In *Tarasoff v. Regents of the University of California*, 551 P.2d 340, the court held that the defendant psychotherapists, who allegedly had knowledge of their patient's intentions to kill the plaintiffs' decedent, could not

---

[4]Certain religious sects do not permit shaving. If an employee was a member of such a sect, and requested exemption on the basis of a sincerely held religious belief, the employer would probably be required to accommodate the exception by assigning the employee to a different work unit if possible.

escape liability "merely because [the victim] herself was not their patient." According to the court, "[w]hen a therapist determines, or pursuant to the standards of his profession should determine, that his patient presents a serious danger of violence to another, he incurs an obligation to use reasonable care to protect the intended victim against such danger." *Id.* "The discharge of this duty may require the therapist . . . to warn the intended victim or others likely to apprise the victim of the danger, to notify police, or to take whatever other steps are reasonably necessary under the circumstances." *Id.*

The court in *Tarasoff* recognized an exception to the general rule that "one person owed no duty to control the conduct of another . . . nor to warn those endangered by such conduct," where "the defendant stands in some *special relationship* to either the person whose conduct needs to be controlled or in a relationship to the foreseeable victim of that conduct." (Citations omitted; emphasis added.) *Id.*, 343.

The court held that the relationship of the defendant therapist to either the intended victim or the patient, who confided his intention to kill another, will suffice to establish a duty of care on the part of the therapist to warn the intended victim or take other appropriate action. *Id.*, 342-43, citing 2 Restatement (Second), Torts § 315 (1965).

Accordingly, the court concluded that *"once a therapist does in fact determine, or under applicable professional standards reasonably should have determined, that a patient poses a serious danger of violence to others, he bears a duty to exercise reasonable care to protect the foreseeable victim of that danger."* (Emphasis added.) *Id.*, 345. "[T]he therapist has no general duty to warn of each threat."

Only if he "does in fact determine, or under applicable professional standards reasonably should have determined, that a patient poses a serious danger of violence to others, [does he bear] a duty to exercise reasonable care to protect the *foreseeable victim* of that danger." *Thompson v. County of Alameda,* 27 Cal.3d 741, 614 P.2d 728, 734, 167 Cal.Rptr. 70 (1980). "[I]n each instance the adequacy of the therapist's conduct must be measured against the traditional negligence standard of the rendition of reasonable care under the circumstances." *Tarasoff v. Regents of the University of California, supra,* 551 P.2d 345.

The court made an analogy to cases that have imposed a duty upon physicians to diagnose and warn about a patient's contagious disease and concluded that, " by entering into a doctor-patient relationship the therapist becomes sufficiently involved to assume some responsibility for the safety, not only of the patient himself, but also of any third person whom the doctor knows to be threatened by the patient." *Id.*, 17 Cal.3d at 437, 131 Cal.Rptr. at

24, 551 P.2d at 344, quoting Fleming & Maximov, *The Patient and His Victim: The Therapist's Dilemma*, 62 Cal. L.Rev. 1025, 1030 (1974).

The court also considered various public policy interests determining that the public interest in safety from violent assault outweighed countervailing interests of the confidentiality of patient therapist communications and the difficulty in predicting dangerousness. *Id.*, 17 Cal.3d at 437-43, 131 Cal.Rptr. at 24-28, 551 P.2d at 344-48.

As a general rule, hospitals have a duty to protect third persons from harm when they know of specific and credible threats. An analysis of Emma Turner's case against Nashville psychiatrist Harold Jordan is illustrative of this concept.

In March of 1993 Emma Turner, a nurse at Hubbard Hospital in Nashville, was attacked and severely beaten by Tarry Williams, a psychiatric in-patient at the hospital. The defendant, Harold Jordan, M.D., was the attending psychiatrist for Williams.

Williams, who had been diagnosed as bipolar and manic, had been a patient at Hubbard on five prior occasions. Three of these times he was found to be a danger to himself or others and was committed to the Middle Tennessee Mental Health Institute. On one occasion, in April of 1990, Williams tried to attack Dr. Jordan with a table leg, but the hospital staff intervened.

On March 4, 1993, Williams was admitted to Hubbard's psychiatric ward and examined by a resident physician. Williams's history indicated that he had not taken his prescribed lithium, which was used to control his bipolar disorder, for over a week. Williams also reported that he had met with "Gorbachev and Saddam Hussein" and that he had "classified information" about space flights and nuclear science. The resident physician determined that Williams had illogical and disorganized thinking, flight of ideas, grandiosity, and delusional thinking. Lithium was prescribed, which takes five to seven days to reach a therapeutic level.

The next day, on March 5, 1993, Dr. Jordan reviewed and approved the resident physician's orders. He and members of a treatment team then attempted to interview Williams, who refused to cooperate and left the interview. The treatment team then discussed the case for 30 to 45 minutes, after which Dr. Jordan wrote:

This patient presents no behavior or clinical evidence suggesting that he is suicidal. He is aggressive, grandiose, intimidating, combative, and dangerous. *We will discharge him soon by allowing him to sign out AMA [Against Medical Advice].*

That evening, according to notes, Williams, although quiet and non-disruptive, had an "angry and hostile" affect. Around 11:30 p.m., after requesting a cigarette and asking the nurse, Emma Turner, about being discharged, Williams attacked Turner, inflicting severe head injuries.

Thereafter, Emma Turner sued Dr. Jordan for medical negligence, alleging that he violated his duty to use reasonable care in the treatment of his patient, which proximately caused her injuries and damages. At trial, Dr. David Sternberg, a psychiatric expert witness, testified that Jordan's failure to medicate, restrain, seclude or transfer Williams fell below the standard of care for psychiatrists. He explained:

> *The standard of care in a case like this requires, first, an evaluation of whether the patient is a danger to himself or others. And, indeed, Dr. Jordan determined, it seems to me from the record, both his deposition and from the records from the hospital, that the patient was, indeed, dangerous. Then the standard of care requires, if a patient is found, in fact, to be dangerous, that the patient be prevented from acting on that dangerousness; that staff be informed, of course, about the patient's dangerousness; that the patient be medicated, if necessary, to prevent acting on the dangerousness, or be restrained or secluded; or that the patient be transferred to another treatment setting which could handle a patient who is of that severe dangerousness.*

In his own defense, Dr. Jordan testified that he did not remember Williams or any information about his dangerousness prior to the attack on Emma Turner. He agreed that had he known about Williams' prior dangerousness, he would have discharged him. However, Dr. Jordan's discharge summary written after the incident said:

> *Realizing that this patient had been hospitalized on this issue before and exhibited some hostile and violent behavior and questioning the veracity of his statement that he was suicidal, we wrote an order indicating that [Williams] could be encouraged to sign out and be allowed to sign out on request.* We considered discharging him outright because of his history of violent behavior.

In addition, Linda Lawrence, nursing coordinator at Hubbard Hospital, testified that Williams' past violent behavior, including the attempted attack on Jordan in 1990, had been discussed during the treatment team meeting on March 5, 1993.

After the completion of the proof, the trial court instructed the jury on the law of comparative fault, and it provided the jury with a verdict form indicating it could allocate the fault, if any, between the alleged negligence of Dr. Jordan and the alleged intentional conduct of patient Williams. The jury returned a verdict for the plaintiffs, Emma and Rufus Turner, allocating 100 percent of the fault to defendant Jordan.

In upholding liability against Jordan, the Tennessee Supreme Court said:

> *We stress that we are not requiring psychiatrists or physicians to possess per-fect judgment or a degree of clairvoyance in determining whether a patient poses a risk of harm to a third person. Instead, we merely hold that a duty of care may exist where a psychiatrist, in accordance with professional standards, knows or reasonably should know that a patient poses an unreasonable risk of harm to a foreseeable, readily identifiable third person. The courts below cor-rectly held that the facts in this case met this standard.* **Turner v. Jordan,** *957 S.W.2d 815 (Tenn. 1997)*

Other courts have not been so quick to expand the doctrine and have nar-rowly construed it to situations where a medical professional has knowledge of a specific threat to a specific individual, and not some generalized knowl-edge of a potential for harm.

H. IS THERE A DUTY TO PROTECT EMPLOYEES?

Yes. State Workers Compensation law imposes on employers a duty to protect their employees. The Occupational Health and Safety Administration (OSHA) requires employers to protect workers from certain known dangers. An employer has an obligation to ensure that working conditions are safe and that he has complied with all applicable OSHA standards.

Failure to comply with OSHA standards, where they exist (e.g., blood stan-dards, sharps standards, radiation exposure standards) usually results in fines or civil money penalties.

The OSHA standards governing health care are too diverse and too lengthy to include here. Employers should, however, be fully aware of those that apply. When they are not, tragedies occur. As an attorney, I've been per-sonally involved investigating industrial accidents that resulted from failure to adhere to OSHA regulations. The liability risk for organizations is too se-vere to underestimate.

I. HOW DO EMPLOYERS AVOID UNFAIR LABOR PRACTICE CHARGES?

When an unfair labor practice charge is filed with the NLRB, an investiga-tor is assigned. The investigator contacts the organization and takes state-ments from those who are believed to be responsible for the unfair labor practice.

The best way to avoid these charges is to provide counsel to any manager that the NLRB wishes to interview or obtain a statement from. This is particularly true when an individual who files a charge with the NLRB was terminated or demoted under conditions that might suggest an unfair labor practice.

The fact is that many employees use the NLRB as the court of last resort. In the Waggoner case, the employee first went to the EEOC charging discrimination on the basis of age and gender. The EEOC was not fooled, and refused to enter a probable cause statement.

The employee sought an attorney to file an EEOC action. No attorney ever entered an appearance. But the NLRB represented the employee, free of charge, and proved that, as is frequently charged, it is the last refuge for the scoundrels in the workplace.

The NLRB will not only contact managers and supervisors, normally through counsel, but will also contact "back door" employees. It will come onto the premises and meet with employees, frequently on work time, and interview them. Once it finds one or two who will support the claim made by the employee, the NLRB will file a formal charge against the institution.

It cannot be overstated how important it is for counsel to be engaged as quickly as possible once an NLRB charge is filed. Under no circumstances should the manager or supervisor accused of an unfair labor practice start calling in employees and suggesting what they should say to the NLRB. In fact, the less said the better.

Under the National Labor Relations Act, it is an unfair labor practice to interrogate an employee about his union sympathies or union interest. The NLRB is apt to file an interrogation charge if employees are questioned about what they said to the investigator.

For this reason, competent counsel who have defended NLRB actions should be engaged immediately to investigate and prepare a defense. This counsel should be involved from the minute the NLRB notifies the organization that it has filed a complaint.

Similarly, if any of the actions of an employee that lead to his or her termination could legitimately be called protected concerted activities under the National Labor Relations Act, care must be taken to document the termination carefully and prepare for any claim of unfair labor practice that might later be filed. Managers, or in some cases, counsel, should be careful to take statements from employees about what happened and who said what at the time of the termination. These statements may be very useful later if the NLRB investigator pressures different statements out of employees when it conducts its "investigation."

In the Waggoner case, the employer had seven current and former employees testify to the bad conduct of the employee, Waggoner, and it simply disregarded that information in reaching its determination that XYZ committed an unfair labor practice. For this reason, a seasoned manager will tread very carefully in the area of labor relations, and will go to whatever lengths are necessary to avoid dealing with the NLRB.

I. HOW DO EMPLOYERS AVOID DISCRIMINATION CHARGES?

Of all the duties given to a hospital department head or manager, the primary duty is to make sure that those who are employed to give treatments give those treatments in a safe and effective way. That calls for management skills, communication skills, and for a willingness to follow up with individual employees.

There is no science in management. Management and motivation are art. But just as there are rules to follow in any art, there are rules to follow in the area of management and motivation.

1. Is Management Responsible?

Although it should be clear after four decades of civil rights law, there is no place in any organization for a bigot. Someone who makes personnel decisions on the basis of skin color, religion, national origin, or sex is not an effective manager. An effective manager is someone who gets things done within the law. A bigot is someone who manages to escape the law while practicing his craft.

Make no mistake, every hospital has a closet bigot somewhere in the organization. Although there have been steady efforts to rid organizations of these managers, they still exist. An organization that tolerates such a manager will soon make itself a lawsuit target.

The first rule of management is that there are some things that are just not funny. Stereotypes are one form of bigotry. All Hispanics talk with an accent. African-Americans like watermelons. Irishmen are all drunks. Chinese all have trouble saying the letter "l" in conversation. On the basis of these stereotypes, thousands of jokes have been written. I would be dishonest to say that, before I understood the implications of them, I had not told them. Similarly, I would be dishonest to say that I had not laughed at some of them before I understood their impact on victims of discrimination.

But in today's world, management cannot tolerate that kind of humor. First, Irish, Chinese, Hispanics, and African-Americans do not find the matter humorous.[5] They regard the remarks as offensive just as most any member of any definable group is offended when made the butt of a joke. Most Caucasians have never seen a plantation and have never owned a slave. They consider slavery to have been a barbarous wrong. They do not wish to be associated with it. And if an African-American says his family came to the country in chains, you can bet a white person's first thought is "no one in my family owned any slaves." White people, speaking from personal experience now, often feel insulted to be lumped into the same category as whip-toting overseers from the 1800s.

And yet, it is precisely that kind of stereotyping that occurs when racially-themed jokes are told. The fact is, racist jokes are not funny, and should not be permitted. The quickest and most effective way to get sued for creating a hostile work environment is for management and supervisors to be guilty of sharing in the fun of a stereotypical joke session aimed at a defined racial, ethnic, or religious group.

Many would bemoan a loss of a sense of humor and say it is sad that we can't laugh at ourselves. But we can laugh at ourselves—we just can't laugh at racial stereotypes. It must be a zero tolerance rule in the workplace, and that is true whether there are any employees of a particular race in the department or not. This is because the danger is not in the color of an employee's skin, but in the content of the management's character.

Management must take a dim view and enforce the rule because doing otherwise encourages the behavior. And, while it might be fun to make fun of Asians when there are none in the department, it might be very hard to explain to a physician or visitor who overhears the bigotry and is offended by it.

The second rule management and supervisors should practice in motivating employees is to forbid clinicians to complain about patients on the basis of racial stereotypes. While a little blowing off of steam is a good thing, and clinicians should be encouraged to pass along relevant information to the next shift, references to patients by their identifying racial characteristics should never be permitted. A hospital should never have black patients, white patients, or patients denominated by racially-charged names like wop, spic, or mick. It should have patients who are being treated for a disease condition or surgical condition, and the other factors should not matter.

---

[5]Lawyer jokes remain constitutionally protected free speech, much to the chagrin of lawyers who often bring them on themselves.

Just as jokes with racial stereotypes are forbidden, so are jokes with sexual overtones and stereotypes. While these jokes frequently appear to be just a way of good-naturedly blowing off steam, they can come back to haunt management. In this regard, it doesn't matter who starts them. If a woman starts making lewd and salacious comments in the work room, and the manager hears and joins in, the employee's recollection might later be tainted by a strong desire to win cash and prizes in court. Zero tolerance ends the inquiry.

If you tolerate jokes of a sexual nature, even if all the women and all the men join in making them, there will always be the possibility that one employee will be offended and will claim, later, that management created a hostile work environment by not taking action.

The third rule is to have in place a plan for dealing with complaints about any form of bigotry. If a woman or man is being harassed by co-workers, there must be a way for that employee to bring that fact to the attention of the boss. Once that conduct is brought to attention, there should be immediate interdiction. That does not necessarily mean discipline. A simple word to the wise may be sufficient to solve the problem without blowing the matter out of proportion. But action must be taken and must be documented.

2. Is Follow-Up Important?

Just as important as the action is the follow-up. The manager or supervisor must follow up, within a month, with the employee who complained so as to ensure that they are satisfied, and that the harassment or hostile environment has been abated. Simply paying lip service to a complaint, ensuring action, and then documenting that an employee was counseled is not enough to prevent a claim of sexual harassment based on hostile work environment.

Instead, there must be demonstrated sensitivity to the issue, and it begins with a follow-up within a reasonable amount of time to ensure that the problem has been solved.

Frequently, the problem is not a case of sexual harassment so much as a case of discordant personalities in conflict. Often, it is necessary to remove one of the persons from the environment in order to quell the disturbance. Sometimes disciplinary action is required to deal with the harassing individual.

One thing is vital: documentation. Every step in the process should be documented. The key factor in sexual harassment cases is that both the complainer and the person being complained about should be regarded as potential litigants. More than one good manager or supervisor has been fired because he or she failed to consider this fact.

My advice to managers is to write their memoranda involving these matters as if they were going to be published on the front page of the daily newspaper, because some day, they may well be.

3. Can Employees Receive Recognition?

Every employee likes to be rewarded and recognized for what he or she does. When engaging in employee recognition, keep in mind that people tend to recognize the good things in others that they feel are good in themselves. As a result, if there are African-American managers in a department, they may tend to recognize other African-American employees disproportionately to other races. The same can be said for any race.

When these managers recognize persons who look and sound like they do, they are practicing not so much a subtle form of discrimination as a narrowing of their focus. We tend to see the good in people who look like us and talk like us. We do not tend to see the same things in those who look differently.

For that reason any departmental recognition program that recognizes employees should be based on input from other departments, other employees, and patient surveys. Stated more bluntly, if patients and visitors wish to heap praise on people who look and sound like them, they are entitled to do so, and may do so without violating the Civil Rights Act. But if a manager who is white tends to give recognition only to white employees, such that only white employees get selected for promotions and new positions, that becomes a problem for the employer.

Another tool that can be good, so long as it does not become a tool for racism, is the peer review. If employees rate each other in certain areas, the results may tend to be a more honest and objective measure of the contribution of an individual team member than a manager's rather subjective analysis. However, if all good marks go to persons in identifiable racial groups, and minority groups tend to be under-recognized, that can be a problem that results in litigation.

Another frequent problem is recognition of borderline employees. If an employee is borderline, a recognition of good work might go a long way toward making him or her a team player. It might also show up, at the NLRB hearing, as evidence that he or she was a good worker and was being unfairly singled out. Recognition of employees should be based on exceptional conduct.

4. Must Managers Enforce a Rule No One Likes?

Managers may choose which regulations they enforce; however, the application of their discretion must be uniform. If we excuse tennis shoes for one worker, we have to excuse them for others unless there is a rational basis (like disability) for making the determination. Another important policy for department managers is that all policies should be enforced uniformly. If the hospital policy is that no employee will clock in early, and Jane has done it for six years, it begins to look like a lie if Harold is fired for violating this work rule.

Rules must be enforced not only against the bad employees, the ones who are constantly late, but the good employees too, when they violate those rules. Consider the hypothetical example below:

Katie is a good therapist. She does excellent work. She has been working at the hospital for two years with excellent evaluations every year. Recently her husband, a police officer, has been transferred to the day shift. Since that time, Katie has had several instances of being late to work. In addition, an employee who never called in sick in two years has now called in sick three weekends in a row. The manager wants to cut Katie a break and not write a written warning and put it in her file. Should he?

In this case, the employee should be counseled as non-judgmentally as possible. She should be told she is a valued employee that the hospital needs for her to be there every day. She should be told that coming in late is not acceptable, and that she should do what she needs to do to ensure that the problem is fixed.

5. Is "Tough Love" Appropriate?

Frequently, managers make the wrong decision for the right reason. They sense that an employee is really trying, and they want to help them through a rough time. In speaking with Katie, the manager learns she is having marital troubles with her husband. He also notices a bruise on Katie's arm. He concludes Katie has enough problems, and just encourages her to come to work on time.

Over the next month, the problem gets worse. Katie misses eleven days in six months. The manager gives her a written warning. Katie misses another week of work when she is hospitalized for what she reports to be a fall down the stairs at her apartment. During the fall, Katie broke her nose. Her manager visits her in the hospital, and she swears she will be a more dependable employee.

When the problem doesn't improve, a suspension for three days is imposed. Four weeks later, Katie files for divorce. Her attendance improves. She later says that if the hospital had not been tough on her, she would not have had the courage to be tough on her ex-husband and end the cycle of violence. She tells her manager that she was hospitalized not from a fall, but from being beaten by her husband.[6]

Unfortunately for managers, when they make exceptions to the rules for employees they like, they are also making exceptions for all the employees they do not like. If a manager waives a work rule for one employee, there is no reason why he could not, or perhaps, should not waive it for another employee. When the manager fails to waive it, the first charge asserted is discrimination. For this reason, rules are not meant to be broken, and all must be enforced uniformly.

6. How Is a Discrimination Case Handled?

To most people, the whole idea of discrimination is foreign. The idea that a hospital or some other employer would discriminate on the basis of color seems hard to swallow. But employers are routinely charged with it. And one of the reasons, frankly, is that there is a very low hurdle to cross in filing a discrimination charge.

In *McDonnell Douglas v. Green,* 411 US 792 (1973), the United States Supreme Court dealt with the issue of how the burden of proof must be allocated in a case involving a charge of discrimination under the Civil Rights Act. The Civil Rights Act stated that an employer may not discriminate, but also allowed an employer to terminate an employee for a bona fide occupational reason, like tardiness, absenteeism, or violation of work rules.

What happens when the employee makes his case of discrimination, and the employer puts forth a basis for firing the employee? Does the jury decide?

In *Green,* the Supreme Court decided on dancing the two step. The first part of the two step is called the prima facie case, and that is made by showing that the employee is in a protected class (in this case, he was an African-American) and by showing that he suffered a loss of pay or benefits, or some

---

[6]During 13 years as a therapist, and 8 years as a manager, I saw this scenario occur several times at hospitals all over the country. Employees with absentee problems almost always have some ongoing serious pathology including domestic violence, gambling addiction, or alcoholism.

other change in the conditions or terms of his employment (in Green's case, termination). Once the employee can show that he is a protected worker, and that he suffered an adverse job action, the employer gets to introduce evidence of the employee's wrongdoing.

In Green's case, he was accused of committing violations of the law, and McDonnell Douglas (now Boeing) didn't want him back. The district court allowed the case to be disposed on the employer's word that they had fired him for work violations, and the Supreme Court said "not so fast." It said:

> *Petitioner's reason for rejection thus suffices to meet the prima facie case, but the inquiry must not end here. While Title VII does not, without more, compel rehiring of respondent, neither does it permit petitioner to use respondent's conduct as a pretext for the sort of discrimination prohibited by 703 (a) (1). On remand, respondent must, as the Court of Appeals recognized, be afforded a fair opportunity to show that petitioner's stated reason for respondent's rejection was in fact pretext. Especially relevant to such a showing would be evidence that white employees involved in acts against petitioner of comparable seriousness to the "stall-in" were nevertheless retained or rehired. Petitioner may justifiably refuse to rehire one who was engaged in unlawful, disruptive acts against it, but only if this criterion is applied alike to members of all races.*

McDonnell Douglas v. Green, 411 US 792 (1973)

As can be seen from the McDonnell Douglas case, all a civil rights plaintiff needs to show is: (1) membership in a protected class (race, sex, age, disability, national origin, color, or pregnancy), and (2) an adverse job action (refusal to hire, firing, demotion, non-promotion). Once he does, the burden then shifts to the employer. The employer must show a legitimate non-discriminatory reason for the job action.

The employee, or applicant, however, gets one more bite at the apple. The employee can show that the employer's reasons are pretextual. How does the employee do this?

Simple. The employee shows that other employees with similar transgressions were treated differently. For example, while the Hispanic employee was terminated for three late attendance issues in one pay period, Randy, a white employee whose father is a physician at the hospital, was allowed to be late six times in one pay period without any disciplinary action.

In effect, the Supreme Court made the rebuttal evidence the most powerful part of a plaintiff's case, and allowed the employee to show how other employees were treated. But for *McDonnell Douglas v. Green,* this information might not even have been legally relevant. However, now it is a large part of every civil rights case.

It is for this reason that work rules must be enforced uniformly.

K. MUST A HOSPITAL PROTECT PATIENTS AND VISITORS FROM BAD EMPLOYEES?

As set out more fully in Chapter Two, patients have a right to expect that they will not be attacked, abused, or injured in the hospital as the result of the criminal acts of third persons. A hospital should be a safe zone. One way to ensure this is for every hospital to do background checks on all individuals who are admitted into the patient care areas.

1. How Important Are Background Checks?

As stupid as it may sound, there are still hospitals where a background check is not a mandatory part of the hiring process. There are hospitals that expose their patients to former convicted felons and persons with violent histories without ever knowing it. In many cases, the employer never learns of the employee's criminal past.

2. What Can We Learn from the Strange Case of Mike Swango?

Mike Swango, a former physician and convicted murderer, is one living, breathing example of how hospitals often fall short of their duty to protect the public and their employees.

Swango was a paramedic before he left Quincy, Illinois, to begin medical school. After a stellar medical education, Swango took a residency in Neurosurgery at Ohio State. After only a few months, the nurses began to notice that when Swango was around, things didn't always go well for their patients. Swango was suspected in the deaths of several patients at Ohio State, and was discharged from the residency program. He returned to his home town of Quincy, Illinois. He was hired by the Adams County Emergency Medical Service and not by the hospital, but his duty required him to work out of the hospital on most days.[7]

---

[7]No criticism is intended of the hospital or the Adams County EMS. Neither entity knew of Swango's background, and had no reason to know.

Unable to set up a medical practice in Quincy because he had not finished a residency, Swango did the next best thing. He applied for an Illinois medical license with the idea of doing a residency at the Illinois Veterans Home. The Veterans Home had few physicians on staff, and was willing to take a home town boy and former valedictorian of the local Catholic high school into their family of practitioners.

But as his license application pended, he needed funds, and he got them by serving as a paramedic with the Adams County EMS. Soon enough, paramedics began to realize that when Swango was around, things got strange. When the mad gunman shot up the McDonald's restaurant in San Ysidro, California, Swango was heard to remark, "every time I get a good idea someone goes and steals it." If that wasn't strange enough, it seemed that whenever anyone went out on a call with Swango, they got sick. Whenever Swango brought treats or soda pop to the hospital, people got sick.

One day Swango was left alone with a jug of iced tea. His co-workers, now suspicious of him, decided to lay a trap. When Swango left on a call, the jug of tea was sent for analysis. The paramedics, tired of becoming sick when Swango worked, took the tea to the laboratory and asked a professor to check it. They found it contained large amounts of an arsenic-based ant poison.

Swango was arrested and charged with aggravated battery. On conviction, he was forced to give up his Illinois license and sentenced to five years in prison.

If hospitals did their jobs, that would be the end of the story. But it isn't. Swango tried to get a job in a Virginia hospital, but was denied after a background check. It didn't stop him from trying to find another medical job. A few years later, Swango got a job at the University of South Dakota, and began serving as a resident. He distinguished himself, until he got a little too cute. When he applied for membership in the American Medical Association, the fact that he did not have a medical license and had been barred from practice in Illinois was found during a routine check. The AMA called the judge in Quincy, Illinois, who sentenced him. The judge called the hospital in South Dakota, and the poisoner was quickly discharged from employment.

That didn't stop him, however, from applying to the University of New York at Stony Brook, where he was admitted to a psychiatric residency. Swango's background wasn't discovered until patients again began to die. When they did, the FBI got involved.

The FBI sought a warrant against Swango, but Swango eluded them, traveling to Zimbabwe in Africa. There, he went to work for the Lutheran hospital and over the next several years managed to kill several more patients.

Before he was arrested and charged with fraud, and later murder, Swango is estimated to have killed between 30 and 60 patients in hospitals across the country and around the world.

Swango was an expert forger who cooked up his own documents and letters of reference. He was a talented liar who convinced people to believe him and not bother checking the court files. His tale of serial murder is all the more illustrative to respiratory therapists because of what happened with Efren Saldivar.

3. What Can We Learn from the Saldivar Story?

Saldivar was a popular respiratory therapist at Glendale Adventist. Using paralytic drugs, he admitted to committing six murders and was suspected of being involved in between 40 and 50 homicides at the facility over his tenure there. Even though the hospital knew there was someone killing patients, it took them a long time to figure out who was doing it. The internal investigation conducted by the hospital was criticized by attorneys for victims because the hospital looked as if it was more concerned for its reputation than for patient safety. In the end analysis, the investigation was fruitless because the therapists did not cooperate with the hospital. One of the reasons was that therapists did not feel comfortable reporting their suspicions to the hospital administration.

Saldivar's actions in killing patients brought discredit on the department and on all the therapists. However, it also caused the California Board for Respiratory Care to tighten up the process of granting licenses, and caused hospitals to be more careful about whom they recruited for critical care positions. Of course, Saldivar also unleashed a liability deluge on Glendale Adventist Hospital that may take years to sort out.

The lesson to be learned from Swango is that hospitals must conduct background investigations on new employees. The lesson in the Saldivar case is different. Hospitals need an anonymous way for employees to bring wrongdoing to the attention of decision-makers.

While hospitals have a duty to protect patients, they generally do not have a duty to protect others, including visitors, from criminal attack. A patient has a special relationship with the hospital, and is owed a duty. A visitor is there to see the patient, is not a customer of the hospital, and is not owed a duty.

Of course, hospitals still have to keep their hallways safe and free from spills to prevent falls because they do owe a duty to visitors to make their hospital safe from dangers that are known or easily discovered. Likewise, they have a duty to fence off dangerous areas of property on hospital grounds, and light their parking lots so as to permit safe travel to vehicles.

Therapists have a duty to protect patients and visitors from the dangers of oxygen. Therapists routinely hang signs saying "Danger—Oxygen in Use" in rooms where patients are using oxygen. Similarly, therapists should always make sure that oxygen tanks are secured in holders that do not allow them to become damaged. Oxygen tanks become high-speed undirected torpedoes when their valves are damaged.

Similarly, therapists have a duty to warn visitors about the substances they use. Therapists should be sure to tell visitors what medications they are nebulizing and delivering in their equipment. In the event the nebulizer disconnects or the substance is aerosolized in the room, a visitor who is allergic to the substance will want to be informed.

4. How Does This Affect Employment Law?

If there is one place where a hospital is caught on the horns of a dilemma, it is the situation where an employee is thought to be injuring or harming patients through active abuse or neglect. In that situation, the needs of employment law must bow to the needs of the greater threat to the organization.

If an employee is wrongfully terminated the harm to the hospital is normally limited to a requirement to pay that employee back pay and reinstate them. Even if an employee who takes his case to the NLRB and wins is not going to cause a significant financial hit on the organization.

A wrongful death lawsuit, or a lawsuit where a child is rendered paraplegic as a result of active abuse or negligence, is certain to produce a verdict in the millions of dollars. If it is disclosed that the abuser was known to be abusing, but the facility had not taken action against him, that is a situation where punitive damages may be awarded. Thus, there is a significant threat to the institution where there is an employee suspected of causing injury.

Any employee so suspected should be immediately suspended, with pay, and an investigation started. The investigation, if it clears the employee, can return the employee to work without sanction. If it fails to clear the employee, but does not provide sufficient basis to initiate prosecution or termination action, then the employee must be monitored.

Under no circumstances should an employee who is arrested and charged with any form of violence (including domestic violence) be permitted to return to a patient care environment until adequate testing has been done to rule out a threat to patient safety.

L. CORPORATE COMPLIANCE PROGRAMS AND THE LAW

1. Why Have a Compliance Program?

One of the first reasons to have a compliance program is that hospitals and private employers are being hit with lawsuits by the federal government and whistleblowers to recover funds that they may have been wrongfully paid. The last several years have seen the United States Department of Justice recover an average of $300,000,000 per year in overpayments and penalties.

In addition to the Department of Justice, the State Attorney General has the power to recover Medicaid funds, and each insurance carrier has a "Special Investigative Unit" or SIU program that allows them to try to recover funds wrongly paid.

What constitutes wrongful payments? Any payment where the documentation and systems do not exist to prove that the patient was provided the services and that those services were of benefit.

Hospitals, then, can be exposed to civil lawsuits by private insurance companies, and to whistleblower lawsuits filed in federal court if they engage in conduct that is false or fraudulent. But what about mere error? Suppose a hospital or a home care company makes an honest mistake in how it codes a procedure, and that coding error causes an overpayment. Can the entity be liable?

The answer, unfortunately, is yes. The facility can be liable if its forms are merely false in the sense that they are wrong. No specific intent to defraud the government must be found in order to prosecute a False Claims Act Lawsuit.

It is for these reasons that Compliance Plans exist.

2. Can You Avoid Whistleblower Suits?

It probably goes without saying that the way an employer avoids liability for whistleblower lawsuits is to avoid committing fraudulent acts in the first place. Indeed, the first line of defense against claims of fraud is hiring competent, honest, ethical managers who put the health care organization's good name and reputation ahead of their own.

Unfortunately, no matter how great a health care organization's screening process, and no matter how diligent the background check, there are still ways for a hospital to acquire employees who put their own interests above those of the health care organization. When an organization does so, those in top management may not know it. But you can bet that somewhere out in the rank and file there is someone who does know what's going on, and who would report it if there were no chance it would affect their employment.

Employees are self-interested. Most live from paycheck to paycheck and count as heavily on the next one as the last one they received. As a result, anything that makes them choose between doing the right thing and getting fired, and doing nothing and continuing to draw a paycheck, will cause the employee to choose to do nothing.

For many, it is a peculiar form of what psychologists call "cognitive dissonance"—the belief that "it can't happen to me," that lets employees continue to violate the law, even though they know it is wrong.

It is said that criminals who abduct children frequently tell them that their parents have abandoned them, or that they will kill their parents if the children attempt to go home. As a result, the children, even though paralyzed with fear, remain with their abductors. It is frequently that way when a particular supervisor or manager directs employees to commit unlawful, dishonest, and illegal acts. They know that it is wrong, and they want to stop, but they lack the means because doing something will almost always get them fired.

3. Why Do You Care About Sentencing Guidelines?

Several years ago, Congress proposed and the federal court system implemented the federal sentencing guidelines. Sentences in federal cases have become formulaic. The crimes have ranges of months of incarceration, and the federal judge has discretion to choose where to impose a prison sentence. In the now famous Martha Stewart case the federal judge imposed five months of prison, five months of home confinement, and a period of probation.

Most people think, therefore, that sentencing guidelines apply only to those individuals unlucky enough to be caught breaking the law. But that is an erroneous belief.

Although it may seem difficult to accept, corporations can break the law, too. When they do, unless specific officers or directors took part and profited directly, the corporate officers cannot be punished. Thus a company that, because of negligence, allows some temporary workers to violate the Clean Water Act is guilty of a federal misdemeanor. Individual corporate officers may have taken no part in the crime, and had they known, would not have permitted it. But a breakdown in communication results in a federal crime, and the federal agents can't find a single person to blame or punish. What do they do?

Corporations are "virtual persons." In other words, when a corporation is formed, a legal existence just like that of a person is created under state law. That legal existence can be punished. Licenses can be suspended or revoked. Fines can be imposed. And, the fact is, the most common way that corporations are punished is through imposition of fines.

When the sentencing guidelines were being debated, however, someone took notice of the fact that in most cases of corporate fraud there was someone in the know inside the organization who kept quiet for fear of his or her job. What if, the drafters thought, we made it possible for those people to come forward without fear of sanction?

The feds cooked up a little carrot and stick approach to encourage companies to improve their compliance with federal laws. If a company has a good "corporate compliance program," then the company gets a significant break on any fines or penalties that are imposed. If it doesn't have a corporate compliance program, then the company pays the entire fine, even if that means the company must go bankrupt in the process.

4. How Corporate Compliance Programs Work

The Health Care Organization's Board of Trustees is charged with directing and developing the corporate compliance program. The corporation's officers are charged with implementing the program. A good program has seven elements. They are:

- A Code of Conduct covering officers, directors, employees, and independent contractors. As part of the development of the code of conduct, the organization should review all of its policies and procedures for compliance with federal and state regulatory guidelines.[8] During the process of creating the code of conduct, policies and procedures will need to be re-written and revised with an aim toward total compliance with federal and state law. These policies should be considered an integral part of the program.

---

[8]For example, while developing the code of conduct, the organization should pay particular attention to compliance with both state and federal law, at both the criminal level and the civil level. In doing the review, the organization policies should be evaluated as much for their impact on federal criminal law as for impact in the area of employment discrimination. The code of conduct should be all-encompassing.

- Corporate Compliance Officer and Compliance Committee: The Board of Directors should ensure that a corporate compliance committee is formed and chaired by officers and directors of the corporation. A separate corporate compliance officer, with twin reporting responsibilities to the CEO and the Board of Directors, should be hired and should be trained.[9]
- Compliance Training: Every employee with responsibilities in patient care, billing, management, and supervision will be trained on the code of conduct and on the duties and responsibilities of the Compliance Committee. Special training should be given to employees whose job functions place the organization at greatest risk of liability for fraud.[10]
- Hotline: Every organization with a compliance program needs an anonymous hotline where the CCO can receive complaints confidentially. The anonymous reporting procedure is meant to reduce the possibility of retaliation. When a report is not made anonymously, the CCO must still protect the reporter's identity, even from members of the Board and CEO, if the reporter requests it.
- Enforcement: The organization should set up an appropriate mechanism for the enforcement of its code of conduct through disciplinary actions against employees, physicians, or on-site agents or contractors who violate the organization's compliance policies, applicable laws, or federal health care program requirements. Attention to due process for employees suspected of wrongdoing, and a meaningful opportunity for those employees to contest their guilt, will be provided.[11]
- Monitoring: Simply setting up the program is not enough. The CCO and the Compliance Committee must perform regular audits and risk assessments in order to identify problems and prevent individuals from engineering around the compliance system. Monitoring should be ongoing wherever there is an identified problem area.
- Self-Disclosure and Remediation: The CCO is responsible for the investigation and remediation of identified compliance problems and the

---

[9]Although nothing requires the compliance officer be an attorney, it is a good idea for the CCO to be an attorney. In the course of his job he will come across information that, if divulged, could hurt the organization. An attorney is enjoined by the attorney client privilege from divulging the information.

[10]Janitorial personnel have responsibility for compliance with disposal of infective material. Literally every employee in the organization will have the need to attend compliance training. Training should be conducted by training professionals, not by hospital personnel, and should be tailored to each individual department's compliance needs.

[11]When an employee is terminated for failure to comply with federal guidelines, he may retaliate by filing a False Claims Act lawsuit. Thus, sometimes it may be wiser to impose discipline judiciously.

development of appropriate corrective action plans to remediate such problems. If self-disclosure to the government agencies is required to mitigate harm to the organization, the CCO is required to take such steps as are necessary to protect the organization.

5. Code of Conduct

In setting up the compliance program, the first and most daunting task is to write a code of conduct. Here is a model code of conduct that can be adapted for use by an organization. In addition, model compliance plans and codes of conduct can be found on the website of the Office of the Inspector General of Health and Human Services, www.hhs.gov.

Code of Conduct

Here at _____ we believe in principled, ethical decision-making. We provide this Code of Conduct to assist individuals in compliance with federal and state laws. Although the Code of Conduct cannot cover every situation in the daily conduct of the organization, neither can it substitute for common sense, individual judgment or personal responsibility. It is the duty of each member of this organization to adhere, without exception, to the principles set forth as follows:

1. **Compliance with Laws**

   It is the duty of this organization and each team member to uphold all applicable laws and regulations. Every employee must be aware of the legal requirements and restrictions applicable to their position and duties. We demand that each of our employees and team members refrain from engaging in activity which may jeopardize the name, reputation, or tax exempt status of the organization.

   We shall implement programs necessary to further such awareness and to monitor and promote compliance with such laws and regulations.

   Questions about the legality or propriety of any actions undertaken by or on behalf of this organization should be referred immediately to a supervisor, the Organization Compliance Officer (CO) or Legal Counsel. To enhance such communication, we have implemented a hotline. Any member of the organization who has confidential information about compliance violations should call _____ and report that information.

---

2. Business Ethics

This organization and all of its employees and team members shall conduct all patient care, business, and personal activities in accordance with the highest ethical standards of the community and their respective professions. Making false, inaccurate, or misleading statements to any patient, visitor, investigator, federal or state enforcement agent, or law enforcement officer is strictly forbidden.

3. Conflicts of Interest

We are a non-profit organization dedicated to the provision of health care. All members of this organization will conduct their duties for the benefit and interest of the organization and those it serves. All employees and team members have a duty to avoid conflicts of interest. Team members and employees may not use their positions and affiliations with this organization for their personal pecuniary benefit.

4. Quality of Care

This organization's mission is to provide health services of the highest quality. All care will be delivered in accordance with the professional standards of care of each profession represented in this organization. Patient care shall be properly documented as required by law and regulation, payor requirements and professional standards.

5. Equal Opportunity and Respect

We are committed to providing healthcare, education, and employment for all persons, without regard to race, color, nationality or ethnic origin, religion, gender, sexual orientation, disability, or veteran status. Discrimination in any form or context will simply not be tolerated.

6. Confidential Information

This organization complies fully with all standards set out in the Health Insurance Portability and Accountability Act (HIPAA), and will safeguard all patient care information. No confidential patient information shall be shared with any individual or entity unless such sharing meets the standards set out in HIPAA and its governing regulations.

7. Respect For Payors

All requests for payment for healthcare services provided at this organization must be:

(a) reasonable, necessary and appropriate; and

(b) provided by properly qualified persons, and

(c) the claims for such services shall be billed in the correct amount and supported by appropriate documentation.

When an individual or entity cannot make full payment of health care costs, this organization is committed to work with them to prevent financial ruin.

8. Honesty and Integrity

There is no room for anyone in this organization who is not honest and forthright. Errors and omissions occur and will be corrected promptly. Falsification of records, including destruction of patient care records, is forbidden. Any individual questioned by state or federal regulators is expected to provide that agency with accurate and truthful information. There are no exceptions to this rule, other than for patient confidentiality, as set out above. If there is a question as to patient confidentiality, it will be resolved before disclosure of any information to any investigative source. If any inquiry is made at any time to any individual, by any investigative body, such inquiry will be reported to the Corporate Compliance Officer and the employee will be provided with legal counsel at the expense of the Organization.

9. Safety

We are committed to compliance with all OSHA and state safety regulations, as well as all applicable environmental laws and regulations.

10. This Code of Conduct Governs

The Code of Conduct exists for the benefit of this institution and its employees, patients, visitors, and team members. It will be updated periodically when the need arises. It is the duty of every employee to know the provisions of this Code of Conduct and to practice their professional responsibilities with its core principles firmly in their methods and results.

6. Should Employers Encourage Anonymous Reporting?

There is some debate about whether organizations should allow anonymous reporting of information that can lead to discipline against an individual. In most cases the line is drawn in the employee's favor. If an employee will not commit her story to paper, there is some substantial doubt, and rightly so, about the truth of that story.

The corporate compliance area, however, is the one exception to the issue of anonymous reporting. The rationale is clear. While employees might lie about an employee cutting corners in the ICU for the sole purpose of seeing that employee terminated, most would not lie about a manager misappropriating funds, or a supervisor engaged in inappropriate sexual conduct with patients.

If Glendale Adventist Hospital had had a good corporate compliance program at the time that Efren Saldivar began killing patients, there might be a few patients up and walking around today who are not. While no one wanted to go up against Saldivar on something murky like personal suspicions, a compliance report would have alerted investigators much sooner.

In a compliance program, the anonymous report to the Corporate Compliance Officer (CCO) does not trigger discipline, it triggers investigation. Consider, for example, an employee's report that an ICU nurse is taking prescription drugs meant for her patients. The tip is anonymous, but identifies the purported drug diverter.

The CCO works with hospital security to place a hidden camera in the medication room. Those tapes are reviewed on a daily basis. After two weeks of surveillance the nurse is not found to have diverted any drugs. To be on the safe side, the CCO adds her name to a list of employees who are required to take "random" drug tests. She tests clean.

The CCO has not revealed any information to the ICU nurse manager, and has not revealed any information to anyone other than the director of security. The ICU nurse reported anonymously is never subjected to the enmity of her peers, and guilt by suspicion.

Without a CCO, the report would have been made, probably by anonymous note, to the ICU nurse manager, who would then take it upon herself to investigate. Frequently this would involve asking other nurses if the suspected nurse was doing anything different or "acting funny." Employees would begin to suspect the nurse, who would suddenly sense a change in her peers. Because a rumor as good as a drug-diverting nurse can never be kept within management, before long the entire hospital would "know" that the nurse was a drug diverter. The damage to her career and reputation would be enormous.

Thus, the Corporate Compliance system works well to protect employees who are suspected, but not actually guilty, of wrongdoing.

More importantly, it protects someone who is a line employee from retaliation or termination by a manager if they anonymously report to the hotline that their boss is routinely billing for testing and therapy that wasn't done in order to inflate his department's statistics.

Reports like the latter are difficult for the employee to make in the first place. Once made, however, the paper trail created by the false billing will lead to immediate and punitive action against the manager. It may also require the hospital to self-disclose the billing error and make restitution to Medicare and Medicaid. While this is painful, carrying with it a penalty, it is much better than nondisclosure, which can result in treble damages (i.e., a $100 claim becomes a $300 claim).

M. KEY POINTS

- Courts give employers leeway to hire and fire employees as they see fit, within certain parameters.
- One of those parameters is discrimination on the basis of age, sex, national origin, gender, race, skin color, and disability.
- An employee may generally be fired for any reason, or no reason, but not for an unlawful reason.
- Employers must adhere to nondiscrimination policies in all phases of employment.
- Advertising should include an affirmation that the employer is an equal opportunity employer.
- Advertisements should be screened for sexist and potentially racist language.
- Interview questions should stay away from topics that might lead a prospective employee to think that you are evaluating criteria on the basis of any protected status.
- Employees who have engaged in protected concerted activity (like union organizing, etc.) should be treated very carefully to avoid sanction by the NLRB.
- Documentation is the key to defending against claims of employment discrimination.

- Employers have a duty to protect employees as well as visitors.
- Employers have a duty to protect patients from employees, and must exercise that duty before any concern is given to employment law issues.
- A corporate compliance plan is a means to avoid litigation and federal penalties for false claims.
- An effective corporate compliance program enforces a code of conduct.
- The code of conduct should be endorsed by the board of directors.
- Good Compliance programs prevent damage to innocent employees while protecting the organization.

N. SUMMARY

The employer must be very careful to protect itself from claims of violations of the law, including violations of state and federal employment laws. The best way to do that is with managers who understand the risk and know where the land mines are in the hiring process.

Documentation is another key step in protecting the employer from claims of discrimination. When an employee is terminated or an applicant rejected, good notes about the reasons and rationale are helpful.

The best protection comes from a well-informed, well-motivated, and well-trained staff of managers and supervisors who understand their obligations under the law. Managers and supervisors must never tolerate the trappings of discrimination, or conduct that demeans an identifiable group of employees on the basis of race, sex, religion, age, or national origin.

CHAPTER 7

Essentials of Tort Law

*I can't do literary work for the rest of this year because I'm
meditating another lawsuit and looking around for a defendant.*

Mark Twain

A. INTRODUCTION

If you ask a therapist about his or her greatest legal worry in providing
care, you're often going to find that it is a fear of being sued for negligence.
The myths that have built up around lawsuits suggest that professionals routinely lose houses, cars, and jobs when they are sued. This is mostly just
myth. When professionals are sued, generally the lawsuit involves a claim of
tort law. Tort law is the branch of law that deals with redressing civil (as opposed to criminal) wrongs. Most of these lawsuits are settled and most judgments and settlements are paid by insurance without the loss of any homes,
cars, or life savings.

This chapter describes the tort law generally, focusing on the many different causes of action that exist for personal injuries. Many are directly applicable to health care. This chapter does not focus on medical negligence, however. Understanding medical negligence depends on understanding the basic
concepts of tort law presented here. In Chapter Seven we will look more
closely at medical negligence law, and how it affects therapists and hospitals.
This chapter deals with all the areas of tort law that do not directly relate to
medical or professional negligence, but provides an understanding of the design and goals of the tort system and the different causes of action.

There are three general types of torts. There are intentional torts—torts that
arise out of acts of intentional conduct, as the name implies, and negligent
torts—torts which arise as a result of a failure, at one level or another, to meet

the standards of reasonable people. Also, there are "strict liability" torts. These are torts where, irrespective of how careful a person was, the law says he or she must bear the responsibility for any harm they caused. In this chapter we'll look first at intentional torts, and later, at negligent torts and strict liability.

1. Who Is This Reasonable Person (and Do I Know Him)?

In discussing tort cases, one thing that helps is to understand the concepts of the reasonable person, and the terminology of tort law. The "reasonable person" is a creation of the law and lawyers. It is a shorthand way of saying that conduct is objectively reasonable. Reasonable simply means that under a given set of circumstances a person faced with the choices at issue would choose the most reasonable path. This reasonable person, however, is a fictional character. He doesn't exist in real life. The decision with respect to what is or was reasonable at a given time is a retrospective decision and is the ultimate form of "Monday Morning Quarterbacking."

Of course, the plaintiff wants to paint one set of conduct as reasonable, and another set as unreasonable. There is a great deal of room for argument on the concept of reasonable, and the general concept of the reasonable person.

In a recent case, a truck driver was driving at 59 miles per hour down an interstate highway inside a large metropolitan city. He could see that traffic was slowing ahead of him, and he could see the orange barrels and "Give 'Em A Brake" signs denoting a construction area. He could see cars "jumping over" from one lane to another. In spite of this heavy traffic, the driver decided to take a few seconds to check his load by focusing not on where he was going, but on the load that was behind him.

A fellow traveler on the road that day was clipped by another car, and pushed into the truck driver's lane. The truck driver hit her and killed her. The truck driver contended that the first accident created an emergency that he could not have reasonably expected. The lawyers representing the driver of the car said that if he had been moving at an appropriate speed (he initially told police officers and testified in a deposition that he was going 50 miles per hour) he would not have hit the driver. When the plaintiff discovered "black box" evidence that he was really going 59 miles per hour, they were able to paint the driver as a liar who was knowingly going too fast for conditions.

The jury found that a reasonable person in the position of the driver should have been going only 50, and held the driver responsible. While their view is logical, and supported by the evidence, there is an equally valid countervailing argument that the truck driver just picked a bad time to check his mirrors, and really could not have anticipated the first accident.

For obvious reasons, the test of a "reasonable person" is usually very fact specific, and often difficult to understand.

In tort law, a person who commits a tort is a tortfeasor, and law refers to the person injured as the victim in most cases. In the pages that follow, a reference to a tortfeasor means the person who is alleged to have acted wrongly.

B. WHAT ARE INTENTIONAL TORTS?

Intentional torts are those where someone does an intentional act that produces an injury or causes legal damages.

"An intentional tort is one in which the actor intends to produce the harm that ensues; it is not enough that he intends to perform the act."[1] This principle of law seems to conflict with the "natural and probable consequence" language used by courts. However, courts say that a plaintiff must prove that "the harm as well as the act" was intentional before there is tort liability. As one court said, "A voluntary act may result in injury to another, but it is only when the harm is intentionally inflicted that there is a "willful" tort."[2] It is "the intent to injure and not merely the intent to act that must be proven."[3] Like all statements of the law, the devil is in the details.

1. How Is Intent Decided?

Courts look beyond the intent expressed by the individual inflicting the harm, and look instead to the circumstances of the injury. "[The person causing the harm] is treated as intending that consequence [harm] if he knows or believes that the consequence is certain, or substantially certain, to result from his act."[4] "When an intentional act results in injuries that are the natural and probable consequences of the act, the injuries as well as the act are intentional."[5]

In other words, intent is determined after the fact by looking at the action taken, and what the natural and probable consequences of that act are. Of

---

[1]Restatement (Second) of Torts § 870, comment b (1977)

[2]*Rector v. Tobin Construction Company,* 377 S.W.2d 409, 414 (Mo. banc 1964).

[3]*Wilt v. Kansas City Area Transportation Authority,* 629 S.W.2d 669, 672 (Mo.App.1982).

[4]Restatement (Second) of Torts § 870, comment b (1977)

[5]*Truck Insurance Exchange v. Pickering,* 642 S.W.2d 113, 116 [1] (Mo.App.1982).

course, looking back, through the "retrospectoscope"—and lawyers are always guilty of this—everything seems logical and predictable. Moreover, a jury is apt to decide the issue of foreseeability on the basis of emotion, not on the basis of logic.

Suppose a therapist is tired of a particular patient's whining. He decides to have a little fun at the patient's expense, and substitutes Mucomyst in the nebulizer (without a physician's order) instead of Albuterol. The therapist has great fun, watching the patient cough and complain about the smell, until the patient begins to wheeze and gasp for breath. Emergency care is rendered, but not before the patient suffers anoxic brain injury.

The therapist acted outside the scope of his practice by administering a drug that was not ordered. He intended to "have a little fun"—not to inflict injury. Is his act intentional or negligent?

A court would most likely hold it to be intentional, given the fact that he knew or should have known that Mucomyst would produce bronchospasm, and since he knew that the natural and probable consequences of bronchospasm can be anoxic injury.

2. How Does Intentional Conduct Differ from Negligent?

Sometimes the line is hard to draw. For example, suppose a therapist intentionally withheld medication for a patient in order to steal that medication for his own use or resell it. For example, suppose he had a need for Albuterol, and administered saline to patients who, in his opinion, didn't require any therapy. One of those patients is a young asthmatic who, absent her medications, suffers a severe bout of bronchospasm and dies.

Is the therapist's act intentional, or negligent? It is a far tougher call because the natural and probable consequences for the asthmatic of not getting ordered medication include bronchospasm, and possibly death. Here, however, the therapist clearly had no intent to harm or "have fun with" the patient. Thus, a court would probably have a more difficult time with the issue of intent. Negligence, of course, is another issue.

Keep in mind that there are frequently different rules for individuals who cannot form an intention to act. The elderly, the demented, the insane, and children too small to appreciate the gravity of their conduct most likely do not commit intentional torts. Also remember that an involuntary act, like withdrawing your hand from a hot stove, or other reflexive actions do not constitute intentional torts in most instances.

As a general rule, all intentionally tortious acts begin with an intention to produce harm or injury, and end when a judge or jury decides what level of damages to impose. For this reason, it is very important to understand the elements of different torts so as to avoid any suggestion that you may have committed one.

This chapter looks at the most common forms of intentional tort. They are Assault, Battery, Intentional Infliction of Emotional Distress, Fraud, Tortious Interference with Contract, Invasion of Privacy, Libel, and Slander.

3. What Is an Assault?

Assault is defined by courts as "any unlawful offer or attempt to injure another with the apparent present ability to effectuate the attempt under circumstances creating a fear of imminent peril."[6] What a mouthful! And what does it tell you? Certainly it doesn't tell you enough to protect yourself, because therapists are routinely exposed to situations in which this particular tort can arise.

Assault is simply the act of putting someone in fear of an unlawful or unpermitted touching. Like most aspects of the law, the law of assault is best clarified by looking at a few examples.

Suppose a therapist is very frustrated with an elderly woman with dementia. She is 89 years old, weighs 98 pounds, and wears mittens to avoid pulling out her IV lines. Our elderly patient calls our therapist some very vile names and threatens to "knock his teeth in." Is this patient committing an assault under the civil law?

Most likely she is not. First, there probably is no intent, given that the woman is demented and cannot truly form the intent to act. More importantly, an able-bodied therapist probably has little to actually fear from a 98 pound octogenarian, and so any fear would not be reasonable.

Now suppose the therapist, frustrated by a workload he cannot meet and the mean attitude of this patient, responds to the "knock your teeth in" statement by drawing his hand back rapidly, as if to slap the woman. She recoils in horror and screams. Is this assault?

Most likely, yes. Here, the therapist has drawn back his hand as though he wants to do physical violence to the patient. The patient has seen this, experienced fear, and reacted. Under the definition in the law, she has been placed

---

[6]*Geiger v. Bowersox*, 974 S.W.2d 513, 516 (Mo.App. E.D.1998).

in anticipation of a harmful or wrongful contact. The patient believed she was in imminent peril, and the therapist certainly had taken all the steps necessary to effectuate a battery on the patient. The tort of assault has probably been committed.[7]

More importantly, his conduct, judged from the standard of a reasonable person, would seem to be a desire to cause just that reaction in the patient. Even though there was no actual touching, the elements of assault are complete in this case.

4. How Is Assault Different from Assault and Battery?

A battery is a completed assault. Swinging at someone is an assault. Hitting them is a battery. Swinging is wrong and constitutes the tort of assault. Actual contact is even more wrong, and establishes the tort of battery.

While cases of assault unaccompanied by the physical contact of battery are rare, it is not impossible to prove assault without physical contact. An example of one such case is *Hickey v. Welch*, 91 Mo.App. 4, 14, 1901 WL 1547 (1901), where the defendant was found to have committed an assault. He pointed a loaded pistol at the plaintiff and threatened to shoot her, but did not fire the weapon. By putting the plaintiff in fear of present violence the defendant was held to have committed "an inchoate battery."

Generally, a plaintiff must prove the following: (1) defendant's intent to cause bodily harm or offensive contact, or apprehension of either; (2) conduct of the defendant indicating such intent, and (3) apprehension of bodily harm or offensive contact on the part of the plaintiff caused by defendant's conduct. If the plaintiff can prove these elements, then the tort of assault is complete, and the issue is whether the plaintiff was damaged as a result of the assault.[8]

5. What Is Battery?

A battery is the intentional and wrongful or offensive physical contact with another without the consent of the victim. Where there is physical contact between two individuals, and one of those two individuals initiates the

---

[7]If you take nothing away from this book, understand that threatening patients or actually hitting them is a certain ticket to the end of your career.

[8]While an assault case is still technically a tort, it isn't a very popular one where the victim suffers no contact or mental anguish. It is hard for a jury to get worked up and award damages when the most that happened was that, for an instant or two, a person was afraid. Still, the law recognizes the tort, and therapists should remember that care of the elderly and infirm requires an infinite amount of patience.

contact intentionally, without the consent of the other person, there is battery. A shorthand way of thinking about it is that battery is an assault that has been completed.

A person who pushes past others in a line essentially causes a battery, but isn't likely to get sued because there simply isn't any damage associated with it. But the example fits the definition of an unpermitted application of trauma by one person upon the body of another person.

Put another way, battery is the willful and harmful or offensive touching of another person, which results from an act intended to cause such contact. To constitute offensive contact for purposes of a battery claim, the contact must be offensive to a reasonable sense of personal dignity. For example, intentionally spitting upon another person is a battery. At least one court has defined "battery" as any unconsented to touching of another person. For battery to be actionable, there must be damages (either economic or non-economic) that result from the contact. For example, a patient is pushed by a visitor in the hospital and falls and breaks a hip. That is a battery with damages.

6. Can Clinicians Commit an Assault or Battery?

Battery is a tort with significant import for clinicians. Almost all touching in a hospital, with the exception of an occasional backrub, is intentional, and generally unpleasant. In most cases, it is not wrongful or offensive in that the patient has, at least implicitly, consented to the touching by coming to the hospital. Almost all hospitals now routinely include a Consent to Examine and Treat in their admission paperwork to cover the odd patient who might consider an examination by a person of a different gender to be offensive.

7. How Important Is Consent?

Consent, and particularly informed consent, is vital to the practice of the craft of the respiratory therapist. See Chapter Two, regarding the importance of consent.

Of course, consent, like any other form of permission, can be withdrawn. When a patient refuses an intervention, unless the patient is not of sound mind and has a guardian appointed for him or her, the therapist must adhere to his or her wishes. If he or she refuse the treatment, there is no consent to the treatment, and any touching is a battery.

8. How Important Is Informed Consent?

Only consent that is informed is actually consent. If you materially misrepresent what will happen, what the risks and benefits are, and what the alternatives are, you commit either an assault or a battery if you go forward with the procedure without informed consent.

Is the situation below informed consent?

Therapist	Hi, my name is Mike, and I am here to do a blood gas.
Patient	What's that?
Therapist	It's a blood test. No big deal. You'll feel a little sting down here.
Patient	Yeouch! A little sting? $#$%* I was shot in Vietnam and it didn't hurt that much!

Of course the scenario above is not informed consent! Informed consent would have gone something like this:

Therapist	Hi, my name is Mike, and I am here to do a blood gas.
Patient	What's that?
Therapist	It's a blood test where we put a needle into your artery in your wrist, and we draw out a sample of blood and analyze it for oxygen, carbon dioxide, and acid.
Patient	Geez, that sounds painful.
Therapist	Well, to be honest with you, it can be. But we need the information to plan how we're going to care for you.
Patient	Well, can't you get the information some other way?
Therapist	Yes, we can get some parts of the information. We can use different methods to monitor your oxygen and carbon dioxide,

but they're indirect and not nearly as accurate as this test. It is painful, but the procedure is necessary, and we hope you'll consent to this.

Consent in a hospital always means informed consent. Consent is informed if the information a reasonable person would need to know in order to consent to the procedure is provided, along with all the risks and benefits of the procedure. Taking shortcuts with informed consent is dangerous.

While Battery is a serious civil tort, keep in mind that accidental or inadvertent contact, even if harmful and offensive, doesn't rise to the level of a battery. Thus when someone is not watching where he or she is going and knocks down a passer-by, that is probably negligent, but not intentional. It may be a negligent injury case (where liability is based on the failure to exercise ordinary care for the protection of another person), but it isn't a battery because there is no intent to cause harm.

9. What Is Intentional Infliction of Emotional Distress?

It is the intentional act of causing someone to suffer mentally. To be actionable, it must cause damages (like psychiatric or medical treatment).

It is said the law does not concern itself with trifles, and hurt feelings are not the concern of the law. Everyone experiences an occasional bruised ego and has their feelings hurt by comments or actions of others.

But sometimes the harm caused by intentional acts, acts intended to extract a toll in human misery, is so significant and so severe that the law will recognize the injury and provide recompense. The tort is called Intentional Infliction of Emotional Distress, and in some jurisdictions, the tort of outrage.

To recover damages for intentional infliction of emotional distress, a plaintiff must prove that: (1) the defendant acted intentionally or recklessly; (2) the conduct was extreme and outrageous; (3) the actions of the defendant caused the plaintiff emotional distress; and (4) the resulting emotional distress was severe.[9] In addition, "[a] claim for intentional infliction of emotional distress cannot be maintained when the risk that emotional distress will result is merely incidental to the commission of some other tort." Accordingly, a claim for intentional infliction of emotional distress will not lie if emotional distress is not the intended or primary consequence of the defendant's conduct.

---

[9]*Standard Fruit & Vegetable Co. v. Johnson,* 985 S.W.2d 62, 65 (Tex.1998).

10. What Is an Example of Intentional Infliction of Emotional Distress?

Consider the infamous Tonya Harding case. Harding arranged to commit a battery on Nancy Kerrigan. When Kerrigan went down with a smack to the kneecap, it no doubt produced extreme emotional upset and trauma. But the intent of the attack was to batter Kerrigan, and Kerrigan could recover for her damages in battery. Thus, even though the attack did produce extreme mental anguish, Kerrigan couldn't maintain an action for Intentional Infliction of Emotional Distress because she had a complete remedy in the law of battery.

But suppose a supervisor in a small department continually engaged in repeated instances of humiliation, degradation, abuse, and intimidation. Suppose that supervisor used foul language and physically threatened the employees. Suppose the situation was so bad that the employees could not do their work and sought medical help for stress. Would that constitute intentional infliction of emotional distress? One court in Texas thought so. In **GTE Southwest Inc. v. Bruce**, 998 S.W.2d 605, (Tex. Civ. App. 1999), the defendant company employed a supervisor who had received numerous complaints about his violent temper and abusive nature. He was placed in supervision of several employees whom he continually abused and harassed.

Eventually, a jury found that the company that employed the supervisor had committed the tort of intentional infliction of emotional distress, and the Texas courts agreed:

> We recognize that, even when an employer or supervisor abuses a position of power over an employee, the employer will not be liable for mere insults, indignities, or annoyances that are not extreme and outrageous. Restatement (Second) of Torts § 46 cmt. e (1965). But Shields' ongoing acts of harassment, intimidation, and humiliation and his daily obscene and vulgar behavior, which GTE defends as his "management style," went beyond the bounds of tolerable workplace conduct. See Travis, 504 S.E.2d at 423; White, 585 So.2d at 1210. The picture painted by the evidence at trial was unmistakable: Shields greatly exceeded the necessary leeway to supervise, criticize, demote, transfer, and discipline, and created a workplace that was a den of terror for the employees. And the evidence showed that all of Shields' abusive conduct was common, not rare. Being purposefully humiliated and intimidated and being repeatedly put in fear of one's physical well-being at the hands of a supervisor is more than a mere triviality or annoyance.

GTE Southwest, *998 S.W.2d at 617.*

11. What Is Extreme and Outrageous Conduct?

It is conduct that is outrageous in character and extreme in degree—so much so that anyone would think so upon hearing of it.

It is the element of extreme and outrageous conduct that presents plaintiffs the most difficult hurdle in such a case. To be extreme and outrageous, conduct must be "so outrageous in character, and so extreme in degree, as to go beyond all possible bounds of decency, and to be regarded as atrocious, and utterly intolerable in a civilized community."[10] Generally, insensitive or even rude behavior does not constitute extreme and outrageous conduct. Similarly, mere insults, indignities, threats, annoyances, petty oppressions, or other trivialities do not rise to the level of extreme and outrageous conduct. In determining whether certain conduct is extreme and outrageous, courts consider the context and the relationship between the parties.[11] "[S]ome States consider the context and the relationship between the parties significant, placing special emphasis on the workplace."[12] "The extreme and outrageous character of the conduct may arise from an abuse by the actor of a position, or a relation with the other, which gives him actual or apparent authority over the other, or power to affect his interests."[13]

If a clinician were to act toward a patient with utter disregard for that patient's interests, for example, by falsely telling them that they had lung cancer and had better get their affairs in order, the relationship between patient and caregiver would most likely cause a court to view the conduct as extreme and outrageous. But if the caregiver made a mistake and simply had the wrong patient file, and did not purposefully cause this upset, there is little likelihood a court would find for the plaintiff on an Intentional Infliction of Emotional Distress theory. Negligence, again, would be another matter.

It is rare for patients to bring a claim of intentional infliction, but it does happen. For example, when patients sued Robert Courtney, the Kansas City pharmacist, for diluting their cancer drugs, most included a claim for intentional infliction of emotional distress. Clearly the act of diluting life-saving medicine well below any therapeutic level was within the scope of the tort.

---

[10]*Natividad v. Alexsis, Inc.,* 875 S.W.2d 695, 699 (Tex.1994) (quoting *Twyman v. Twyman,* 855 S.W.2d 619, 621 (Tex.1993)); Restatement (Second) of Torts § 46 cmt. d (1965).

[11]See *Atchison, Topeka & Santa Fe Ry. v. Buell,* 480 U.S. 557, 569, 107 S.Ct. 1410, 94 L.Ed.2d 563 (1987)

[12]*Wilson v. Monarch Paper Co.,* 939 F.2d 1138, 1143 (5th Cir.1991) ("The facts of a given claim of outrageous conduct must be analyzed in context. . . .")

[13]Restatement (Second) of Torts § 46 cmt. e (1965).

Another variant of the outrage tort is where a person inflicts harm on one person, and a third person sees and is emotionally harmed as a result. For example, where a child is thrown to the floor by a store security guard and placed in a headlock while the child's mother looks on and begs for officers to stop. If the child did nothing wrong, and the store officers were not within their rights to assault him, they could be liable to him for assault and to the mother for intentional infliction of emotional distress.

12. What Is Invasion of Privacy?

It is similar to libel, except that personal or private things are disclosed.

In libel, a person is held to account for telling lies about a person. In Invasion of Privacy, a person is held to account for telling the truth, when the truth should, by all accounts, remain secret.

It is generally accepted that the invasion of privacy tort consists of four distinct wrongs: (1) the intrusion upon the plaintiff's physical solitude or seclusion; (2) publicity which violates the ordinary decencies; (3) putting the plaintiff in a false, but not necessarily defamatory, position in the public eye; and (4) the appropriation of some element of the plaintiff's personality for a commercial use.[14]

Invasion of Privacy claims are infrequently seen, but do happen in the health care context. In one recent case, a hospital performed an HIV test on a patient and disclosed those results to third parties even though they did not have authorization to do so. The results to the patient were devastating, and the lawsuit was equally devastating to the hospital.

13. What Is False Imprisonment?

False imprisonment, sometimes called false arrest, is the direct restraint of personal liberty. In other words, stopping someone from going where they want to go is unlawful. There need not be any actual force used for false imprisonment to occur; the restraint may be from the fear of force, as well as from force itself. Words alone are frequently sufficient to bring about the actual restraint of a person's liberty.

For this reason, false imprisonment may be committed by words alone, by acts alone, or by both and by merely operating the will of the individual. There

---

[14]*Norris v. Moskin Stores, Inc.,* 272 Ala. 174, 132 So.2d 321 (Ala.1961), citing W. Prosser, *Law of Torts,* pp. 637-39 (2d ed. 1955).

need be no formal declaration of arrest. It is not necessary that the individual be confined within a jail or prison or that he or she be assaulted or touched.

Suppose that a patient comes into the Pulmonary department for a bronchoscopy. After signing the paperwork to allow the procedure, the patient has an IV started by the nurse, and his hands are secured to the bed by restraints because it has been the experience of the bronchoscopy team that sometimes people react differently to the sedating agents used.

After a few minutes of waiting for the pulmonologist to return, the patient decides he no longer wants the procedure done. He tells the nurse to take off the restraints and let him leave.

"I can't let you leave until the doctor sees you."

"I want to go now."

"I can't let you go. The doctor hasn't discharged you."

"I want out of these restraints!" The patient begins to yell and shout. The nurse confers with the therapist who tells her to go ahead and give him some Valium and calm him down.

This is false imprisonment. In most cases, it isn't actionable because there are no damages. Here, the hospital team has not only engaged in false imprisonment, they have also committed a battery by giving a sedative that the patient did not want. The only proper conduct in this case is to let the patient go. The patient becomes responsible if some harm befalls him as a result of his conduct, not the caregivers. Retaining him against his will is unlawful.

14. What Are Slander and Libel?

Slander is telling a lie about someone, which causes them injury. Libel is publishing that lie.

If fraud cases are hard, Slander and Libel cases are almost impossible. Slander and Libel fall under the heading of defamation torts.

Defamation is an invasion of the interest in reputation and good name. It consists of a complex set of rules developed over a period of centuries in the common-law courts of England and later refined in the state court systems of America.[15] Defamation is made up of the twin torts of Libel and Slander—the former being written and the latter being oral. The standards for the two torts being the same, we'll confine our discussion here to Libel. Libel has been defined as the "malicious publication, expressed either in printing or in writing,

---

[15]*See* Note, *Iowa Libel Law and the First Amendment:* Defamation Displaced, 62 Iowa L.Rev. 1067, 1068 (1977).

or by signs or pictures, tending to injure the reputation of another person or to expose [that person] to public hatred, contempt, or ridicule or to injure [the person] in the maintenance of [a] business."[16]

To establish a prima facie case of libel, the plaintiff must show that the defendant published a statement that was defamatory of and concerning the plaintiff, and resulted in injury to the plaintiff.

Under the traditional rule, malice is not an element of libel and will be presumed from the publication.[17] The only exception is if the defendant claims to have acted under a privilege, and then the plaintiff must plead and prove that there was actual malice involved.

15. Do Different Rules Affect the News Media?

It is hard to sue the media. Our constitutional form of government grants special protection in what is called the "fourth branch of government."

A series of United States Supreme Court decisions has reshaped the law of defamation as it relates to lawsuits against the news media. Beginning with *New York Times Co. v. Sullivan,* 376 U.S. 254, 84 S.Ct. 710, 11 L.Ed.2d 686 (1964), the court for the first time afforded first amendment protection to defamation concerning the official conduct of a public official. The court held that a public official may not recover damages for a defamatory falsehood relating to his or her official conduct without first proving the statement was made with actual malice. Actual malice was defined as knowledge or reckless disregard of whether a statement was false. On the heels of *New York Times,* the court extended actual malice protection to "all discussion and communication involving matters of public or general concern, without regard to whether the persons involved are famous or anonymous." *Rosenbloom v. Metromedia, Inc.,* 403 U.S. 29, 43-44, 91 S.Ct. 1811, 1819, 29 L.Ed.2d 296, 312 (1971)

The court retreated, however, from the *Rosenbloom* standard in *Gertz v. Robert Welch, Inc.,* 418 U.S. 323, 94 S.Ct. 2997, 41 L.Ed.2d 789 (1974). Instead, the court prescribed two levels of protection. Speech concerning public officials and public figures was still protected by the actual malice requirement. For speech concerning private parties, however, the states were free to interpret their own law.

---

[16]*Plendl v. Beuttler,* 253 Iowa 259, 262, 111 N.W.2d 669, 670-71 (1961).
  [17]62 Iowa L.Rev. at 1068 n. 10.

C. TORTS BASED ON NEGLIGENCE

In torts based on intentional conduct, the foundation for liability is the intentional conduct itself. If there is an intention to cause harm, it only makes sense for the person causing the harm to be liable for it. The law recognizes that acts that spring out of a desire to inflict harm are themselves morally blameworthy, and that anyone harmed by that act should be granted recompense because (in most cases anyway) there is no blame attached to their conduct.

Negligent conduct is different. Here, the liability is founded on the failure to use ordinary care. The liability attaches because if the person had been paying attention, and doing his job, he could have avoided the injury to the third person, and for that reason, he should make that person whole.

1. How Are Negligent Torts Different from Intentional Torts?

Negligent torts take a different view from intentional torts. While intentional torts are based on the principle of righting a wrong, negligent torts are based on the principle of making people safer by placing the strongest incentive on the person who can best ensure the safety of others.

The economic principle behind negligent torts is that the person who has the most to lose if his or her conduct injures another person, is the person who will have the greatest incentive to maximize safety and minimize the harm. Consider, for example, the manufacturer of a lawnmower. If the lawnmower sells for $100, and costs $50 to build, the manufacturer can get a $50 return on each lawnmower. If the manufacturer knows that a person using the lawnmower could get hurt and sue, he will take extra precautions to avoid that, perhaps by warning the end user or by fitting the device with blade guards, so that he is not subject to a lawsuit for damages. As one court put it:

> The imposition of strict tort liability is justified on the grounds that the manufacturer or seller is almost always better equipped than the consumer to endure the economic consequences of accidents caused by defective products. Everything in the marketplace has a price, including profits. Economic responsibility for the debilitating consequences of injuries caused by defective products is but one of the many costs associated with doing business and earning profits. All things considered, we find no unfairness in holding manufacturers and sellers economically and socially responsible for injuries actually caused by the products they place for profit in the stream of commerce.

Nesselrode v. Executive Beechcraft, 707 S.W.2d 371 (Mo. banc 1986)

Of course, like most other theories in the law, this theory breaks down in terms of reality. The manufacturer is going to do its best to cut corners and make the cheapest product it can get away with. Because it is cutting corners, it buys insurance to cover its liability.

If there are one or two cases over ten or twelve years, the premiums generally keep pace with inflation. If there are a large number of claims, the manufacturer either redesigns the product or loses his insurance. In the real world, the jury verdict has less impact on the manufacturer than the rise in insurance premiums.

2. Is Public Policy Important?

Negligence law is the branch of the legal system that deals more often with economics and public policy than it does with compensating injured persons. As a result, there are many interesting and sometimes competing policies that affect how courts decide cases. We can see some of those policies at work in the cases in this section.

3. What Is Negligence Generally?

While negligence is founded on the concept of the reasonable man, and what that reasonable man would do in a given set of circumstances, the fundamental concept that underlies all negligence law is the concept of duty. In order to hold a person accountable under the civil law, the first thing that has to exist is a duty on the part of the tortfeasor.

But, what accounts for duty? Where does it arise? How is it analyzed? For this, we must turn to the case law.

4. What Is Duty?

Duty arises out of foreseeability. Foreseeability simply means the ability to predict harm based on the circumstances. As one court suggested, "The touchstone for the creation of a duty is foreseeability. A duty of care arises out of circumstances in which there is a foreseeable likelihood that particular acts or omissions will cause harm or injury."[18]

If you are driving down the road and suddenly decide to drive on the left side, instead of the right side of the road, it is certainly foreseeable that you

---

[18]*Lowrey v. Horvath,* 689 S.W.2d 625, 627 (Mo. banc 1985).

might cause an accident. You would have a duty to persons on the road (and to bystanders walking along the road) to act as a reasonable person and drive on the right side of the road.

Similarly, if you leave a huge hole open in the middle of a field, you might not consider that to be a big deal. After all, it is your property, and you get to say who comes onto it. You might figure that a trespasser walking across the property ought to be watching where he is going, and so you might think that you'd have no duty to protect him.

In some jurisdictions that is still the rule, but in many more the rule is that you have a duty to protect people who are reasonably foreseeable to come onto your property. So if you have knowledge that sometimes people come onto the property to hunt, or to cut through as a short cut, you have a duty to put up a fence or barricade around the hole so as to protect those trespassers.

5. What Is This Concern with Foreseeability?

If it sounds as though everyone has a duty to everyone else, that is not the intent of this section. Duty arises on foreseeability, and there are some things that are not foreseeable. For example, it could certainly be argued that the attack on the World Trade Center was not foreseeable, and hence, it was not foreseeable that visitors to the Trade Center that day would be injured by the acts of the terrorists.[19]

Likewise there is no duty to rescue another person. If you are an Olympic-qualified swimmer who has had six summers of life-saving practice, you have no duty to attempt to rescue a passerby who falls into a river. Even though you probably could perform the rescue, you have no duty to do so. This is because the law does not require you to imperil your life in order to save the life of another.[20]

The duty issue often plays itself out in the context of new or novel applications of old court doctrines. For example, in most situations a business owner is not liable for the criminal acts of third persons against persons who come to the place of business.

---

[19]For purposes of argument, it is also foreseeable, based on the prior attack on the World Trade Center, that the attack was foreseeable, and that better escape equipment should have been provided. At present, cases that make these claims have not been resolved through litigation.

[20]In one case, a boat owner rented his boat to a man who took it out on to the lake and proceeded to fall overboard without a life jacket. The owner sat down on his chair, lit up a cigar, and watched the man drown. The court imposed no liability.

In a case this author argued on appeal, the issue was whether the business owner was under a duty to provide for the safety of the plaintiff. Dwight Bowman was a college student who owned a fast and fancy car. He drove to a section of Kansas City that was known to have had numerous gang attacks. He had stopped at a McDonald's restaurant where he was planning on a snack, when another car pulled in behind him. Two men jumped from the car and gave chase to him. McDonald's employees saw that the men had guns, and locked their doors. Bowman refused to give up his car keys, and was shot in the back and paralyzed.

Bowman sued McDonalds. At issue was whether McDonald's had any duty at all, given the fact that there had been no violent crimes on the premises of the restaurant. There were numerous crimes in the area, and the court allowed some of these crimes to come in. The trial court allowed the case to go to the jury.

McDonald's, for its part, argued forcefully that it was not to blame, and convinced the jury that when you drive in a bad part of town you get what happens to you.

In the Bowman case, however, the key holding of the trial court was that McDonald's was under a duty to protect its customers.

The bottom line of duty is that it is determined after the fact, and the analysis is based not only on what a person or institution actually knows, but on what they could have discovered if they had tried.

As mentioned earlier, in 2001, Kansas City pharmacist Robert Courtney admitted to FBI agents that he had diluted the medications of hundreds of cancer patients. Lawyers quickly learned, however, that Courtney did not have funds to pay a judgment, and that his insurance company would refuse to pay any claim brought against it.

As a result, they went after the two major drug companies who supplied drugs to Courtney's pharmacy for the treatment of cancer. Those two companies were charged with negligence, not because they actually knew that Courtney was diluting cancer medications, but because with the exercise of reasonable care, they could have learned.

One company used an external consultant to provide it with marketing data. The consultant polled pharmacy records and clinical records and provided to the manufacturer the number of units of cancer medication sold in the local area. The drug company monitored this evidence very carefully.

A drug representative for the company was responsible for selling the drugs to hospitals and physicians. He made frequent contacts with physicians pushing his products, and yet was not seeing any increase in the amount of sales associated with a group of doctors at Research Medical Center. While there were several oncologists, two groups in particular did a lot of business with the cancer drug that the drug rep sold.

He would show the reports to the doctor's accounting people, who would show him their records demonstrating that they had delivered thousands of doses of his product. The rep would send this proof in to the company to get credit for these sales.

Over and over he did this. And over and over he questioned his company about why his sales were missing. The company asked several individuals to investigate, and they decided it was not important enough and placed it "on the back burner."

The company that sent the "back burner" memo, also lobbied Congress heavily with regard to the importation of foreign drugs. They complained to Congress that only American drug companies could ensure the quality of their product and protect the public from the scourge of diluted, adulterated, and misbranded drugs.

Within the hour of the ink drying on the petition, lawyers for the drug companies, represented by two national law firms with national reputations in the area of pharmaceutical law, filed motions to dismiss based on an absence of duty.

In essence, the drug companies said "you can't hold us responsible because (1) the patient is not our customer, the doctor is; (2) we had no knowledge of the dilution; and (3) we do not owe patients any duty to protect them from the criminal acts of third persons.

Kansas City Judge Lee Wells, the trial judge who shepherded the case through its settlement, held that the drug companies did have a duty to protect the public, and were responsible because in the exercise of reasonable care, they could have discovered the dilution if they had acted reasonably.

Eventually, the drug companies settled the case with the more than 300 plaintiffs who sued for damages. One of the reasons that the plaintiffs accepted a very small settlement from the drug companies is that there was a real likelihood that any verdict against the drug companies would have been reversed on appeal. The lawyers on the case all believed that the drug companies might well have escaped on the issue of duty because the drug companies had no idea who the patients actually were, and thus, had no way to actively warn them about the dilution.

6. What Is Considered to Be a Breach of Duty?

Once a duty exists, negligence begins with any breach of the duty to the victim of the tort. In the example of the person driving on the left side of the road, the breach occurs at the moment that the driver goes into the left lane. The breach of duty occurs when the owner of the land discovers a hole, and doesn't fence it off or place a warning sign. The breach of duty allegedly occurred in the Bowman case when McDonalds didn't hire security to protect its patrons. The breach of duty occurred in the Robert Courtney/Drug Company case when the drug company, armed with information that it couldn't explain, and regarding the misappropriation of a life-saving cancer drug, placed the investigation "on the back burner."

7. What Is Negligence Per Se?

There is another way to breach a legal duty. And that is to violate a statute or regulation enacted for the protection of the public. Sometimes referred to as "negligence per se," the doctrine arises out of a violation of a statute. The law imposes a duty on the truck driver to stay within the posted speed limits. When the truck driver exceeds the posted speed by driving at 85 mph, and rear-ends a vehicle going the posted speed of 45 mph, he not only violates the criminal law, he commits a breach of the duty imposed on him by the civil law.[21] Even if the plaintiff does not elect to proceed under a theory of negligence per se, he can still assert that the criminal law establishes the duty to the plaintiff.

8. What Defines Injury?

Have you ever run a stop sign? Most of us have. If you run a stop sign, and nothing happens, you may have been negligent, but you didn't inflict any injury, and hence, the element of a negligence cause of action that requires injury has not been satisfied.

Injury is not always physical. Sometimes emotional injury can suffice for this element in a negligence tort. Injury can be economic, but it can also be non-economic.

---

[21]Although negligence per se essentially relieves the plaintiff of proving the elements of negligence if he proves the violation of the statutory duty, the most essential effect of proving a breach of the criminal law standard is that duty is established.

9. What Is Proximate Cause?

Proximate cause is another way of saying that the law requires that the negligent act of the tortfeasor be the true cause or at the very least a true contributing cause of the injury to the plaintiff. In the example above, if the truck driver runs the stop sign and plows into the side of the car carrying the plaintiff, there is little doubt that the negligence of the driver in running the stop sign caused or contributed to causing the broken ribs and punctured lung of the plaintiff.

The law makes proximate cause an essential element of any negligence action. Proximate cause is defined as "that which in a natural and continuous sequence, unbroken by an independent cause, produces the event and without which the event would not have occurred."[22] At some level, foreseeability becomes a part of the proximate cause equation in much the same way that it comes into the duty question. The foreseeability of an injury as a result of the negligent act is an essential element of proximate cause. The question of proximate cause becomes one of law when there is no evidence from which the jury could find a causal nexus between the negligent act and the resulting injuries. The failure to establish that Defendant's negligence was the proximate cause of the harmful event is fatal to Plaintiff's claim.

What then, does the plaintiff have to show? First, that the injury was the foreseeable result of the negligent act. For example, some injuries are so attenuated that they cannot be said to have resulted from the negligent act. Like most of the legal issues in this book, this one begs for an example:

> Fred leaves Jimmy's Jigger, a popular metropolitan bar, and sets off down the state highway on his motorcycle. Ahead of him he sees bright flares of light about every ten seconds. He is watching for the next flare of light when a blue car turns in front of him, causing him to collide with it, and fly over the top of the car, landing in the field. He breaks his neck, rendering himself quadriplegic. He sues the driver of the car and the oil company and contractor that was doing the flaring, alleging that absent their use of blinding light, he would not have collided with the car.

Is a motorcycle collision foreseeable? Certainly it is when you turn your car in front of it, and so proximate cause as to the driver of the car would be easy to establish. However, proximate cause against the oil company is more

---

[22]*Gaines v. Providence Apartments*, 750 P.2d 125, 126-27 (Okla.1987).

difficult. While the blinding lights of the gas flaring operation might excuse Fred, and negate any negligence on his part (for example, it might help reduce his own fault for having a .128 blood alcohol content), it does not explain why the driver turned in front of Fred. It was the car turning in front of Fred that produced the accident; the gas flaring did not set that turn in motion, and therefore is not the proximate cause of Fred's injuries.

10. What Kinds of Damages Exist?

There are three kinds of damages: economic, non-economic, and punitive. In most health care cases, there are only economic and non-economic damages. In other kinds of tort cases all three kinds appear.

11. What Are Economic Damages?

Economic damages are damages that can be quantified in economic terms. Lost wages, lost fringe benefits, insurance payments, medical bills, funeral expenses, and similar costs paid directly by family members are obvious examples of economic injuries. Anything that can be replaced with a checkbook is an element of economic damage.

Some economic damages, however, you may not have thought about. For example, when a husband and father loses a wife of six years, he loses more than the mother of his two children. He loses a cook, a housekeeper, and a second wage-earner.[23] We know that if we go to Merry Maids, we can replace the housekeeper for a fixed amount of $78 every week. We know that if we have six meals a week cooked outside the home and brought to the home, that it would cost us roughly $30 per meal. We know that the wife in the relationship brought in a salary of $16,000 per year and had health and dental insurance benefits that the husband did not. All of these are elements of economic damage.

Frequently, economic damage is easy to present in a tort lawsuit. If the accident produced medical bills, the plaintiff can show the medical bills. If the accident resulted in the need to modify a person's home for wheelchair access or to hire a full-time on-site registered nurse for 24-hour care, all of those are elements of economic injury that can be proved with simple evidence of the costs.

---

[23]Economic damages are almost always greater when a wife is involved. While a husband may perform valuable economic services around the home, they cannot be as easily quantified as the services a wife traditionally performs. Of course, every family, and every marriage, is different, and in some cases the sweeping generalizations above may not be accurate.

In many cases, however, a specialized expert, usually a nurse, is called in to prepare a "life care plan" that is then used to justify the economic damages. The nurse uses commonly available statistical models and information from the medical record to prepare a life care plan to show how many hospitalizations will occur in the future, and how much money will be spent on drugs, doctor bills, and other costs.

This information is then passed along to a specialized expert—the economist—to "discount" for the jury. The reason for discounting is simple. Although the damages are sure to occur over time, the bill for those damages in the future is not presently due. Thus, if a person invests $20,000 today at 10% interest (or whatever interest rate is practical to use), that return on the investment is "discounted" against the amount of money a jury needs to award to compensate the victim. So if it will cost $100,000 over ten years, the jury should award the sum of money that, when invested today, will yield $100,000 in six years (a sum of between $85,000 and $95,000, depending on which economist is used).

12. What Are Non-Economic Damages?

The chief difference between economic and non-economic damages is that while we can measure or approximate the economic costs of damages for a housekeeper and cook, we cannot do the same with things like pain and suffering.

Pain, suffering, disability, disfigurement, loss of mobility, loss of independence, loss of enjoyment of life, loss of love, care, comfort, and guidance are all non-economic damages.

We know that if we want to hire a housekeeper, we have to pay approximately $10 per hour. We know that it will require 10 hours a week. We have an economic model that we can show for figuring out exactly what the loss of housekeeping services is worth.

But how do we value the love, nurturing, and affection that a mother provides to a child? How do we measure the amount of time she would have spent on the first day of school, getting little Timmy ready for the school bus? What kind of economic model can we create that will show us the value of a burn victim's pain?

Simply stated, we cannot put those things into a nice equation and render a reproducible result.

Because it is impossible to create an economic model for what are essentially non-economic harms, jurors are asked to award such a sum of money as they believe will adequately compensate a victim for his or her injuries.

13. What Are Punitive Damages?

Punitive damages are damages imposed on someone who has engaged in conduct that is morally blameworthy. When a jury, by clear and convincing evidence, finds that a tortfeasor has acted with reckless indifference, or has acted in a willful, wanton, or callous manner toward a victim, jurors are entitled to impose punitive damages.

Jurors are told to award such sum of money as will adequately punish the defendant and deter that defendant, and others like him, from similar conduct in the future.

To support a claim for punitive damages, there must be clear and convincing evidence that the defendant either knew or had reason to know that there was a high degree of probability that the defendant's conduct would result in injury. The defendant's conduct must be tantamount to intentional wrongdoing where the natural and probable consequence of the conduct is injury. With such a showing, a plaintiff can recover punitive damages based upon the defendant's complete indifference to or conscious disregard for the safety of others. Courts often refer to this kind of behavior as similar to "firing a rifle into a passing train."

In the context of a negligence case, the "high degree of probability of injury" and "complete indifference or conscious disregard" standards are somewhat ambiguous. They don't give a jury a clear definition of what it must find to hold a defendant responsible. From the negligence cases in which punitive damages have been disallowed, however, factors that assist in identifying when submission of such damages is permissible can be distilled. Weighing against submission of punitive damages are circumstances in which prior similar occurrences known to the defendant have been infrequent. Similarly, where the injurious event was unlikely to have occurred absent negligence on the part of someone other than the defendant, punitive damages may not be proper. If the defendant did not knowingly violate a statute, regulation, or clear industry standard designed to prevent the type of injury that occurred, then punitive damages may not be proper.

Conversely, punitive damages are proper where there is clear and convincing evidence that a defendant acted with reckless disregard of the rights of others. It is a high standard, and in the last several years courts have cut back steadily on what constitutes a proper case of punitive damages. Look for this area of the law to change even more in the years to come.

14. What Is Premises Liability?

Premises liability means imposing liability for a dangerous condition on property. There are numerous types of premises cases. When a visitor slips on spilled IV fluid in the hallway, falls, and breaks a hip, that is not a medical negligence case, it is a premises liability case. The business, in this case the hospital, has the same duty to make its premises safe for people it invites onto its premises as does Wal-Mart. It must use all reasonable care to make its premises safe from known dangers. So if the fluid had been on the floor for more than a few moments, and if someone employed by the hospital knew it was there and took no action to either warn (by placing a "wet floor" sign in the hallway) or clean up the fluid, then the hospital is liable for the damages.

Premises liability is based on negligence. There must be a negligent act, such as to create a dangerous condition on the property. For example, a hole in the sidewalk that goes unrepaired, is a dangerous condition on the property. An oily spot on stairs or a wet spot on a polished floor also qualifies. Negligence is generally proved by showing the existence of the dangerous condition along with knowledge, on the part of the business, that the condition was present.

15. How Is Knowledge Proved?

Sometimes the knowledge is easy to show. A hole in a sidewalk generally does not happen in a matter of moments. In other cases, knowledge is more difficult to prove, for example, in a restaurant where a customer may spill a liquid and not report it to management.

Direct proof of knowledge, because it is a mental state, is seldom available and is usually inferred from circumstantial evidence.[24] "Knowledge, of course, is also a state of mind and, like intent, is rarely susceptible to direct proof."[25] "Mental elements which establish that a defendant knowingly did an act may be proved by indirect evidence and inferences reasonably drawn from circumstances surrounding the incident."[26]

---

[24]*State v. Turner,* 623 S.W.2d 4, 7 (Mo. banc 1981).

[25]*State v. Seeger,* 725 S.W.2d 39, 44 (Mo.App.1986).

[26]*State v. Abercrombie,* 694 S.W.2d 268, 271 (Mo.App.1985); **State v. Fuelling,** 2004 WL 1607052 (Mo.App. W.D.).

In other words, suppose a plaintiff wishes to establish that a company had knowledge of a large gap in its sidewalk. It could introduce evidence that the defendant's employees drove to work, parked in the same lot he had parked in, and walked along the very same sidewalk that plaintiff fell on. The jury could infer that by walking down the sidewalk, the employees would have had to know that there was a six-inch gap between pieces of the sidewalk. This would be sufficient to prove knowledge.

16. What Is Causation?

In addition to showing negligence, the plaintiff must show that he or she was injured, and that his or her injuries (damages) are the direct and proximate result of the negligence. In most cases, that is easy; however, it can sometimes be problematic.

For example, Al, a 48-year-old lawyer, has gout. He has pain in his knee on a regular basis. One day at Total-Mart he trips over a cart left sticking out in an aisle, and breaks his left leg at the knee. His leg heals, but his knee pain grows worse, and he now requires treatment for chronic pain associated with the injury.

Is his injury directly and proximately related to the fall?

Although the defendant will argue that the injury was pre-existing, the rule in tort law is that a defendant takes his victim as he finds him. It is called the "egg-shell tortfeasor" rule. In essence it means that if the tortfeasor's victim has brittle bones, and a normal person wouldn't break a bone in the fall, but this victim breaks six bones, the tortfeasor has to pay for all the harm he caused.

While some types of lawsuits are generally disfavored in the courts, the most disfavored of all is the premises case based on a "slip and fall." Where the plaintiff alleges that there is a dangerous condition on the property, courts have gone to great lengths to excuse the defendant's failures. If a dangerous condition on property is "open and obvious" such that a person exercising ordinary care for his or her own safety would see it and avoid it, then in many jurisdictions the plaintiff may not recover.

17. What Is Comparative Fault?

John pulls out onto Interstate 95 from a rest area. He merges flawlessly into the far right travel lane, when all of a sudden his car engine fails. His speed begins to fall below 60, and John tries furiously to restart his car as it slows to a halt in the travel lane. John is busy trying to restart his car when a pickup truck rear-ends him. John is severely injured.

John sues the driver of the truck for damages. The truck driver claims that John was negligent, and asks for "comparative fault" instructions. In essence, he asks the jury, if he was negligent for not keeping a careful lookout and running into John, to give some percentage of fault to John for not having the sense to move his car to the shoulder.

Suppose John's damages are $100,000. The jury finds that the truck driver is 68% at fault, and that John is 32% at fault. John will recover $68,000 from the truck driver.

In some states comparative fault is a complete defense if the fault of the plaintiff is more than 49%. Suppose in the situation above, John sued the truck driver and the gas station that sold him watered gas and caused his car to stop. John puts on his best case, and the jury finds him 60% responsible, and the gas station 20% responsible, and the truck driver 20% responsible. In most states John will recover $40,000 from the two defendants.

But in some states, such as Kansas, the fact that he was more than 49% responsible for the accident will mean that he won't recover anything.

18. What Is Joint and Several Liability?

Just as comparative fault would allow the truck driver to find John partially at fault, most states also have a mechanism for regulating the amount of fault between defendants. In the case above, if John is only 10% liable, and the gas station is 10% liable, then the truck driver will have to pay $80,000.

If the truck driver doesn't have the money, what happens?

In a state with "joint and several" liability, the gas station will be on the hook for the entire judgment of $90,000. It must pay its share (10%) and the share of the other defendant (80%), and it can collect the $80,000 from the other defendant in a "contribution" action.

In states like Kansas, where there is no joint and several liability, the gas station would pay its $10,000, and the plaintiff would have to chase the defendant who owed the $80,000 for the money.

D. WHAT IS STRICT LIABILITY?

Strict liability imposes liability without a finding of negligence on the basis of some inherent danger in conduct. There are numerous types of strict liability. There is strict liability for defective products (a key portion of the chapter here) and for carrying on abnormally dangerous activities. Here we will first examine abnormally dangerous activities and then product liability. This is because product liability has the most application in the field of respiratory care.

Strict liability depends on an inherent danger. For example, storing natural gas involves inherent danger because the gas is explosive. If the gas leaks and explodes, the nature of the harm is so great that the courts impose "strict liability" for all harm that is the natural and probable consequence of the activity. Many activities are exposed to strict liability, including the storage of gas, transmission of electricity along power lines, and the like. Another kind of entity exposed to strict liability is anyone who manufactures a product. If you make a product, you essentially make a promise that you have taken pains to ensure that it is reasonably safe when used as specified. Thus if someone uses a leaf trimmer the way it was designed to be used, and cuts off a finger in the process, there is a potential claim that the product was responsible.

1. What Are Abnormally Dangerous Activities?

When a person undertakes an abnormally dangerous activity, he is responsible for whatever harm he causes. The American Law Institute says it this way:

(1) One who carries on an abnormally dangerous activity is subject to liability for harm to the person, land or chattels of another resulting from the activity, although he has exercised the utmost care to prevent the harm.
(2) This strict liability is limited to the kind of harm, the possibility of which makes the activity abnormally dangerous.

What does this mean? Well, first, it is important to understand what constitutes an abnormally dangerous activity. Courts apply a variety of tests. For example, they consider whether there is a high degree of risk of harm to a person, to land, or to personal property of other persons. They look at the likelihood of how catastrophic the harm will be if it results. They consider whether it is possible to eliminate the risk by taking proper precautions, and whether the activity is a matter of common usage or practice. The courts examine whether the activity was appropriate to the time and place where it was carried on, and the extent to which it provided a value to the community. Value to the community is offset somewhat against the risk.

2. What Is Strict Product Liability?

Although it is often lost in the greater scheme of medical negligence, product liability is a significant problem for makers of medical equipment, and therapists should be alert for dangerous and defective products.

According to the American Law Institution, a product is defective when "at the time of sale or distribution, it contains a manufacturing defect, is defective in design, or is defective because of inadequate instructions or warnings."

That laundry list covers a multitude of manufacturing and design sins. It is helpful to examine these issues one at a time.

3. How Do Manufacturing Defects Lead to Liability?

A product contains a manufacturing defect when the product, as it reaches the consumer, is different from, or in some material way departs from, its original or intended design. This is true even if all possible care was exercised in the preparation and marketing of the product. In other words, negligence or intentional conduct is not an element of a product liability claim for a manufacturing defect. As with many principles, this theory of liability is easier to understand if illustrated by examples.

S. S. was a 38-year-old woman who had bowel dysmotility syndrome. She was experiencing severe pain as a result of her disease, and her physician was worried about drug dependency. He was also worried about her multiple small children, and their ability to get their hands on their mother's very powerful pain-killing medication. He called a local home care company to find out if he could place a patient controlled analgesia (PCA) pump in the home.

State pharmacy regulations required that the patient be terminal, and this patient was not terminal. Nevertheless, the pharmacist averred that he would get the woman a PCA pump, and the physician thought no more about it. Without the physician's knowledge or consent, the pharmacist wrote "terminal patient" on the prescription.

The patient was ordered to receive Meperidine HCL by IV, and hyperconcentrated Meperidine was placed into her PCA pump. The home care company did not know (because the pump manufacturer had not issued a recall) that the PCA pump had a serious defect. If the drug cartridge were not properly seated and locked, the pump could cause a free-flow event. In essence, if the pump were not properly engaged, the lock-out mechanism on the pump would fail to function, and any time the pump was higher than the heart, the patient would get a massive bolus of drugs.

S. S. had her drug cartridge replaced on a bright summer morning, and went to take a nap. A few seconds after lying down she stumbled out and asked her daughter to call 911. Moments later she collapsed. The code at the hospital lasted for an hour and a half, with the physician unable to explain the prolonged and refractory metabolic acidosis. After she was pronounced dead, the home care company made immediate arrangements to pick up the PCA pump.

The patient's death was due to a deviation from the original design, introduced in the manufacturing process, that caused the lock on the unit to function at a half-stop. The unit appeared to lock, but did not engage the fail-safe lock inside the unit that prevented a free-flow of medication.

The device was fatally flawed, and ultimately it was recalled by the manufacturer.

In the preceding case, not only was there a product liability claim against the manufacturer, there were also claims against the home care company for failing to follow proper steps in placing the device. However, it was the product liability claims that resulted in the bulk of the settlement.

4. What Is a "Design Defect"?

What accounts for defective design? A design is defective when the foreseeable risks of harm posed by the product could have been reduced or avoided by the adoption of a reasonable alternative design, and the design used is unsafe.

G. R. is a 48-year-old executive with IBM who enjoys weekend boating trips. On a particularly hot spring day, he is fueling his boat in his garage when he gets a telephone call and goes back into his house. He leaves his uncapped gas can in the garage. The garage is not air conditioned. After 40 minutes in the house on the phone, G. R. returns to the garage to finish fueling his boat for an afternoon run. When he enters the garage, however, he realizes that the heat in the garage has vaporized a lot of the gasoline in his gas can, and in response to the smell of the gasoline he pushes the switch to turn on the garage door to ventilate the garage. A spark in the motor causes the gas vapors to ignite. The explosion burns G. R. over 93 percent of his body, and he expires the next day in the burn center.

An expert examines the motor and finds that there was an alternate design that should have been used in view of the fact that the motor was used in an area where flammable vapors are likely to be encountered (the garage), and that the current design is unsafe. Plaintiff has made a case for strict liability based on design defect.

5. What Is a Failure to Warn?

Sometimes a product is reasonably safe, but if improperly used, can be unsafe. Strict liability attaches for failure to warn when the foreseeable risks of harm posed by the product could have been reduced or avoided by reasonable instructions or warnings. For example, a saw when used to cut wood may be perfectly safe, and may be dangerous if used to cut metal. A warning on the blade of the saw discharges the manufacturer's duty to the public. Although failure to warn has its roots in negligence law, it is now well-recognized that a product may be defective or unreasonably dangerous under strict liability when it is not accompanied by an adequate warning of the danger attending its use.

In *Williams v. Brown Manufacturing Company, Inc.* (1968), 93 Ill.App.2d 334, 360, 236 N.E.2d 125, 139, rev'd on other grounds (1970), 45 Ill.2d 418, 261 N.E.2d 305, it was stated:

> *In the absence of adequate warning, liability may arise from use of an instrumentality not otherwise defective, since failure to warn may itself be the defect which causes injury.*

In *Frisch v. International Harvester Company* (1975), 33 Ill.App.3d 507, 516, 338 N.E.2d 90, 97, the court said that "(P)roducts otherwise not defective unaccompanied by proper warnings are covered under the theory of strict liability."

In recent years, product liability claims for failure to warn have become such an issue that Claymore mines sold to the military now contain the warning "front toward enemy, do not eat." A dozen other stupid warnings can be found on power tools. But, in many ways, such warnings do contribute toward keeping people safer. While the world might be a safer place if people who needed to be told not to operate an electric hair-dryer in the bathtub were never sold one, the law favors making them responsible for their own harm. If they drop the device in the bathtub and electrocute themselves, their families cannot claim they were not warned.

E. WHAT IS MASTER-SERVANT LAW?

Perhaps no area of the law is so poorly understood as the law of Master and Servant. In part, the law is poorly understood because no one wants to think in those anachronistic terms. A "master" is a term that should have

gone out of style with the 13th Amendment, but in the law the term continues to be used. A master is no more than an employer. A master is someone
who has the right to control the actions of an employee.

A master controls his or her servants. A servant is under the direction and
control of the master. An employee has no discretion as to whether to obey
the boss. If the boss says "get this pizza downtown in 20 minutes or less," the
employee is going to do everything he can to comply. When the employee
runs over a 90-year-old woman in a wheelchair on his way to deliver the
pizza, is it fair to blame the employee alone for this act, or more fair to blame
both the employee and the employer who commanded the employee to perform the act?

A master-servant relationship exists between employees, and that is the relationship between a hospital and its employees. But, unless the hospital employs and pays a physician, that physician is not a servant of the institution.
This is true even in the Emergency Department. This is because unless the
hospital has a right to control how the physician does his job, the relationship
is one of contractor and independent contractor. A contractor is not responsible for the torts of an independent contractor. So a hospital is not responsible
for the actions of an independent physician.[27]

1. What Is *Respondeat Superior*?

Under the doctrine of *respondeat superior,* an employer is liable for the negligent acts or omissions of his employee. In order for the employer to be liable, however, the employee must be acting within the scope and course of
his employment.[28] Liability based on *respondeat superior* requires evidence
that a master-servant relationship existed between the parties.[29] Usually this
is not challenged in cases where the employee is an hourly employee doing
routine work. What often is challenged is that the employee was somehow
acting outside the scope and course of his employment.

Several years ago, a respiratory therapist in an Oregon hospital raped a
surgical patient while she was still sedated. The patient then sued the hospi-

---

[27]This may not always be the case. For example, where the medical director in a pulmonary function lab
reads pulmonary function test results, and the hospital bills for his services and receives payments for
those services in its own name, the physician may be an ostensible agent of the hospital, and the hospital may be liable. The law is varied and different on this issue across the fifty states.

[28]*Light v. Lang,* 539 S.W.2d 795, 799 (Mo.App.1976).

[29]*Usrey v. Dr. Pepper Bottling Co.,* Poplar Bluff, 385 S.W.2d 335, 337 (Mo.App.1964).

tal for assault, battery, and intentional infliction of emotional distress. The therapist was arrested and convicted of sexual assault. He had no assets. The plaintiff, if she was to recover at all, had to recover against the hospital.

The hospital lawyer, however, had a better idea. He explained that the therapist had not been acting to further the interests of the hospital when he raped the plaintiff, and thus the defendant hospital could not be held responsible for the conduct of the therapist. The Oregon Supreme Court sided with the hospital and found he was acting outside the scope and course of his employment.

2. What Determines Master-Servant Relationships?

The test to determine if *respondeat superior* applies to the particular tort of a particular employee is whether the employer had the right or power to control and direct the physical conduct of the employee in the performance of the act. Here, the act that the courts look at is the act leading to the injury. So, for example, in the pizza delivery example, the employer has the right to direct the time frame by when the pizza will be delivered. As such, it is responsible for the negligence arising from that conduct. On the other hand, if the pizza delivery driver puts rat poison on the pizza in order to cause problems for his employer, the employer is most likely not personally liable under *respondeat superior*.

The rule is that if there is no right to control, there is no liability; those rendering services but retaining control over their own movements are not servants.[30] The master-servant relationship arises when the employer has the right to direct the method by which the employee's service is performed.

An additional inquiry is whether the employee was engaged in the prosecution of his master's business and not simply whether the accident occurred during the time of employment.[31] Whether a party is liable under the doctrine of *respondeat superior* depends on the facts and circumstances in evidence in each particular case, and no single test is conclusive of the issue of the party's interest in the activity and his right of control.[32]

---

[30]If McDonald's hires a concrete contractor to pour a driveway, and the concrete truck runs over a customer's foot, it is the concrete company and not McDonald's that is liable under *respondeat superior*, because McDonald's does not have the right to control how the concrete company pours the driveway.

[31]*Gardner v. Simmons*, 370 S.W.2d 359, 364 (Mo.1963).

[32]*Sharp v. W. & W. Trucking Co.*, 421 S.W.2d 213, 220 (Mo. banc 1967).

3. What Is Ostensible Agency?

It is said that sometimes perception is reality. This is sometimes true in the law. When a person appears to be something more than they are, the results are often a conversion. For example, when Doctor Smith's lab coat says "Our Lady of Perpetual Billing Staff Physician" and his name badge looks exactly like Nurse Sprocket's, a patient might well believe that Doctor Smith was an employee of the Hospital. This is particularly true when the hospital has signs up all over town that say "Our ER Doctors are the Best in the World," and "Your Heart Would Choose Our ER Doctors if It Knew What Was Good for It." The hospital is "holding out" the ER doctors as employees of the hospital. More importantly, the bill for the physician's services comes from the hospital. The discharge instructions say "Our Lady of Perpetual Billing" at the top, and below that say "Your Doctor's Discharge Instructions."

Under the law of agency, the hospital is giving the doctor apparent authority. It is saying to the public that the doctor can act on its behalf. The doctor is giving the hospital authority to act for him by billing for his services and paying him for his services. Under agency law, each is the "ostensible agent" of the other.

A hospital cannot control the professional behavior of a physician. How a physician exercises his judgment (the essence of a malpractice claim) is solely his decision. The hospital has no right to control, and hence, there is no liability under the doctrine of *respondeat superior.* But there can be liability under the doctrine of agency. The hospital is just as liable for the acts of its agents as it is for its employees.

Ostensible agency presents itself in the respiratory care context too, particularly where the hospital uses part time and agency staffing. Agency staffers usually dress no differently and have no different identification than do regular hospital employees. They conform to the same dress code, and generally are not permitted to identify themselves any differently. As a result, when an agency staffer commits a tortious act, there is a good chance that the hospital will have actual liability under the doctrine of ostensible agency even if the employee's status as an independent contractor can be proved.

F. KEY POINTS

- Intentional torts are torts where the individual intends the consequences of his action.
- An intentional tort requires the plaintiff to prove the "culpable mental state" of intent.

- Intent is usually proved by the application of common sense to the problem. If a man picks up a softball bat and swings at another man, his intention is not to play softball.
- Intentional torts carry with them some aspects of intentional evil motive.
- Fraud is an intentional tort that deals with deceit.
- Assault and Battery are intentional torts that deal with causing violence or harm.
- Consent is a defense to Assault or Battery, and is necessary before touching patients.
- Consent always means informed consent.
- Intentional Infliction of Emotional Distress is an intentional tort that deals with causing mental suffering.
- In addition to intentional torts, there are negligent torts.
- In a tort based on negligence, the plaintiff does not have to show that the person committing the harm or negligent act intended to hurt anyone.
- Negligence deals with duty, breach of duty, injury, and damages.
- Duty is the key to all negligence cases.
- Breach of duty is determined by the facts and circumstances.
- Not only must the act of the wrongdoer cause harm, it must be the cause in fact and legal cause of the person's damages.
- There are three kinds of damages: economic (things that can be replaced with money), non-economic (things that do not have an economic value, like pain and suffering), and punitive (damages imposed to punish wrongful conduct and to deter future wrongful conduct).
- Punitive damages are very rare.
- Comparative Fault makes it possible for a defendant to require plaintiffs to take responsibility for their own faults in any accident.
- Joint and Several Liability means that a person who is only responsible for 10% of the damage might still be responsible for 100% of the judgment.
- In addition to intentional and negligence torts, there are strict liability Torts.
- Strict liability is based on an abnormally dangerous activity or the manufacture of a product.
- Under strict liability, negligence does not need to be proved.

G. SUMMARY

The law of torts is varied. There are intentional, negligent, and strict liability torts. There are hundreds of ways to get sued for failing to act as a reasonable person. There are numerous ways to get sued for acting intentionally to harm another person or entity. And, there are even ways to get sued without being negligent or acting intentionally, if you are engaged in the manufacture of products or in ultra-hazardous activity.

In the next chapter, we'll take a close and careful look at the law of medical negligence, and how that law affects therapists.

CHAPTER 8

Essential Malpractice Law: Consequences of Medical Error

What's happening all across this country is that lawyers are filing baseless suits against hospitals and doctors, and they're doing it for a simple reason: They know the medical liability system is tilted in their favor.

George W. Bush, January 5, 2005[1]

A. A GENERAL INTRODUCTION TO THE CONCEPT OF MEDICAL LIABILITY

Of all the things you can say to a clinician, perhaps the most offensive is to accuse a clinician of malpractice. Most clinicians not only take pride in what they do on a daily basis, they regard their work more as a calling than a profession. Thus, when you suggest malpractice, you attack the very core of who they are.

Medical malpractice lawyers on both sides will tell you that the parties in an automobile case are a lot easier to deal with than the parties in a medical malpractice case. The physician, nurse, therapist, or other clinician accused of wrongdoing reacts emotionally to the incident, and it often takes years of work by counsel to even get a small recognition that they may not have met the standard of care. Plaintiffs are outraged that someone they paid to take care of their loved one didn't do what he was trained to do, and often they want blood more than money.

---

[1]"Congress should not be giving a free pass to big drug companies at a time when millions of Americans may have had their health put at risk by pharmaceutical giants." Democratic Senator Harry Reid, January 5, 2005.

As a result, many medical malpractice cases go to trial, and trials are won more often by the defendant health care provider (75%) than they are by the plaintiff. This is because most cases of malpractice where the error is documented and easily proved are settled before trial.

In this chapter, we'll look at the definitions of malpractice, what has to be proved to establish a claim of malpractice, and we'll finish with an explanation of the things you need to do to protect yourself from just such a claim.

1. What Is Medical Error?

Simply put, medical error is a failure to perform an intended diagnostic or therapeutic action that was correct, given the event or circumstances and the information available at the time. Medical error can occur only if there was or should have been an appropriate intention to act in a correct fashion, and the action taken (or lack of action taken) is incorrect or improper.

2. Is an Adverse Outcome Automatically an Error?

No. An error is not defined by an adverse or negative outcome. A bad outcome may occur with no error. Heart attack patients die. Trauma patients die. Spinal cords are torn and fail to function. Negative outcomes happen, and when they do, they are not routinely traceable to medical error. This is because if the intention of the caregiver was the proper one, the action was properly executed, and the outcome was not dependent completely on the propriety of that action. A negative outcome is not medical error; it is the end result of a sequence of events and nothing more.

3. Does Error Always Produce Negative Outcome?

No. Medical error can produce no negative or adverse outcome whatsoever. A patient can be given the wrong antibiotic without harm. A patient can be given a chemotherapy agent in a dose that will not affect the cancer, and no immediate harm will come to the patient as a result.[2] But the absence of immediate or negative outcomes does not, in any way, lessen the impact of medical error.

---

[2]Of course, the long-term harm could be horrible, as patients who received diluted chemotherapy from Kansas City pharmacist Robert Courtney found out in the Fall of 2001.

4. System Errors?

Usually medical errors are accidental byproducts of systems. What is an accident? An accident is an unplanned, unexpected, and undesired event, usually with an adverse outcome. An adverse outcome after an error, by this definition, must be construed to be an accident. No one plans an error; no one expects an error; no one desires an error. This is one reason that medical error and medical liability do not always walk hand-in-hand.

5. What Is the Cost of Medical Error?

What is the cost of medical error? Medical error produces horrific results. As the Institute of Medicine said in its 2001 Report:

Two large studies, one conducted in Colorado and Utah and the other in New York, found that adverse events occurred in 2.9 and 3.7 percent of hospitalizations, respectively. In Colorado and Utah hospitals, 6.6 percent of adverse events led to death, as compared with 13.6 percent in New York hospitals. In both of these studies, over half of these adverse events resulted from medical errors and could have been prevented.

When extrapolated to the over 33.6 million admissions to U.S. hospitals in 1997, the results of the study in Colorado and Utah imply that at least 44,000 Americans die each year as a result of medical errors. The results of the New York Study suggest the number may be as high as 98,000. Even when using the lower estimate, deaths due to medical errors exceed the number attributable to the 8th leading cause of death. More people die in a given year as a result of medical errors than from motor vehicle accidents (43,458), breast cancer (42,297), or AIDS (16,516).[3]

Imagine that: medical error, if the results of the Institute of Medicine Study are to be believed, account for more deaths in a given year than motor vehicle trauma. The numbers are amazing, as are the costs. Total national costs (lost income, lost household production, disability and health care costs) of preventable medical errors are estimated to be between $17 billion and $29 billion, of which health care costs represent over one half.[4] This, of course,

---

[3] *To Err is Human,* Institute of Medicine, 2001.
   [4] Id.

does not factor in the costs of the litigation system, and the drain on productivity accompanying it.

6. Should Medical Error Be Disclosed to Patients?

Perhaps the hardest thing for clinicians to understand is that medical error does not always mean medical negligence. But the culture of fear in this country—the fear of being sued or of losing a job because of making a serious medical error—has caused hundreds of patient deaths that, with timely disclosure and appropriate clinical intervention might never have occurred.

Here is what the president of the Joint Commission for the Accreditation of Health Care Organizations told Congress about disclosing medical error:

> The first task is the creation of a blame-free, protected environment that encourages the systematic surfacing and reporting of serious adverse events. Fear of reprisals, public castigation, and loss of business will continue to impede the reporting of serious errors unless we provide incentives for making mistakes known to accountable oversight bodies. Today, the blame-and-punishment orientation of our society drives errors underground. Indeed, we believe that most medical errors never reach the leadership level of the organizations in which they occur. For the typical caregiver involved in a medical error that leads to a serious adverse event, the incentives to report are all negative—potential job loss, humiliation, shunning. It is a small wonder that we know so little about this terrible problem. If we are to get a handle on the epidemiology of medical errors, we must create a protected, blame-free environment that will lead to a more accurate understanding of their scope and nature.[5]

But what about the lawyers? That always seems to be the rationale recited for hiding, burying, and not reporting medical error to the family or patient. "The lawyers will use the information against us." But frequently this concern is overblown, because it fails to take into account the driving force of most medical negligence lawsuits.

Most lawsuits don't arise because someone had something bad happen and they'd like to get rich over it. Rather, they occur because someone suf-

---

[5]Dr. Denis O'Leary, JCAHO, February 22, 2000, Testimony before the Health, Education, Labor and Pensions, U.S. Senate and the Subcommittee on Labor, Health and Human Services, and Education of the Senate Committee on Appropriations.

fered an adverse outcome, and can't seem to get a straight answer about what it was that happened and why it might have happened.

When medical error is disclosed in a straightforward way, the liability risks are small and the risk-management benefit is great. The patient tends to trust someone who tells them the truth. The patient is likely to be forgiving. Even patient's families are likely to forgive the loss of a loved one if the error is explained in a calm and reasonable manner.

Worse, when patients are stonewalled, the inevitable result is exactly what the stonewalling attempts to prevent. In 1996, I had the good fortune to try a medical negligence case involving gross pulmonary medical negligence. The medical error was committed by a pulmonologist and surgeon.

During opening statement, the defense counsel made a lot of hay over the fact that we chose to sue "these good doctors" and told the jury it was all about money. On direct examination of the plaintiff, counsel tried to deal with this issue:

Q. *Jim, I just have a couple more questions to ask you.*
Someone asked a question of one of the witnesses about whether
you stand to gain financially over this lawsuit. Do you remember that?
A. *Yes.*
Q. *Is that why you filed this lawsuit, to gain financially?*
A. *No.*
Q. *Why did you file this lawsuit?*
A. *I wanted accountability. I wanted to find out what happened. And that's*
why I chose to look into what happened—what transpired that week.
Q. *Has this case ever, in your mind, been about money?*
A. *No.*
Q. *Do you care really what the jury decides with regard to*
compensation?
A. *No. I just—as I got into it further and listened to depositions,*
whenever we had had the records submitted to other doctors
and their testimony or their feedback as far as what they
thought there were problems with from what I consider to be
unbiased—I mean, you sent them out, and that's—I want
accountability. I don't want this to happen to anybody else
again. It's—I've lost the most important thing I can lose.
And there is no money that can ever replace that.

Trial Transcript, ***Pollard v. Whitener.***

There are few good reasons not to disclose error, and many good reasons to disclose the error. But this is a decision best made together by risk managers and clinicians at the time of the incident. The time and place to disclose the maximum benefit to be gained and limit the harm to be done should be chosen.

Still, the one main reason that seems to drive people away from disclosure is fear of being sued. In most respects, this is because most clinicians do not understand what the plaintiff has to show in order to prevail in a medical negligence action. The burden is quite high, and medical malpractice cases are difficult to prosecute.

B. WHAT IS THE PLAINTIFF'S BURDEN IN MALPRACTICE?

In order to prevail in a medical negligence case, a plaintiff has to prove three things. He must prove that the defendant was negligent, that the negligence caused or contributed to cause the damages, and he must prove how much the damages are.

Lawyer shorthand for these three "elements" of the cause of action are negligence, causation, and damages.

1. How Do Courts Define Negligence?

Courts issue "instructions" to juries, and those instructions frequently contain the most useful definitions of legal terms. They are, therefore, good guides for explaining what, exactly, a plaintiff has to show. In Missouri, the state from which most of these examples are drawn, the instructions define medical negligence. Missouri Approved Instruction 11.06 states: "The term 'negligent' or 'negligence' as used in this instruction means the failure to use that degree of skill and learning ordinarily used under the same or similar circumstances by the members of defendant's profession."

That pithy statement is the sole definition a jury gets in deciding whether a physician, nurse, therapist, or other health care worker is liable for negligent conduct. It isn't much guidance, and as a result, the jury is forced to listen to what usually amounts to two competing views of the evidence from two competing teams of attorneys.

Courts allow lawyers and witnesses to discuss medical negligence in terms of "the standard of care" and the breach of that standard. For purposes of this book, a better definition of medical negligence or medical malpractice is "a deviation from accepted standards of care that causes or contributes to cause injury or death to another."

What is "the standard of care"? It is a shorthand way of saying "what a person of the defendant's profession would do under the same or similar circumstances."

In other words, the standard of care is what we expect a clinician to do in a given situation. Therapists intuitively understand this concept. When a therapist is taught to give a standard aerosol treatment, he is taught to wash his hands before touching the patient, assess the patient, review the medical record for order changes, and give the therapy according to the physician's written orders. All of these steps are steps that are written into policies and procedures for the benefit of the patient. The handwashing prevents the spread of pathogens from one patient to the next. The assessment and review of the chart is there to inform the judgment of the therapist. The therapist should see and review the physician's order (and not merely rely on the "treatment card" or "cardex" for his order) because orders change and errors occur.

Thus, when a therapist dashes into the room, slaps a mask on a patient without an assessment, and fails to wash his hands, it is a given that he has deviated from accepted standards of care.[6]

2. Who Sets the Standard of Care?

By definition, deviating from an accepted standard of care is negligence. But who sets that standard? Is it a local or national standard? In most states, it is a national standard (although some states, like Kansas and Tennessee, require experts to be drawn from contiguous states). No one thinks that a patient in Kentucky is less deserving of good medical care than a patient in Alabama. But the medical community protects itself by restricting experts from institutional powerhouses like Harvard and the Mayo Clinic from testifying.

The real answer to this question in terms of medical negligence is that the expert obtained by the plaintiff is the person who sets the standard of care for your hospital and for you as a professional.

That probably sounds scary—that someone you do not know and could not locate on a search on the internet—can set the standard of care for your doing your job. But most states require that an expert need only be qualified by skill and training and experience to testify as an expert. Thus, anyone who holds the same qualifications can testify as an expert against you. It stands to reason, of course, that a person with superior qualifications, for example, a physician, can testify against a therapist. Likewise a nurse (in most localities) can testify as an expert on your standard of care, even though they may know much less than you do.

---

[6]Some institutions have institutionalized medical negligence by insisting that practitioners stack treatments, give medications when they are not in the patient room, and that they do not thoroughly assess patients in order to meet "productivity" guidelines. This approach seems to assume that if everyone does it that way, no one will be guilty of negligence. This is a fundamentally risky approach.

When an expert testifies to the standard of care, he does so to assist the jury in determining whether the therapist or clinician made clinical errors that were negligent. As one example:

Q. *After Dr. Whitener saw the patient and did all the things that you indicated that he should do, what would have been the appropriate diagnosis at that point in time?*

A. *Postoperative atelectasis, due to acute and chronic bronchitis, and probably early pneumonia.*

Q. *What would have been, according to the appropriate standard of care, what would have been the appropriate thing to do by Dr. Whitener after he saw Judy Pollard at 11:30 in the morning?*

A. *To immediately transfer her to medical intensive care unit, culture her up, start her on antibiotics, and to order intensive respiratory therapy.*

Q. *Was it a departure from appropriate standards of care for Dr. Whitener to fail to transfer Judy Pollard to the intensive care unit at about noon on the 18th of September, 1991?*

A. *In my opinion, it was.*

Q. *And did, to a reasonable degree of medical certainty, did that failure to transfer her to the intensive care unit at approximately noon on the 18th of September cause or contribute to cause her death?*

A. *I believe it contributed to her death.*

***

Q. *Doctor, you've indicated that there would be a certain type of monitoring that would be regularly and routinely available in an intensive care unit?*

A. *Yes, sir. I can't conceive of an intensive care unit that wouldn't have those facilities.*

Q. *And as you look at the orders given by Dr. Whitener, was there any order that would provide for Judy Pollard the type of monitoring that an intensive care unit can give at any point during the afternoon of the 18th?*

A. *No, sir, there wasn't.*

***

Q.   Dr. Expert, let me just back up for a moment here. In your opinion, if Judy Pollard had been transferred to the intensive care unit, would she have received more intensive respiratory therapy?

A.   Yes.

Q.   Would she have been evaluated following the respiratory therapy?

A.   Yes, by both nurses and the therapists.

Q.   And how soon should the respiratory therapy treatment have been instituted?

A.   Immediately.

Q.   Would there have been more likelihood of one-on-one nursing?

A.   Far greater likelihood. Indeed at least initially, she would have probably had one-on-one nursing.

Q.   And would there have been more intensive monitoring in the intensive care unit for her respiratory status than on the floor?

A.   Yes. At a minimum, she would have had continuous electrocardiographic monitoring and probably pulse oximetry.

Q.   Now, Doctor, earlier you testified that the failure to transfer Judy Pollard to the intensive care unit in your opinion caused or contributed to cause her death. Do you recall that?

A.   Yes, sir.

Q.   And can you tell us why transferring her to the intensive care unit at about noon on the 18th would in your opinion have prevented her death?

A.   Well, as indicated previously, she would have had more intensive respiratory care. She would have had much closer and more sophisticated monitoring by much more sophisticated personnel, who are used to dealing with seriously ill patients. And they would have picked up— the nurses would have picked up what I feel to an overwhelming probability would have been a continued deterioration in her status throughout at least the latter parts of the afternoon and early evening, and the *nurses would have been aware of that and that they would have been able to contact Dr. Whitener and she would have been able to be intubated and placed on a ventilator, which would have prevented her arrest and her brain death.*

Q.   *You mentioned the respiratory therapy. Are you aware that Dr. Whitener ordered IPPB treatments?*

A.   *Yes.*

Q.   *And that the first treatment was not done until 4:32?*

A.   *That's my understanding, yes.*

Q.   *4:32 in the afternoon.*

A.   *Right. It was ordered about noon.*

Q.   *Should there have been a reevaluation of her status after that first IPPB treatment?*

A.   *The first IPPB treatment should have been given at noon and should have been immediately reevaluated. She should have been immediately evaluated by the nurse and therapist.*

Q.   *Since it wasn't done at noon and also wasn't done at 1:00, 2:00, or 3:00, but rather was done at 4:32, should there have been a reevaluation at that time?*

A.   *Yes, sir.*

Q.   *And when the next respiratory therapy treatment was done at 7:06, should there have been a reevaluation done after that treatment?*

A.   *Yes, there should have been. And of course there should have been several treatments in between.*

Q.   *Okay. And is that all part of the care and monitoring and treatment that she would receive in the ICU?*

A.   *In my experience, yes, sir.*

Q.   *Now was there any reason on the morning of the 18th or around noon on the 18th to wait before placing Judy Pollard in the intensive care unit?*

A.   *No, sir.*

Q.   *Was there anything that would be deleterious to her health in terms of waiting to transfer her to the intensive care unit?*

A.   *It would have been potentially deleterious to wait. It was not deleterious to immediately transfer her over there.*

Q. *Now what is your second opinion concerning Dr. Whitener's departure from appropriate standards of care? And we'll go to the evening now.*

A. *Well, it was his failure to intubate, have Miss Pollard intubated and placed on a ventilator at 9:10.*

Q. *Is that 9:10 p.m.?*

A. *Yes. 2110 hours, yes. 9:10 p.m.*

Q. *In your opinion, if Dr. Whitener had either ordered or come in to the hospital to intubate Judy Pollard sometime between 9:10 and 9:30 p.m., to a reasonable degree of medical certainty, could her death have been prevented?*

A. *Yes, sir.*

Trial Transcript, **Pollard v. Whitener** (To protect the expert witness, his name has been removed from this transcript.)

3. How Do Courts Define Causation?

When a malpractice case is serious enough to warrant being filed by a competent attorney, the negligence is usually severe. The mistake or error is more than a simple missed test or error of judgment. Usually someone made a serious error. Because the errors themselves are hard to defend (no one can really defend not doing a chest radiograph when the patient died from a bilobar pneumonia), the area where these cases are defended is causation.

Causation is the shorthand term that lawyers use to describe the situation where the negligence of the caregiver caused or contributed to cause the injury to the patient. It is also the area where most malpractice cases are defended.

Causation simply means that the acts or omissions of the defendant caused or contributed to cause the damages. It is usually established by an expert who testifies that based on his review of the case, he believes it more likely than not that the plaintiff's injuries arise from and were caused by the negligence of the defendants. For example:

Q. *Was it a departure from appropriate standards of care for Dr. Whitener to fail to transfer Judy Pollard to the intensive care unit at about noon on the 18th of September, 1991?*

A. *In my opinion, it was.*

Q.   *And did, to a reasonable degree of medical certainty, did*
     that failure to transfer her to the intensive care unit
     at approximately noon on the 18th of September cause or
     contribute to cause her death?
A.   *I believe it contributed to her death.*

Trial Transcript, **Pollard v. Whitener**

In many ways, causation is critical because it can be analogized to the stop
sign example earlier. Causation arises in the context of medical negligence
because it is frequently difficult to say with any degree of precision exactly
what caused or contributed to cause a patient's injury.

4. How Do Courts Define Damages?

In medical negligence cases, damages are awarded for past and future injury, and for economic and non-economic harm (see Chapter 6). Clinicians often assume that a wrongful death case, based upon malpractice, is the worst
of all possible types of malpractice cases. But from a damages point of view, it
is by far the best. At the moment of death, damages are fixed. Although there
can be recovery for lost future wages, lost fringe benefits, and other elements
of economic and non-economic harm, most wrongful death cases (unless they
involve egregious malpractice) do not generate exceptional verdicts.

Rather, the worst malpractice victims are the ones brought close to the brink
of death, and who will require, for the remainder of their lives, custodial and
nursing care. These cases often bring exceptionally large verdicts because the
cost of care (calculated by a life-care planner) is added to any non-economic
harms. A child born with cerebral palsy because of a botched neonatal resuscitation, for example, could easily generate a $30,000,000 verdict given the cost
of continuing care. A mother of three children paralyzed from the neck down
because intubation was attempted before her cervical spine was stabilized,
who has custodial care issues for both herself and her children, might generate a similarly large verdict because the economic costs of care are so large.

For this reason, therapists who practice in the emergency department, intensive care unit, neonatal intensive care unit, pediatric intensive care unit, or
who perform transport duty should consider having an insurance policy
with a liability limit in excess of $5,000,000.

Keep in mind that damages do not require expert witnesses (although
sometimes a plaintiff will call a life care planner and economist to testify). So
in a wrongful death case, where there are no other or additional economic
damages that require economic calculation, the plaintiff proves his or her

damages by testifying about the relationship that the decedent had with them, and how much they will be missed.

This is usually very emotional testimony.

> MR. JOHNSON: Okay. Your Honor, we would like to offer that. And we'd like to have Mr. Kissner read it, please.
> THE COURT: Is there an objection, Mr. Lewis?
> MR. LEWIS: No objection.
> THE COURT: Any objection, Mr. Carlton?
> MR. CARLTON: No objection.
> THE COURT: Exhibit 53 is admitted.

***

> Plaintiff's Exhibit 53 admitted into evidence.

***

Q. Can you read that for us, Jim, please?

A. Can I explain what —

Q. Yes, you may explain what it's all about and then —

A. Can I show — I have it with me.

Q. Oh, you have — yes, you may show the actual one, yes. You carry it with you all the time?

A. In my car. It's been out of it because I've had to change cars recently. But, yeah, I carried it in my car for a long time, up until just recently.

Q. Did it come in this little box?

A. Yes, it did.

Q. And is this the note right on top?

A. Yes. That was the actual note that was on there.

Q. Okay.

A. Christmas morning it was on the Christmas tree. And it was the last gift given.
    (Witness crying.)

Q. Let me read it.

A. I can read it. Could I have a drink of water?

Q. Sure. Sure. I'm sorry.

A. "This is a very special gift that you can never see. The reason it's so special, it's just for you from me.
    Whenever you are lonely, or even feeling blue, you only have to hold this gift and know I think of you. You

> *never can unwrap it, please leave the ribbon tied. Just hold the box close to your heart. It's filled with love inside." And at the bottom, it says, "I love you, mom."*
> Q. *When did you open that box?*
> A. *On Christmas Day. It was given on Christmas Day.*
> Q. *Okay.*
> A. *In 1990.*

Trial Transcript, **Pollard v. Whitener**

Damages also include medical costs, doctor bills, pharmacy bills, and the same. Those are proved by showing the invoices and having someone testify that he or she was paid.

5. What Is the Evidentiary Standard?

Under the law, a defendant in a medical malpractice case doesn't have to prove anything. The only person who has any burden of proof is the plaintiff. But how much evidence does the plaintiff have to offer to meet his burden of proof?

Most states say that the plaintiff must prove his case by a "preponderance of the evidence." Like so many legal bits of jargon, this phrase is decidedly unhelpful in defining how much evidence a plaintiff needs to produce. But it basically requires the plaintiff to show that it was more probable than not that the events occurred and that the standard of care was breached in the malpractice action.

Some courts and commentators phrase this standard as "51%" but that is probably misleading, particularly in the area of medical negligence. Jurors normally favor the health care worker over the plaintiff in a medical negligence case, and unless the evidence is more like 80% to 20%, the verdict is going to go in favor of the defendant.

Jurors want a great deal of evidentiary certainty before they hang a clinician out to dry. They want that certainty because they recognize the importance of what they are asked to do, and do not regard it lightly. For this reason, when a plaintiff proves up a medical negligence case, he may need two or more experts for each point of medical error that he proposes to prove in order to convince the jurors.

A defendant doesn't have to offer any evidence. The defendant can merely poke holes in the plaintiff's theories:

> *Doctor, what are you charging to testify here today?*
> A. *$340 an hour.*

Q. What did you charge when I took your deposition in
    Denver?
A. $340 an hour.
Q. You were even going to charge us $340 an hour to drive to
    the deposition, didn't you?
A. If you asked me to go out to the airport, I would have
    charged you for that trip, yes. I charge for the time
    away from my office.
Q. Do you think ventral hernia surgery is a dangerous
    operation?
A. Yes, sir.
Q. Do you think people have difficult times afterwards?
A. I know people have a difficult time afterwards because
    it's one of the operations, that and gall bladder
    operations, are the ones that we had the most difficult
    time in taking care of in post-op care. Now admittedly my
    experience is biased because we wouldn't be involved with
    patients who weren't at high risk of developing
    complications, but we as a—my group as a whole, we had
    our toughest problems postoperatively with gall bladder
    surgery and ventral hernia repairs.
Q. Have you been told that Mrs. Black has been categorized,
    or classified prior to this surgery, as a physical time
    bomb? Have you heard that?
A. I haven't heard that statement, but, in view of the fact
    that she has severe arteriosclerosis, that would not be
    an unfair characterization.
Q. You knew she had prior surgeries.
A. Yes.
Q. You knew she had diabetes.
A. Right.
Q. You knew she smoked.
A. Right.
Q. You knew she was obese.
A. Yes.
Q. You knew the doctors tried to talk her into quitting
    smoking.
A. Yes, sir. Dr. Vogel testified at length about that in
    his deposition.
Q. And even though a while ago I think you said something

about life expectancy of two years, I think, as I recall
in your deposition, you said her life expectancy was one
to two years; is that correct?

A.   To a probability, one to two years. Less probable at two
than one, but still more likely than not. And
possibilities after that.

Q.   You also said that there were a lot of different things
that could happen to her; isn't that right?

A.   Right.

Q.   She could have a heart attack?

A.   Yes.

Q.   She could have a stroke?

A.   Right.

Q.   She could have a pulmonary embolus?

A.   Sure.

Q.   In fact, you even flippantly told me in the deposition
that she could get hit by a meteorite and die, didn't
you?

A.   That was not in that context. That was in a different
context.

Q.   You said that, didn't you?

A.   You were talking about what—you were in the context of
what possibly could happen to her.

Q.   You said she could get hit by a meteorite?
     MR. JOHNSON: Your Honor, I would request he be
allowed to finish his answer.
     THE COURT: You need to answer the question and then
you may explain your answer.

A.   It was in the context when you were I think pushing a
question to the extreme, and I answered you in kind.

Q.   Well, I'm not the one that asked the question.

A.   Well, whoever.

Q.   But that was your answer, wasn't it?

A.   Well, whoever asked the question. Maybe Mr. Lewis.

Q.   Let me make sure I understand exactly what you're telling
us here today. You have no problem with the orders that
Dr. White wrote, except you believe she should have
been in a different room throughout the basis of the
day. Isn't that correct?

A.   *Well, in a different unit. In a room in a different unit, yes.*

Trial Transcript, ***Pollard v. Whitener***

The only thing that the defendant in a medical malpractice case has the burden of proof on is an "affirmative defense," something that, if proved, negates any liability on his part.

6. What Is an Affirmative Defense?

Affirmative defenses are of varying natures. In some instances a defendant may, in addition to denying liability in his or her answer to the petition or complaint, also plead that there are other reasons why the plaintiff cannot recover. These are defenses where the law places the burden of proof on the defendant.

a) Statutes of Limitation/Repose

Every state has a statute of limitations for medical negligence claims. Most also have a "statute of repose" for medical negligence claims. These two statutes are often found in the same piece of legislation, but have radically different effects.

A statute of limitations provides the time frame within which a medical negligence lawsuit may be brought by a plaintiff. The statute of repose cuts off a medical malpractice lawsuit at some future date, if for any reason the statute of limitations might not apply.

The statutes must be raised as an affirmative defense, meaning that the defendant must say that the action is barred by the statute of limitations (or repose). If the defendant can show proof of this defense he can win without a trial on the merits of the claim.

Most state statutes are between one and two years where the patient is a competent adult. Where the patient is a child or incompetent, the statute may be appreciably longer.

b) Governmental Immunity

When a therapist works for a state-owned or operated facility he may have governmental immunity, or official immunity. These doctrines protect some health care workers from liability for discretionary acts taken as a

Statute Time Frame	States
1 year	California, Kentucky, Louisiana, Tennessee
2 years	Alabama, Alaska, Arizona, Colorado, Connecticut, Delaware, Florida, Georgia, Hawaii, Idaho, Illinois, Indiana, Iowa, Kansas, Minnesota, Nevada, New Jersey, North Dakota, Ohio, Oklahoma, Oregon, Pennsylvania, Texas, Virginia, West Virginia
3 years	District of Columbia, Maryland, Massachusetts, Michigan, Mississippi, New Hampshire, New Mexico, New York, North Carolina, Rhode Island, South Carolina, South Dakota, Vermont, Washington, Wisconsin, Missouri (when malpractice results in wrongful death)
4 years	Nebraska, Utah, Wyoming

Table of Statutes of Limitations in Medical Negligence Cases. All statutes have exceptions and state laws change frequently. Only an attorney can advise you on the proper statute of limitations. For a map of state statutes of limitation see http://www.ncsl.org/programs/press/2004/medmalsl.gif.

governmental employee. Like the statute of limitations defense, the defendant must prove the existence of the immunity in order to defeat the claim.

c) Assumption of Risk

The common law defense of assumption of risk appears to have had its genesis in master-servant relationship.[7] Under this early application of the doctrine, if an employee entered into a contractual relationship with his employer with full knowledge of the dangerous conditions associated with his employment, the employee was held to have assumed the risks of those dangers incident to his employment.

A review of the case reveals that the defense has two analytically distinct applications. In one context, the defense refers to those situations where the person who is claimed to be negligent has no duty to protect the other from a risk. This use of the doctrine has been referred to as assumption of risk in its primary sense.[8] When applied in that manner, the defense operates in

---

[7]See, e.g., *Fidelity Storage Co. v. Hopkins*, 44 App.D.C. 230 (1915); *Decatur v. Chas. H. Tompkins Co.*, 58 App.D.C. 102, 25 F.2d 526 (1928); *Baker v. Sterrett Operating Service, Inc.*, 59 App.D.C. 278, 40 F.2d 790 (1930).

[8]See James, *Assumption of Risk*, 61 Yale L.J. 141, 142 (1952).

much the same way as the doctrine of informed consent, thereby relieving the clinician charged with negligence from any liability.

The defense has also been applied in situations where a plaintiff who is aware of the risk created by the defendant's negligence deliberately chooses to encounter that risk.[9] This has been referred to as assumption of risk in its secondary sense. When utilized in these circumstances, the defense of assumption of risk is closely related to the defense of contributory negligence.[10] Nevertheless, the two defenses are separate and distinct; the inquiry into assumption of risk focuses on what the plaintiff actually knew, while the defense of contributory negligence requires a determination of what the plaintiff should have known and acted upon in the exercise of reasonable care for his own safety.

(1) How Is Assumption of the Risk Proved?

Even where there is evidence that tends to show that a plaintiff possessed sufficient comprehension of the risk, the defense won't be allowed unless there is evidence that the plaintiff's acquiescence in that risk (and thereby his acceptance of it) was voluntary.[11] In the words of the Restatement of Torts:

The plaintiff's acceptance of the risk is not to be regarded as voluntary where the defendant's tortious conduct has forced upon him a choice of two courses of conduct which leaves him no reasonable alternative to taking his chances. A defendant who, by his own wrong, has compelled the plaintiff to choose between two evils cannot be permitted to say that the plaintiff is barred from recovery because he has made the choice.

Restatement (Second) of Torts, Supra s 496 E, Comment c.

In sum, the principle elements of the defense are an actual knowledge and comprehension of a danger caused by the defendant's negligence and the plaintiff's voluntary exposure to that known danger.

In a medical negligence case, assumption of the risk normally comes in when the procedure being attempted is something new or novel—an untried operation for example—where science has not validated the procedure and the result is not certain from the outset. If the plaintiff is fully advised that the

---

[9]*Webber v. Eaton,* 82 U.S.App.D.C. 66, 160 F.2d 577 (1947).

[10]Contributory negligence compares the fault of the plaintiff with the fault of the defendant.

[11]See *Martin v. George Hyman Construction Co.,* D.C.App., 395 A.2d 63, 71 (1978); *Kanelos v. Kettler,* supra, 132 U.S.App.D.C. at 137, 406 F.2d at 955; *Dougherty v. Chas. Tompkins Co.,* supra, 99 U.S.App.D.C. at 350, 240 F.2d at 36.

procedure is new, novel, untried, experimental, and uncertain to provide a cure, and undertakes it anyway, she is said to have assumed the risk that the procedure would fail.

This is a frequent source of concern for patients who wish to sue for surgical error. They believe that the consent they signed to have surgery, the document that disclosed that they might suffer everything from croup to gout as a result, renders them unable to sue because they knew the risks of the procedure.

In some cases that is true. So, where the patient goes in for a knee replacement operation, and signs a form that acknowledges that she is having the device implanted with a glue, and that the glue sometimes fails, she cannot later sue the physician when the glue does fail and another operation is required to remove and replace the joint. She was aware of that particular risk, and she assumed that risk when she had the surgery.

She can sue, however, for the failure of the physician to detect the lack of surgical correction, and the damage that was being done by the loose joint. That is not barred by assumption of the risk.

Assumption of the risk is critical in situations where patients are placed on novel treatments like heliox or jet ventilation. Patients should be fully informed of the possible consequences of such procedures and should be asked to assume those risks in consent forms.

d) What Is the Professional Judgment Defense?

A therapist is entitled to use judgment when treating a patient. If a therapist has to choose between two different paths (say, for example, intubating the patient or continuing bag-mask ventilation), and chooses one that turns out in retrospect to be a mistake, that is not medical malpractice in many jurisdictions if the therapist used his best judgment, skill, and learning at the time.

The Model Jury Charge (the instructions given to jurors in many states) instructs the jury that a therapist must exercise the standard of care appropriate to the average member of the profession practicing in that field. The model charge further instructs the jurors that they must rely on expert testimony and "not speculate or guess" about the standard of care applicable to the diagnosis and treatment at issue in the case.

After giving the charge relating to the standard of care, a trial court must decide whether to instruct the jury that defendant's actions may constitute an exercise of medical judgment that would excuse that defendant from liability for a poor result. To constitute a medical judgment, a medical decision generally must involve misdiagnosis or the selection of one of two or more generally accepted courses of treatment. In the latter category, the course of treatment followed by the caregiver must be an "equally acceptable approach" in order not to be considered a deviation from the appropriate standard of care. Otherwise, if the exercise of judgment rule is inappropriately or erroneously applied in a case that involves only the exercise of reasonable care, the aspect of the rule that excuses a physician for "mistakes" would enable the physician to avoid responsibility for ordinary negligence.

This is because, unless he contracts otherwise, a therapist employed to treat a person implies that he possesses that degree of learning, skill, and experience ordinarily possessed by others of his profession practicing in the same field in the same or a similar locality at the same time. He warrants that he will use ordinary care in the exercise of his skill and the application of his knowledge and experience to accomplish the purpose for which he is employed. Also, he makes the representation that he will use his best judgment in the exercise of his skill in diagnosing the condition and in treating the patient.

7. Are Therapists Responsible If Therapy Doesn't Result in Cure or Improvement?

A therapist does not warrant a result or a cure and is not responsible for the lack of success unless that lack results from his failure to exercise ordinary care or from his lack of ordinary learning, skill, and experience. If he possesses ordinary learning, skills, and experience and exercises ordinary care in applying same, he is not responsible for "mistakes of judgment."

This is because a therapist is not bound to use any particular method of treatment with his patient. If, among therapists of ordinary skill and learning, more than one method of treatment is recognized as proper, it is not negligence for a therapist in good faith to adopt and use either of such methods of treatment.

So it is a defense for a therapist, in a malpractice action, to claim that he had to choose between two options: ventilating with a bag-mask, and intubating. He considered the information available to him at the time. The patient was a trauma patient who was brought in by helicopter. She did not need intubation in the field, but had become short of breath and suffered respiratory failure on arrival in the ER. The patient had serious blood loss, and abdominal surgery was indicated. Rather than attempt intubation in the ER, the therapist decided to defer to the anesthesia service in the OR, and transport to the OR using a bag mask. In so doing the patient aspirated and developed pneumonia that ultimately cost the patient her life.

Here, the exercise of professional judgment was sound, does not appear to be in any way related to negligence, and the therapist may avail himself of the defense.

8. What Is the Importance of the Therapist's Independent Duty to the Patient?

Each therapist has an independent duty to the patient, and to discharge that duty each must follow the dictates of his or her profession, and they must adhere to the rules and regulations of his or her employer.

Suppose a physician has written an order for a tidal volume of 1500 ccs on a frail, 90-year-old woman weighing 86 pounds. Let's suppose further, that the therapist thinks this order is inappropriate and dangerous.

Can the therapist escape liability for harm by saying "the doctor ordered it, and I did what he told me"?

No. She cannot. A therapist has an independent duty to the patient, and if she knows that the volume is inappropriate and she carries out the order anyway, she is liable for the harm that results.

Suppose the policy and procedure manual says that she should discuss this issue with the physician, and if the physician will not change the order, that she must call the medical director. Does she discharge her duty to the patient if she merely complains to the ordering physician that the order is wrong?

Again, the therapist is held to the standard of all the other therapists, and if the policy says you have to involve the medical director, you have to involve the medical director or you're liable for the harm.

If the therapist follows the policy and procedure manual and is still required to carry out an order she thinks is wrong, by following the policy and procedure manual and turfing the issue to the medical director, she has made the medical director and the ordering physicians the defendants in any lawsuit to come. She will probably be a witness, and if she is sued, will have a defense that she followed the dictates of her profession and ultimately carried out an order she didn't agree with because she was required to do so.

9. Is Comparative Fault Used in Malpractice?

Although it doesn't seem logical, because it is hard to think that a patient could somehow be negligent, comparative fault is another affirmative defense sometimes applied in medical negligence cases. It compares the plaintiff's negligence in not acting reasonably (for example, not following instructions) with the caregiver's negligence.

For example, Mr. X has a methacholine challenge test done in the pulmonary laboratory and seems to do reasonably well. He is given explicit discharge instructions that tell him that if he has any shortness of breath to call his doctor, or, if it is severe, to call 911.

When Mr. X goes home, he has shortness of breath when he climbs the stairs. He assumes this is due, in large part, to his weight and exertion. He does not call the doctor, but lies down on the bed to rest. The shortness of breath gets worse. He self-medicates with an inhaler. That does not help. The shortness of breath is getting much worse. He finally calls an ambulance and passes out. By the time he arrives in the ER, he is brain dead.

The family brings a lawsuit for negligent instruction by the therapist. The therapist can compare her negligence (which is not apparent here) with the negligence of the patient who ignored written discharge instructions and delayed calling for medical help.

C. HOW DOES A PLAINTIFF GO ABOUT PROVING THE STANDARD OF CARE?

In order to prevail in court, the plaintiff has to prove his case, and he needs an expert to do that. If he claims that John Smith, RRT, is negligent, he needs another RRT or an MD familiar with respiratory care to testify that Smith breached the standard of care. To do that, he has to find an expert who can tell the jury what the standard of care is, how it was breached, and what should have been done. The expert has to be able to explain things clearly and cogently to the jury, and that expert has to be able to withstand withering cross examination.

1. What Is the Standard?

Generally, an expert will define the standard of care in terms of the situation. "When a patient presents in the Emergency Room, generally the standard of care requires that the airway be immediately evaluated." This statement tells the jury what the standard is because that is what a reasonable person would do under those circumstances.

"Here, when the patient was admitted to the ER, he was placed in the room farthest from the nurses' station, and was told someone would be in to see him shortly. For a patient who came to the hospital short of breath, this is not the place to put him. He should have been placed near the nursing station. He then should have received an immediate evaluation of his ability to exchange air by having his lungs auscultated and by having his chest expansion checked. His color and sensorium should have been evaluated, and this information should have been recorded in the patient record."

Now the jury knows precisely what things should have happened for this patient on admission.

"Instead, he was allowed to sit in the back. No one assessed his airway. His airway swelled shut due to an adverse drug reaction, and no one heard his cries for help until he fell from the bed. That is a violation of the standard of care. It caused or contributed to cause the death of this patient."

2. How Is Standard of Care Proved Through Expert Testimony?

Lawyers obtain experts the same way many people look for a good physician or a good employee. They go to published sources and look for someone who has written on the subject. If the issue is the standard of care in the emergency department, they look for a physician who has written on the subject. If the case deals with the drug Flagyl, they may find someone who did initial research on the drug, or alternatively, someone whose research shows problems with the drug.

Lawyers find expert witnesses, retain them, and pay them well. Some physicians command sums in excess of $500 per hour. Therapists often testify for $125 to $200 per hour. The testimonial fees are based in large part on how effective the witness is in delivering information to the jury, how well the jury likes the witness, and how often he or she may have been used.

If an expert only works for the plaintiff or only for the defense, their value is limited. Juries tend to see them as advocates, not independent experts. While some experts testify only for the defense, most experts who testify for plaintiffs also testify for defendants when they can. A witness who appears to be an advocate for one side or the other, instead of a neutral witness explaining the standard of care, harms the side that brings that witness to trial.

3. What Is Meant by *Res Ipsa Loquitur*—The Thing Speaks for Itself?

Not every case requires an expert. Some cases are simply so plain that an expert is not needed. When a former convict beat a nursing home resident with a wheelchair leg in 1998, our office did not offer an expert to testify that the beating caused the death. The photos of the decedent and the bruising shown in the photos did all the talking necessary. It is a very rare case that fits the doctrine, but when the negligence complained of is the kind that doesn't occur without someone making an error, the doctrine of *res ipsa loquitur* comes into play.

Put another way, *res ipsa loquitur* is a kind of rule of evidence whereby the issue of a professional's negligence can be shown by circumstantial, rather than testimonial evidence. That is done by showing a particular kind of occurrence which, because of its character and circumstances, allows a jury of laymen to draw a rebuttable inference, based on their common knowledge or experience, that the cause of the occurrence in question does not ordinarily arise except where someone is negligent.

In one case, the plaintiff filed a claim for relief under the *res ipsa loquitur* doctrine after his deceased wife died during childbirth. The plaintiff alleged in part that the fatality rate of mothers in childbirth is so low as not to be the subject of statistics, that the death of the plaintiff's wife was proximately caused by the negligence and carelessness of the defendant doctor, and that plaintiff did not know the exact nature of the carelessness and negligence because he was not present at the time of treatment. In so doing he tried to take advantage of the *res ipsa loquitur* doctrine.

The Supreme Court disallowed the plaintiff from using the *res ipsa loquitur* doctrine because his case did not involve either a fact pattern: (1) where a patient received treatment for one problem and incurred an unusual injury, or (2) where a surgeon left a foreign object in an operative cavity. The result is that in many states, a plaintiff cannot use expert testimony to establish a *res ipsa loquitur* case in a medical malpractice action. Instead, laypersons must know, based on their common knowledge or experience, that the cause of the plaintiff's injury does not ordinarily exist but for negligence of the one in control.

By way of illustration, incidents where this principle have been applied are all rather unusual. In one case during knee replacement surgery, the plaintiff sustained an injury to her right hand, arm and shoulder. It is common knowledge among laymen that you don't go into the operating room for knee surgery and come out with problems with other parts of your body. In another case, the plaintiff sustained injuries to the back of her right calf following surgery on the top of her right foot. In *Goodenough v. Deaconess Hosp.*, 637 S.W.2d 123 (Mo.App.1982) a patient suffered a neck injury from being improperly positioned on a table for a proctoscope examination. In each of these situations, the plaintiff went in with one problem, and emerged with something different. As such, the doctrine has limited utility in medical negligence cases, but is of particular importance to therapists, because frequently patients go into the hospital for surgery and come out on a mechanical ventilator.

Failure to properly manage that ventilator often produces complications that can form the basis for a claim of negligence predicated on *res ipsa loquitur.*

4. Why Are Affidavits Required in Medical Negligence Cases?

In many jurisdictions, as a response to the smattering of truly frivolous lawsuits, state legislatures imposed the requirement of an affidavit from a health care provider before allowing a malpractice action to be filed. The affidavit requirement generally requires an attorney or a physician to execute a statement, under oath, that a particular physician, therapist, hospital, or health care provider deviated from the standard of care, and that this deviation caused or contributed to cause the injury to the plaintiff.

Some states, like Missouri, allow the attorney to execute the affidavit. Others, like Illinois, require that the plaintiff file the affidavit of the expert with the trial court. If a plaintiff cannot get an expert to certify that a case has merit within a set time frame (usually between 90 and 120 days) the courts will dismiss them.

D. ARE THERE OTHER THEORIES OF MEDICAL LIABILITY?

There are as many theories as there are plaintiff's attorneys to think them up.

While medical negligence is by far the most common form of litigation brought by patients against therapists and hospitals, it is not the only kind. Sometimes patients and their attorneys go to extraordinary lengths to find ways to pursue a recovery from a health care professional. Clinicians are sued for assault and battery in informed consent cases, and can be sued for libel or slander if they write improper statements in the medical record. They can be sued for violation of HIPAA and other state privacy statutes. The number and type of additional lawsuits that can be brought is beyond the scope of this text; however, one should never assume that a wrongful action is safe to take just because it isn't malpractice. It may not be malpractice to take the patient's diamond wedding ring, but it is wrong, and it will get you sued (and most likely, arrested).

1. Are Product Liability Cases Involving Therapists Frequent?

No, but when they happen, they can be devastating.

When a hospital supplies a device (like a PCA pump, a chest cuirass, or similar medical component) to a patient, they may become a seller of a product, and may become liable for product defects that they know or should know about.

Although many states do not allow product liability claims against health care providers, and some states have strictly limited the liability of hospitals and physicians for medically implanted devices, hospitals and therapists should still be concerned because product liability can create professional liability risks.

For example, if a mechanical ventilator malfunctions and catches fire, as happened several years ago in the northeast, the fire and patient injury can produce lawsuits arising from the defective product. Whenever there are issues of product defect, there are inevitably issues related to whether the product was used correctly. In one recent case, the manufacturers of a popular home/nursing home ventilator tried to place the blame for the patient's death on the respiratory therapist. In *Redfield v. Beverly Health Services, Inc.,* 42 S.W.3d 703 (Mo. App. E.D. 2001), the nursing home and ventilator manufacturer both tried to point the finger at the respiratory therapist. The jury didn't buy it, however, and found the nursing home and ventilator manufacturer at fault. As the case clearly shows, when defendants get desperate, they start pointing fingers at any convenient party—including your friendly neighborhood respiratory therapist.

2. What About Premises Liability in a Hospital?

As set out rather extensively in the last chapter, premises liability issues are created when someone at the hospital knows of a dangerous situation (water on the floor, a broken toilet seat, a loose stair railing) and fails to either warn about the danger (with a "wet floor" sign, for example) or remedy the problem.

Patients are business invitees under the law, and that means that the hospital must make the premises safe from known hazards, and expend effort to detect unknown hazards. Visitors to the hospital may or may not be invitees under the law, and may not be able to take advantage of the enhanced level of care required for a hospital, but that doesn't excuse not being vigilant about spills and dangerous conditions.

If a dangerous condition is noted, particularly if it is noted by the therapist in the course of his travels throughout the hospital, he should document the hazard, warn if possible (for example, by placing a "wet floor" sign on the floor), and should take care to ensure that if he reports the problem to a maintenance or housekeeping worker, that the problem gets taken care of, and not forgotten.

Departmental premises also contain hazards. Cidex machines produce fumes. Medical gases in cylinders can fall and become small torpedoes when the top of the tank breaks. Care should be taken to ensure that tanks are secured, walkways are free of obstructions, and patient transport is not impeded by equipment left in the hallways. A patient who breaks a leg because the oxygen supply hose on a Bird Mark V caught her leg is no less injured, and no less able to sue, than someone who falls an a wet patch of floor.

E. WHAT ABOUT MY EMPLOYER'S PROMISE OF PROVIDING MALPRACTICE LIABILITY INSURANCE?

Most health care employers don't actually provide medical malpractice liability insurance, even if they tell you that you are "covered" under their policy. Instead they provide for their own coverage and don't disclose that you are not insured.

1. What Is the Most Common Misconception About Insurance?

The most common misconception is that you are covered under the malpractice liability policy of the hospital you work for. As a general rule most hospitals, either intentionally or because they are woefully uninformed, make the mistake of telling employees that they are covered under the hospital's medical malpractice liability insurance policy. Since most clinicians don't want to shell out in excess of $100 every year for their own protection, they accept this blanket statement and don't worry about insurance until the lawsuit papers arrive.

Unfortunately, when hospitals tell employees that "they are covered" under the plan, what they really mean is that the hospital has bought insurance to protect it from the consequences of their employees' negligent acts. Although the hospital will most likely have an attorney available to defend the employee if a case should arise, the hospital is under no obligation to pay any personal judgment issued against the employee. For that reason, it is clear that the employee is not really "covered" under the hospital's policy, but rather, the hospital is covered for her mistakes.

Importantly, only a "named insured" (a person specifically named or identified in the policy of insurance) is covered by insurance. Only someone with an insurable interest is required to be defended by an insurance policy.

Insurance policies are contracts. The contract in this case is made between the hospital and the insurance company. The named insured on the contract is the only person who is covered or entitled to a defense by the hospital. It is for this reason that often the CEO and other officers and directors will be named insureds under these contracts in order to protect them from personal liability. But John Smith in the Respiratory Department is not named. And, from a practical standpoint, it would be impossible, given turnover, to ever have a complete policy because every employee would have to be named to be covered.[12]

But if Our Lady of Perpetual Billing is sued along with John Smith in the Respiratory Department, and the judgment of $10,000,000 is apportioned based on fault at 10% to the hospital and 90% to John Smith, the insurance company for the hospital has only to pay the $1,000,000 amount in many jurisdictions because the hospital's insurer will not offer coverage to the employee personally. Thus, Smith might well be held liable for $9,000,000 in damages that he would be unable to pay.

2. Why Do Clinicians Need Their Own Insurance?

Because people get sued every day in health care. Motorcycle riders say that there are two kinds of riders: those who've wiped out, and those who will. The same could be said for therapists. There are only two kinds: those who have been sued, and those who will be.

In addition to the fact that the insurer does not owe the clinician a duty to pay any judgment entered against him or her personally, there is another reason why every therapist should have a personal liability policy for medical negligence.

Frequently, errors in patient care are system errors. System errors do not arise with one person. They arise with multiple persons. They begin in the waiting room, work their way through the operating room, into the recovery room, and play themselves out a few years later in the courtroom. Inevitably, the errors that lead to patient injury and death can be traced not to one discrete person, but to a series of persons and events.

For attorneys, this is a gift tied in a bright red bow. Whenever you have more than one person who could potentially be responsible for the error, each one's interest is in minimizing his or her own responsibility. As a result, they tend to minimize the role they played, and maximize the roles others played. The pulmonologist claims that the nurses and therapist did not keep him

---

[12]Some employees have made claims of promissory estoppel against hospitals that told them they were covered and who later failed to honor the promise. This contractual doctrine says that once a person has relied on a representation (in this case, that they are covered by insurance) the promisor cannot refuse to provide the coverage.

informed of patient changes. The nurse claims she did not understand the importance of the changing readings from the ventilator. The therapist complains that he told the physician what was happening, but could not get appropriate orders from the physician. With all three people pointing fingers at one another, the plaintiff is less concerned with proving a case against one person because everyone is pointing figures amongst themselves.

Sometimes defense attorneys attempt to minimize the situation by insisting that everyone have harmonious views of what happened. They will work with individual therapists and explain that if they don't criticize the doctor, the doctor won't criticize them. While this may seem like common sense advice, in many respects it is a perversion of justice because the attorney is using an implied threat to change the testimony of a witness in a case.

Not long ago, this author handled a medical negligence case against a nursing home where a patient died after aspirating pizza. The medical records were sanitized of all references to pizza, and the witnesses were leaned on by management and, we believe, by the attorneys. One witness was told to "choose her words carefully, or you won't be able to work in health care ever again."

When the hospital is represented by one attorney, and when the hospital is not mandated to provide attorneys for its employees, a single attorney is given the task of representing the hospital and the clinicians. When that happens, the attorney owes a duty of loyalty only to the hospital. He does not owe a duty of loyalty to the clinicians, and if it benefits his client to throw a witness to the dogs, he can do so.

Consider the situation where the employee at the time of the incident is now a former employee. Even if the hospital had promised coverage, by virtue of separation from employment, the hospital probably has no duty to supply an attorney. If the former employee is named personally in the lawsuit, and if it benefits the hospital to have the liability decided against the former employee, the insurance company can simply refuse to defend or indemnify her. Since she is not a "named insured" on the policy, she cannot enforce the insurance contract unless she sues her former hospital claiming she relied on their promise.[13]

3. What Does Insurance Provide?

It provides for a fund to pay any judgments, and it provides for defense of the charges by a seasoned attorney with your best interests at heart.

---

[13]This is the doctrine of "promissory estoppel" or "detrimental reliance" discussed earlier in this chapter.

Most people think of insurance as a way of protecting themselves against liability judgments. An insurance policy does provide a fund of money for payment of any judgment, but it also provides something far more important. It provides a fund of money to pay an attorney who is loyal only to you, and who has only your interests at heart. An employee covered by a separate policy of insurance has an advantage over those who are not represented by an insurance carrier. The employee has the ability to deal with only one attorney, leaving the coordination of defenses to the attorney she has received through the insurance company.

The employee doesn't have to worry about being made a scapegoat and being stuck with a judgment against her. Instead, she has a fund of money available to pay a judgment, and more importantly someone to fight for her rights.

4. What is the Dirty Little Secret About Liability Insurance?

a) Indemnity and Contribution

Although you won't find many hospitals talking about it, there is another little secret that defense attorneys use to bring employees into line. Sometimes employees witness horrible acts of negligence on the part of doctors, nurses, and other clinicians. They are horrified at the results, and are ashamed of the conduct of their peers. When a lawsuit arrives, they are willing to tell the truth, the whole truth, and nothing but the truth about what happened. When a defense attorney encounters one of these, some (certainly not all) will suggest that they rethink their recollection of events to be more favorable. The conversation goes like this:

Attorney	*So, what you're saying is that the nurse dumped Ensure down the NG tube into the lungs?*
Therapist	*Yes.*
Attorney	*And you believe this caused or contributed to cause the injuries?*
Therapist	*Yes, and I am willing to say that under oath.*
Attorney	*You know that will hurt the hospital's chances of defending this lawsuit?*
Therapist	*I know it, but they should never have hired that nurse. That nurse was fired by the other hospital here in town for doing the same thing. They knew she was a failure nurse. They knew it, and they still hired her. It's shameful!*

Attorney	Are you aware of the law of indemnity?
Therapist	In who?
Attorney	Indemnity. It provides that if the master is made liable for the torts of the servant, that the servant has to stand good for the loss to the master.
Therapist	Never heard of it.
Attorney	I didn't think so. You see, at least one claim of the plaintiffs is that the therapists in the ICU—and that means you—didn't act fast enough after the aspiration was discovered. If there is a judgment against the hospital, the hospital has the right to pursue you for any money it pays out as a result of your negligence.
Therapist	They can't do that. I'm covered by the hospital's insurance.
Attorney	Not for that you aren't. Now, we don't have to worry about that if you just keep from volunteering your opinions. . . .

Under the law of "contribution" a co-defendant can have part of the amount of her liability offset. Contribution works like this: Plaintiff sues Dr. John and the Hospital for medical negligence alleging that the doctor did not treat her pulmonary condition appropriately, and that the hospital was negligent in not having sufficient nursing staff. At trial, the jury finds for the plaintiff against the doctor, based in part on the testimony of the therapist, Jane, who says that Dr. John ignored her frequent pages regarding the patient.

The jury returns a verdict of $1,000,000, and Dr. John's insurance company turns around and files an action in contribution against Jane. They allege that Jane had an independent duty to Dr. John, and that she breached that duty. The hospital, who is not a party to the lawsuit, refuses to defend Jane. Unless Jane has her own policy of insurance, she could be in a world of hurt for simply telling the truth.

5. Does Insurance Make You a Lawsuit Target?

No. It has no effect on your ability to be sued because most attorneys won't know you're insured. There is no central list or registry of people who have insurance. The lawyer would know only **after** you were sued.

Employees in clinical situations have an absolute right to get their own malpractice insurance. One thing that frequently stops them, however, is a mistaken belief that doing so will make them more likely to be sued. As indicated above, there is a significant likelihood that a therapist could be sued for other reasons, and these reasons alone are sufficient to get insurance.

But understanding how medical liability cases arise may provide some reassurance for those who think that buying insurance is likely to increase their odds of being sued. First, there is no central registry of persons who are insured. When a plaintiff's lawyer sues a therapist, he doesn't know if she has any insurance, let alone if that insurance covers the harms claimed in the lawsuit. For example, while most state laws require a driver to carry insurance, there is no way for a plaintiff to determine if the driver of a particular car was insured or not, and car accidents are much more common than malpractice lawsuits. There is no place for the plaintiff to find out if a particular person is insured.

Secondly, the decision to sue or not to sue is never based on the availability of insurance alone. A therapist may be sued, for example, because he works for a state hospital that cannot be sued for negligence. The hospital, as an entity, has "sovereign immunity" from liability. But individual therapists, nurses, and physicians do not have that immunity, and are subject to a lawsuit. While the institution might maintain insurance to protect those employees, they are certain not to be protected once they leave the employment of the hospital. If they do not have a separate policy, and are no longer employed by the hospital, their defense is in their hands.

F. HOW DO I DOCUMENT AND SAVE MYSELF?

No fact witness accused of medical error or malpractice ever went into a courtroom and said, "Gosh, I sure wish I hadn't written so much." This is because the very nature of lawsuits and litigation frequently spells trouble for most clinicians who generally do not remember patients and what happened to them.

Here's a quick question: do you remember what you had for lunch on August 22, 2003? If that date is a special date in your memory, for example, the day you proposed or your birthday, then perhaps you might well remember. In that case, pick any other day at random on a calendar and ask the same question. For the most part, unless you always eat the same thing every day for lunch, you're going to draw a blank.

That's because the human mind does not have an infinite amount of storage space for unimportant details. A detail is unimportant if, at the time it happens, it doesn't come up on the radar and lock itself into your memory.

Some patients generate that kind of memory. I can still remember my first code, and there are many resuscitation events I went to, much of the detail of which I can recall. But the events leading up to those codes are not as easily remembered. And frequently in litigation it is not what happened during the code that is important, but rather, what happened before the code.

1. What Are the Three Main Reasons for Documentation?

There are three main purposes for documentation. They are:

- For billing purposes
- For communication purposes
- To create a legal record

Billing is certainly important. Without billing and patient accounts, therapists and staff would not be paid. Thus, documenting the treatments and interventions given is important for that purpose alone. It becomes even more important when the auditing process is considered. Auditing is a process that many insurance companies use to match up, on a statistical basis, the medical records and patient billings. Protecting your employer from an audit is one sound purpose for documentation.

Your documentation is also a key tool in communicating with other caregivers. As a general rule, you read what others wrote, and others will read what you wrote. They will rely on your findings and on what you chart that you did. They may have communications with other caregivers where your findings will form an important basis for their plan of care. For this reason, it is very important to chart accurately.[14]

But far and away the most important reason to document and document accurately is the passage of time and the nature of litigation. You need a legal record of what you did at the time that you can rely on in a court of law. Consider the following time line:

---

[14]Therapists may be under the mistaken belief that physicians routinely read their charting. This is seldom true. Physicians are under such intense time demands that they rarely, if ever, read through the nursing or ancillary staff notes.

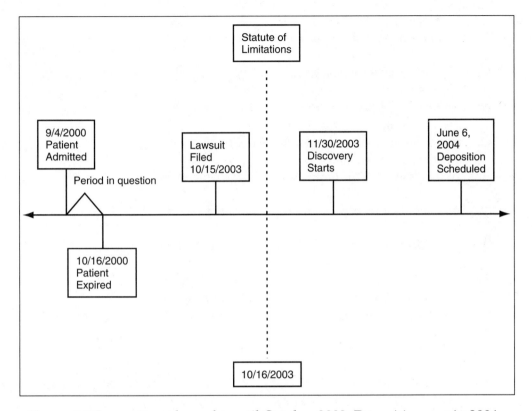

Figure 8-1 Lawsuit not brought until October 2003. Depositions set in 2004. Nearly four years have elapsed since the period in question.

The importance of good documentation when there has been a three- to four-year span of time between the events at issue and the deposition for which you will be summoned to testify cannot be overstated. See figure 8-1.

When asked to testify, a witness needs to be able to tell his or her side of the story. Will a jury trust or believe you if you didn't write down what was important? They might, but they are not required to. Consider the dialog between therapist and lawyer at trial below:

Q. Mr. Coley, could I have you state your name for the
    record, please?

A.   *Laurence Dwayne Coley.*

Q.   *And do you go by Larry or Laurence?*

A.   *Larry most of the time.*

Q.   *Mr. Coley, where do you work?*

A.   *The hospital.*

Q.   *And what do you do there?*

A.   *I'm a respiratory therapy technician.*

Q.   *Okay. Can you tell us generally what a respiratory therapy technician does?*

A.   *We're responsible for the airway of all the patients in the hospital.*

Q.   *And does that involve giving respiratory therapy treatments?*

A.   *Yes, it does.*

***

Q.   *Do you recall taking care of Judy Pollard during her hospitalization in 1991?*

A.   *Vaguely, yes, sir.*

Q.   *Okay. Have you charted any treatments in Judy's Pollard's medical record?*

A.   *Yes, I have.*

Q.   *Okay. I'd like for you to look at the results of therapy from 4:32. And specifically at the heart rates that you have charted. Can you tell me what the heart rate you charted was?*

A.   *Before is 88. After is 92.*

Q.   *So before the treatment it was what?*

A.   *Eighty-eight.*

Q.   *And after?*

A.   *Ninety-two.*

Q.   *All right. Can you look at the results of therapy from 7:06 on the 18th? Can you tell me what the pulse rate was before that you charted?*

A.   *128. 124.*

Q.   *124. All right. And in addition to charting the pulse rates, did you chart the respiratory rates at that time also?*

A.   *Yes, I did.*

Q.   *Okay. And what were the respiratory rates at 4:32?*

A.   *32 before, 28 after.*
Q.   *And at 7:06?*
A.   *32 and 32.*
Q.   *Do you see anything in the 4:32 treatment that would lead
      you to believe that there has been a medication reaction
      that occurred?*
A.   *No, sir.*
Q.   *What about at 7:06?*
A.   *No, sir.*
Q.   *You stated you have some general recollections of Mrs.
      Pollard as a patient?*
A.   *Vaguely, yes, sir.*
Q.   *Do you remember whether Mrs. Pollard was anxious at all
      when you took care of her at 4:32?*
A.   *To be completely honest, no, sir, I really don't.*
Q.   *If I represent to you that in your deposition you stated
      that, would you have any reason to disagree with me?*
A.   *No, sir.*

Trial Transcript, *Pollard v. Whitener*

Here we have a therapist who is treating a woman with a PO2 of 52 on two liters of nasal oxygen, whose respiratory rate is 32, and who cannot tell us with any degree of certainty that the patient was anxious. This fellow's documentation in the medical record was absolutely hideous. It consisted of some check-marked boxes on a form, and some hand-written numbers. Therapy was given by the less-qualified therapists at this institution, and this therapist missed an opportunity to help a patient. He covered his error by claiming a lack of memory.

When you were reading the numbers in the transcript above, it seemed that the therapist knew pretty well what had gone on. The numbers were clear, distinct, and he showed some command of what happened. But when the lawyer started asking about how Ms. Pollard was feeling, and what he remembered of her, this witness was clueless. Amazingly, the therapist didn't apply common sense and say "with a respiratory rate of 32, anyone would be anxious." Instead, he let himself get impeached with what he had testified to previously (and which he apparently had not taken the time to review prior to testifying).

Nothing looks weaker in the eyes of the jury than a clinician who cannot remember what went on. Jurors assume that what goes wrong with them is important to clinicians, even if they may be wrong in that assumption. They assume that everything that happens in a hospital is written down, and many believe what the lawyers tell them, that if it "wasn't charted it didn't happen." So, when a therapist takes the stand and doesn't remember the patient, and doesn't remember what he or she did to the patient, but asks the jury to place trust in them as a caregiver, the jury is rightly suspicious.

2. How Important Is Good Documentation?

It is for this reason that documentation becomes the central focus of every medical negligence case. What is in, and what is not in the charting becomes the very rationale for proceeding against the therapist or clinician. For this reason, documentation cannot be stressed too strongly.

3. What Should I Document?

Good clinical judgment is essential in determining what should be documented on each patient. It would be needless and mindless to chart extensively on every patient receiving a routine nebulizer treatment. However, therapists should remember that part of their job is to be the eyes and ears of the physician and to spot problems before they become crises. For that reason, clinical judgment should include documenting things that appear to have changed between treatments, new problems, or changes in the way the patient is looking or behaving.

a) Document What You Observed

Always chart your observations. Be especially careful to note anything that is out of the ordinary. If the patient's skin color has become more dusky, note it. If their effect has changed, and you suspect it is due to a change in their pulmonary status, chart it. If their position in the bed has shifted from relaxed and reclined to sitting forward, anxiously, these are observations that should be made and recorded.[15] Of course, if you make observations and record them, and then take no action upon these observations, you are setting yourself and your hospital up for a claim that you were negligent. For some reason, there are clinicians who think that not charting things protects them for claims of not doing their job. Nothing could be further from the truth.

---

[15]It goes without saying, of course, that these are observations that should be passed on to the physician as well.

Q. Did you have a telephone conversation with her after her surgery?

A. Yes.

Q. Do you know whether this was the day after her surgery?

A. Yes. It was Tuesday.

Q. Okay. Tuesday —

A. Was the first one.

Q. Okay. Tuesday morning or afternoon?

A. Afternoon.

Q. And who all was involved in that conversation?

A. Everybody at the office.

Q. And did you put it on the speakerphone?

A. We just took turns handing the phone and stuff.

Q. Was there anything about your conversation with Judy on Tuesday afternoon that was of any concern to you?

A. She was having trouble breathing.

Q. And how did you know she was having trouble breathing?

A. You could tell from listening to her.

Q. Had you ever heard her breathe like that before?

A. No.

Q. Can you describe how it sounded at all?

A. It sounded like she was just gasping for air.

***

Q. The next day, which would be Wednesday, did you talk with Judy in the evening?

A. Yes.

Q. And can you tell us about what time you talked with her?

A. It was somewhere between 8:30 and 10:00. I don't remember the exact time. This is the big deal. And I asked her if Larry was there. Are you wanting to know this?

Q. Go ahead. Go ahead.

A. I asked her if Larry was there, and she said, no, he had just left like 15 minutes ago. So I was like — I could tell she was having trouble breathing. I said, "Okay, Judy. I'll just wait and talk to him when he gets in town," because he'll call, because he hadn't called yet. And he would normally give us a report and stuff. And so

*just like five or ten minutes later the phone rang and it
was Larry.*

Q.   *What did Larry say to you?*

***

A.   *Well, when he called, I was kind of surprised that he
called that quick, because obviously Columbia is more
than 15 minutes away from Marshall. And when I told him
that I had talked to Judy, he said, "Well, that's strange."
And it was—I don't really remember if she wasn't supposed
to answer the phone, if the phone was moved across the room,
the nurses were supposed to answer, I don't know.
I just remember something in there about the nurses
were supposed to do something, but I don't remember
what it was. And so—and I was just like, "Well, okay,
what's going on with Judy and everything?" And he just
said, "She is having the same breathing problem." And I
think that he said that they were going to send in a
respiratory therapist or they had sent in a respiratory
therapist. I don't remember whether it was going to or
had been sent in. nd then he was like, "Well, I got to call
everybody else and let them know what's going on and
everything."*

***

Q.   *Could you tell from your conversation with Judy on the
evening of the 18th any difference in her breathing as
you listened to it and as you were aware of her breathing
between the 17th and the 18th? I'm not asking for your
medical opinion. I'm just asking what you thought.
That she was having definite trouble breathing and it was
no better.*

Q.   *Did you say anything to Judy about the difficulty she was
having breathing?*

A.   *No, because I didn't talk to her that long because I
could tell she didn't feel like talking. I just told her
I would talk to Larry when he got to town.*

Q.   *Were you concerned about that, about her breathing?*

A.   *Yes, but can I elaborate on that?*

Q.   *Yes, you may.*

A.   *My mother had had a hernia surgery, and because the incision was really sore, she didn't want to take deep breaths. It hurt. And so when I talked to her on Tuesday, I thought that's what it was. I really did. You know, that's the reason why she is short of breath, is because she is just trying not to move as much as possible. But then on Wednesday, I don't know, it was just different. Yes, I was very concerned.*

***

Q.   *Did you see Judy at all again?*

A.   *(Witness responded by shaking her head from side to side.)*

Patients get visitors. Visitors can come by car, or by telephone, and they see and hear things that go on in the hospital. They can testify to their common-sense impressions of what was happening; as shown above, the judge allowed the witness to testify that the patient was having difficulty breathing based on a telephone call. The failure of the therapist to chart the patient's level of anxiety, her shortness of breath, and her obvious difficulty breathing did nothing to improve his credibility at trial.

In other words, charting nothing doesn't mean that the information about the patient's bad condition, and the therapist's failure to act, won't come in. It just means it won't come in from your records. In many cases, that's worse.

Perhaps more importantly, charting good, accurate information in the record protects the therapist from claims of missed diagnosis, failure to act, and other claims of medical or therapeutic negligence. If a patient arrives at the hospital with pupils fixed and dilated, even if that is recorded in the physician and nursing notes, it should be recorded in your notes as well. When you receive a patient with evidence that brain injury has already occurred, either from another hospital or from the ambulance, and you document it, that documentation prevents a claim that any later negligence at the facility caused that brain injury.

Observations of this nature are important in every case because you never know which cases will wind up in court.

b) Document What You Heard the Patient Say

"I feel like I can't get enough air." If it is something the patient said, and it relates to his or her condition, you can chart it if you believe it to be important.

You are certain to be asked in a deposition what the patient said, how he said it, and anything else you can remember about what the patient said. For these reasons, it is a good idea to chart it.

This is especially true when dealing with patients who, for whatever reason, are violent, abusive, intemperate, drunk, disorderly, harassing, and otherwise unpleasant to deal with. A person who, while sick, manifests these behaviors is likely to be even more ugly in court. An annotation in the record to the effect that you asked the patient to stop referring to you as the male offspring of a female canine, has impact when lawyers review records. When a lawyer reviews a patient's medical record, he wants to make sure that the patient he is representing did not contribute to his own injury. If he did contribute to it, either by consuming alcohol or otherwise, it is important to note that in your records so as to forestall the eventual lawsuits that will follow.

Be careful to report what the patient said exactly, using quotation marks. Do not sugar coat what the patient said. If the patient used a hyphenated string of four-letter words, then use that precise language. Do not paraphrase.

c) Document the Questions You Asked the Patient, And the Answers

If you question the patient about how he is feeling, and what he had to eat or drink, in order to determine what they may have aspirated, or for some other purpose, record the questions and answers as close to verbatim as possible. Accuracy in statements taken from patients is very important and can be crucial to your defense later.

d) Document Your Analysis

Respiratory textbooks used to suggest that SOAP notes (Subjective, Objective, Assessment, and Plan) were appropriate for respiratory care. To a certain extent almost all notes in respiratory care departments now are not so formalized. Nevertheless, there is a sound basis for remembering the SOAP acronym when charting. It is not enough to chart the basics if any component of your job requires you to exercise discretion, analyze data, or plan patient care.

One of the most frequent questions in depositions is "what did you make of that data." In other words, a lawyer not only wants to know what the breath sounds, sensorium, patient affect, patient color, and other objective data were, he wants to know how you perceived them and analyzed them in respect to the patient's condition. For this reason, it is not enough, when caring for a critically ill patient, or one who is taking a turn for the worse, to simply record the data without some analysis. If the data point toward respiratory failure, that should be noted. If you believe the patient is improving, that should be noted. If you believe the patient is stable, that too should be noted. In short, your analysis is an important clue to you, three or four years later, as to what you were thinking at the time.

The same can be said for any plan you develop. Record it in the record. If you plan to follow the patient closely, that is an indication that the patient requires such intervention. This can be critical later on if, for example, a follow-on therapist fails to properly monitor the patient. While the hospital might still be on the hook for his or her failure, you will not be in the position of being party to his or her failures, and you can point to the fact that your plan suggested enhanced monitoring to exculpate you from liability.

e) Document What You Did

Finally, and most importantly, any action you took on behalf of the patient must be documented. Everything, from gathering information through clinical assessment, to delivering medications, should be charted, but special care should be taken to document what you did with the patient.

It is an unfortunate consequence of most medical records that there is no place for a therapist who performs an emergency intubation during a code blue to document what he did, and how he did it. But this is a critical step in the resuscitation, and since the therapist will not have ultimate control over that tube as the patient is moved and transported, care should be taken to document what was done, and when. If an intubation or other emergency procedure is carried out by a therapist, that must be documented to protect the therapist from a later claim that the therapist knocked out a tooth or worse, put the tube in the wrong place.

Documentation regarding what was done is the most important part of documentation. It can be used to "scalp" the lawyer and prevent a case ever being filed.

4. How Can I SCALP the Lawyer?

One of the things I tell students when I talk about the subject of documentation is that they should SCALP the lawyer with their documentation. SCALP is an acronym for Simple, Clear, Accurate, Legible, and Prompt.

a) S Is for Simple

If you normally use ten-dollar words in conversation, then by all means use them in your charting. If not, then your charting should contain short declarative sentences that are short and easy to read. You should chart in chronological fashion, noting everything you did in time order. Charting is not literature, it's litigation prevention. Use the **KISS** method: **Keep It Short and Simple.**

b) C Is for Clear

Clarity in charting is frequently a victim of time constraints. If you do not have time to chart, you may find you have lots of time to think about it when the jury returns a verdict against you. Clear charting is charting that conveys what happened so as to leave no doubt. "Tolerated well" tells the jury nothing. "Patient experienced no adverse reaction to therapy" is much better. It tells the jury you were watching for one, and didn't see one. It takes a few more words, but the time spent is very important in ensuring you do not fall victim to a plaintiff's lawyer.

More importantly, if you don't have time to do it right, why are you doing it in the first place?

c) A Is for Accurate

A military aphorism suggests that "close only counts in horseshoes and hand grenades." It certainly doesn't count in charting. You can't just come close. You have to be accurate. You must record accurate assessments, and you must record accurate data in the chart because if you do not, you run the risk of being impeached by other records. In *Pollard v. Whitener*, the physician attempted to suggest that the patient wasn't really in respiratory distress, and that the medical records made by the therapist and the nurses were not accurate. In reality, he was covering for his own ineptitude. But the following colloquy amply demonstrates why accuracy in medical records is so important.

> Q. *All I asked you was, even if we just base it on the blood gas studies, wasn't Judy Pollard in significantly worse respiratory status at 9:00 on the 18th, in the evening, than she had been at 11:30 when you saw her?*
> A. *Absolutely.*

Q. And isn't it true that there had been a progressive
    deterioration from 11:30 to 9:00 that simply was not
    noted or reported to you?
A. I don't believe that.
Q. Okay. Now were there any blood gas studies between 10:40
    in the morning and 9:10 that night?
A. No, sir.
Q. So would it be safe to say that we don't know what her
    hypoxemia was or what the extent of it was or what her
    respiratory status was in terms of exchanging oxygen from
    10:40 a.m. until 9:20 p.m.?
A. Well, I would expect that the nurses would call me if
    there was a problem.
Q. My question is, Doctor, is the respiration rate of above
    30 for at least eight hours for someone like Judy Pollard
    reassuring with regard to her respiratory status?
A. I don't think her respiratory rates had changed
    significantly over the 17th or the 18th, in my opinion,
    knowing how nurses record respirations, as I have
    explained.
Q. Doctor, my question was, is a respiration rate for
    someone like Judy Pollard of 34, 36, and 32, well over
    30, for a period of eight hours, a reassuring sign with
    regard to her respiratory status?
A. I can't answer the question any more than I could before
    because you are making the assumption—you do not work
    in a hospital, you are not a physician—that those
    respiratory rates are correct—that those respiratory
    rates are as recorded. And I can—if you would like
    for me to tell you what else I think about respiratory
    rates and how they are taken and how they are multiplied
    by four, I will be glad to tell you about that.
Q. Doctor, are you saying that these respiratory rates that
    are recorded on the graphic sheet are incorrect?
A. No, they're not incorrect. They are no more incorrect
    than yours or mine would be if you were in the hospital.
    It's just, in this instance, the numbers are important.
    It doesn't make them any more accurate, though.

Q.   Let me just ask you, if you assume for a moment that Judy
     Pollard's respiration rate was well over 30 for a period
     of eight hours during the afternoon of the 18th, assume
     that that's an accurate respiration rate all for those
     eight hours, is that a reassuring sign with regard to her
     respiratory status?

A.   I have seen patients with restrictive defect, people that
     are obese, people that have pulmonary fibrosis who
     breathe at 25 and 30 all the time and who sit in my
     office and talk to me when their oxygen level on room air
     may be 45.

Q.   Preoperatively her respiration rate was 18, wasn't it?

A.   That's what's recorded.

Q.   Are you saying that that's not true?

A.   I would be very suspicious about that for the reason
     which I have given you, and I'll be glad to go into them
     further if you would like.

Q.   You'll have —

A.   I have a wonderful study for a nursing master student —

Q.   Doctor, all I'm asking you, isn't it true that her
     preoperative respiration rate is recorded as 18?

A.   Yes, it is. And 20.

Q.   18, 20. I'm not going to quibble about 18 or 20.

A.   Yes.

Q.   And wouldn't you agree that 36 is twice 18?

A.   No, it's not twice — well, it's twice 18, yes.

Q.   So were you told the results of the incentive spirometry
     that was supposed to be done at 1:00, 2:00, 3:00, 4:00,
     5:00, 6:00, 7:00, et cetera, when you were called at
     9:10?

A.   No.

Q.   Were you told that the first IPPB treatment was done at
     4:32?

A.   No, but there is a reason for that.

Q.   Were you told of the results of the first IPPB treatment at 4:32?

A.   No. If the respiratory therapist would call me with the
     results of the tidal volume of every IPPB or IS treatment
     I got all day long, I would be on the phone all the time
     just getting those.

Q. *That wasn't my question. At 9:10 —*

A. *No, I was not told that.*

Q. *Were you told that, at 7:06, when the respiratory therapist saw her, that her pulse rate had gone up to 128 I believe? 124.*

A. *I think I have already said I was not told that, that I recall.*

Q. *Were you told of the chest sounds that were found by the respiratory therapist?*

A. *No, sir.*

Q. *Were you told that, at 6:15, Judy had complained of labored respirations?*

A. *No, sir.*

Q. *And that her respiratory rate was 36 and labored?*

A. *No, sir, not that I recall.*

Q. *Were you told at 3:15 that she was complaining of dyspnea and pain while breathing?*

A. *No, I was not told that, but you read those notes. But then a lot of those notes say afterwards, "Demerol given, patient resting comfortably."*

Q. *After she had been given a shot of Demerol.*

A. *That's correct.*

Q. *She would be resting comfortably after being given a shot of Demerol?*

A. *Yes, sir. Sometimes.*

Q. *Were there — you've had a chance now to look at the IPPB treatment notes?*

A. *Yes, sir. I looked at them multiple times.*

Q. *Were the results of those IPPB treatments at 4:32 and 7:06 reassuring with regard to Judy Pollard's —*

A. *I don't think the results as far as the tidal volume that was delivered mean anything. And I would be glad to go into that with you why also if you'd like.*

Q. *I'm just asking whether they were reassuring.*

A. *They were not reassuring nor do they particularly bother me.*

Q. *In your opinion, was Judy Pollard's respiratory status, her respiratory failure and hypoxemia, improved throughout the afternoon of the 18th, right up to 9:00?*

A.   *I made the assumption because I didn't get any calls from the nurses or anybody about that, so I at that time, if I had thought otherwise, I'd have been back over there.*

Q.   *I probably misstated my question. I meant, now that you've reviewed all the records, is it your testimony that Judy Pollard's respiratory condition improved from 11:30 up to the point where you were called — up to the point where she was found confused?*

A.   *I don't know what her status did between 11:30 in the morning and when she was noted to be confused. I would agree with you that, as of 9:10 or 9:20 when those blood gases were drawn, that she was worse.*

Trial Transcript, *Pollard v. Whitener*

Accuracy is important. If you are accurate in your charting, you don't wind up in a position of defending inaction, the way the physician in this case had to.

d) L Is for Legible

The most accurate, simple, clear charting in the world won't help you if no one else can read it. Train yourself to write neatly in your charting, even when in a hurry. The career you save may be your own.

Jurors also like to be able to read what you wrote and not have to take your word for it that the lines that look an aerial map of an Arkansas highway are in fact the words "patient respirations reported to nursing." If you write neatly, you are more professional in the eyes of the jury.

Also, what is clear on Monday is not apt to be clear two years from now. If you can't read it, it isn't charting.

e) P Is for Prompt

The entries in the medical record are hearsay evidence. In other words, under the legal definition of the term, they amount to statements made out of court, when a person is not under oath, and they are not subject to cross examination. As "hearsay" the documents in a medical record are not admissible unless they fall within a hearsay exception.

One exception to the hearsay exception is business records. Business records are considered reliable enough to admit under the hearsay exception, but to gain that reliability they must meet several requirements. They must be routinely made in the normal course of business (a medical record is normally made for every patient) and the events recorded in the record must be recorded at or near the time that those events took place (so things must be recorded in a prompt and timely manner).

Therefore, when information is left out of a medical record, and a therapist makes a late entry, there is a good legal reason to exclude that late entry because it does not fall inside the hearsay exception.

For this reason, charting should be timely.

5. What Should I NOT Document?

Sports trainers and coaches repeatedly emphasize that there is no "I" in team. They do that to underscore that in team sports individual glory isn't important so long as the team wins. It is an apt metaphor for charting and documentation, however, in that it underscores what should not be in medical records. Anything that is inaccurate, irrelevant, inflammatory, illegible, or improper does not belong and should not be included in the medical record.

a) Irrelevant

How do you know when information is irrelevant so as to leave it out of the medical record? One way is by determining whether the information pertains to the clinical situation and would be useful to a clinician who follows you. If what the patient said about her vegetable garden is important (for example, if she was exposed to certain pesticides) by all means include it. Otherwise, leave it out. Only clinically relevant information belongs in the medical record.

b) Inflammatory

Information is inflammatory if it suggests that you were busy evaluating or judging the patient on racial, sexual, or economic bases rather than caring for the patient. While race and religion may be important in the clinical setting, how that information is recorded is important. "African-American male" has import for the standards used for pulmonary function testing, but is not important in describing a patient in the ER with a boil that needs to be lanced.

Sometimes information may be thought important on the basis of safety. You may want to warn your fellow therapists that a person is a member of a notorious street gang. As a general rule, when there is information that must be passed along, or which a clinician wishes to pass along, that should be done verbally, if at all. It is never a good idea to put information in the medical record that a lawyer will later use to suggest you are racist, sexist, or that you discriminate on the basis of how much money a patient has.

c) Inaccurate

It goes without saying that information in the record must be accurate. Respirations cannot be "best guess" measurements. Heart rates cannot be estimates either. It is important to describe a patient's breath sounds properly. Accurate information is to be recorded, and inaccurate information is to be omitted.

The basis for this is clear. If you have charted something different from the nurse, you're going to have to account for the difference, and if what you charted helps your case, and what the nurse charted hurts your case, you can bet the jury will be informed that you have a reason to shade the truth of your recollections.

d) Illegible

Although illegible charting is bad for legal reasons, because it can't be easily read and understood by the jurors, there is another good reason for charting legibly. That is perception. Jurors perceive persons with neat handwriting as careful and accurate and trustworthy. Illegible handwriting is likely to influence a jury negatively toward you.

e) Improper

Bad things happen. Mistakes occur. Other clinicians sometimes intrude onto your turf. Nurses change ventilator settings. Doctors adjust oxygen settings without leaving orders. These kinds of things happen. When they do, they too must be documented, but not in the medical record. That is what an incident report is for. Putting information about errors and mistakes in the medical record is waving a big red flag at the plaintiff's attorney and encouraging him to charge.

If something improper happened, it should be documented, but appropriately:

Good Documentation	Bad Documentation
1:13 p.m. Following 1:00 p.m. ventilator check found dark black water in the Cascade humidifier. When water was removed, strong bleach odor was noted. Metal posts had turned black. Replaced Cascade. Patient alert and oriented. No changes in lung sounds noted. No change in compliance. Ventilator functioning normally. Physician notified.	At 1:00 pm. Replaced water in the Cascade with Dakins Solution that some stupid nurse had left at the bedside and had not marked as not being sterile water. What kind of twit does that? Anyway, the patient did fine once I replaced the Cascade. I told nursing not to leave any more bottles of Dakins on our ventilator shelf where we'd think it was water!

The importance of good documentation cannot be overstated because the effect of bad documentation is often liability. If a jury does not believe that everything was done, if they do not believe the defense that the therapist or hospital acted appropriately, it will be because there is nothing in the records for them to hang their hat on.

Jurors want to find on behalf of the defendant in medical negligence cases. The jury goes in with that predisposition. The plaintiff overcomes that predisposition only where it shows that there are clear deviations from the standards of care, and those deviations are evident only where the record shows them to be.

Ignore documentation at your own peril!

G. HOW IMPORTANT IS TEAM COMMUNICATION?

Of all the things that lead to malpractice lawsuits, poor communication is at the top of the list. Failure to communicate with the patient and with the family when things are going well, and refusal to communicate after things have gone wrong, almost always creates the ripe environment for a lawsuit.

1. How Do I Go About Communicating with the Family?

Although there are practical and policy limits on what a therapist can communicate with a patient and his family, he should remember that basic communication skills are more important than any specific information that is communicated. Said differently, the therapist should remember that how things are said is often as important as what is said.

Consider the patient on a mechanical ventilator after a code. The family is anxious. They are concerned for their family member. They may never have expected to be where they are. The events that led them to this place may be fresh and disorienting. None of them, most likely, expected to be sitting outside the ICU at this particular time. Their lives have been interrupted, and they are being given information, a large part of which they probably do not understand or have not processed.

When dealing with the family, keep this in mind. Keep explanations simple and straightforward. Tell the family what you do, and why you do it. Explain your function. Tell them you are there to help.

If you bridge the gap successfully, the family will come to rely upon you as a resource and will value what you have to tell them. They may have complaints about others at the hospital, but they won't have complaints about you, because you engaged them at a personal level.

The best form of malpractice insurance you can't buy is good interpersonal communications skills. Simple techniques like active listening ("are you saying you're worried about oxygen being used on the ventilator?") and repetition go a long way toward making a family feel like you not only are telling them what they need to know, but are listening to them as well. Good communications often forestall lawsuits because patients will raise their concerns with you, rather than with their lawyer who has an incentive to find your mistakes.

2. How Should I Communicate with Other Caregivers?

The best place, and best way to communicate with other caregivers is in a secure setting, away from other persons.

I was recently in Research Medical Center in Kansas City. My sister was a patient there. In the elevator on the way down to the lobby two nurses were talking about a patient. They were discussing 413 (that is, he was a number, not a name) and his need to call his wife about his medicines. They seemed to think it was funny that his wife had been dead for ten years. As a visitor with a patient in the hospital, I found no humor in it.

While every caregiver has similar experiences, where something strikes the funny bone in an odd sort of way, the right place to discuss that sort of thing is not the hospital elevator. And although I am singling out Research Medical Center because that is where the incident occurred, the same thing happens in hospitals all over this country every day.

Communication with other caregivers is an important part of what therapists do. Doing it properly is a keystone of the clinical duties that therapists perform. If you have to discuss a patient, do it in private, or at the very least, in a place where no one else can overhear. If someone makes use of the information you discuss, it could damage your career and the hospital's reputation.

3. How Important Is It to Investigate Fully?

In the area of malpractice liability, the one thing that seems to cause therapists and other clinicians the most difficulty is a simple little word: assume. Therapists should never assume anything.

4. You Are the Last Line of Defense

Several years ago, I was working with a very good nurse clinician who had a suspicion that a patient had a particular lung problem. She asked me to do some blood gases. I told her I didn't think we needed blood gases because we had gases a few hours earlier and the oximeter had not indicated any change.

She persisted, telling me that in her opinion it was important. So, since the request was on her nickel and not on mine, I did the blood gases and, lo and behold, the nurse was right. The blood gases in terms of oxygenation had not changed markedly, but the blood gases in terms of carbon dioxide had. The patient had gone from normal acid base balance to acidotic, and the CO_2 level had jumped 15 points. It taught me a very valuable lesson about assumptions. They are terrible things upon which to base patient care.

The fact is that your clinical suspicion about what might be going on with a patient is quite often the last line of defense for that patient. You owe an independent duty to your patient to investigate fully and act on the information you obtain.

5. What Do Lawyers Look For?

Finally, no explanation of medical negligence would be complete without an understanding of what a lawyer looks for when he evaluates a medical negligence case. If you understand these factors, it not only makes certain mistakes easier to live with, it also improves the likelihood that when things are the most important you'll do what is in the best interests of the patient.

A plaintiff's lawyer is looking for a clear deviation from the standard of care. He wants that error or omission documented in the record where it can't be said not to have happened. Furthermore, he wants a case to have large amounts of economic damages with a very sympathetic plaintiff.

a) Lawyers Want Clear Deviations

My old boss, Victor Bergman, Esq., used to say that he was waiting for the "perfect case." He defined it as one where the doctor, who was very well insured, was drunk at the time he performed surgery. He wanted the plaintiff to be an NFL place kicker who went in for a wart removal from his thigh, and came out missing his kicking leg. He then said he wanted the physician to come out of OR, be overcome with regret, and apologize for the error in front of three disinterested witnesses, two of whom were clergy.

Suffice it to say that there just are not that many "perfect" cases out there. Rarely are deviations from the standard of care so clear cut as to have the wrong limb removed. Rarely does anyone apologize. It is rarer still for there to be any disinterested witnesses to what happened in the hospital.

But still, deviations do occur. Several years ago our office was asked to evaluate a case for a nursing home patient who was placed on a mechanical ventilator in a nursing home. The nursing home did not have a nurse, aide, supervisor, or other employee in the area where the ventilator patient was for nearly 30 minutes. There was a disconnection and a death as a result. The deviation was very clear from the record.

In another case, the plaintiff's decedent was a lovely lady who was blind and had no teeth. She could not chew her food. She was on a dental soft diet. A nurse gave the woman pepperoni pizza to eat. She tried her best to chew it, since she had Alzheimer's disease, she did not know any better. She choked, aspirated, and shortly thereafter died. The deviation from the standard of care was very clear.

In a recent case we were asked to evaluate, the patient was a woman who, at age 70, had lived a good and productive life, until a truck cut her off and she suffered a car accident. She was airlifted to the hospital with a flail chest. The hospital stabilized her and continued to care for her on a ventilator for about 11 days before a resident physician decided to extubate the patient. Respiratory Care had evaluated the patient and had determined that she was not ready to wean or extubate, but the resident did the extubation herself (it was a teaching facility, and it was early July). The patient started a pulmonary death spiral with increasing respiratory rate and work of breathing, and by the time the resident recognized she was wrong, airway swelling prevented a reintubation. The patient developed brain death and expired. The deviation, in this case, was made all the more clear by the fact that the respiratory therapists charted their findings and the resident ignored them.

These are the kinds of cases that make for good medical negligence cases. They involve very clear deviations from the standard of care. The deviations are obvious from the medical records, and the patient injury is directly tied to the deviation.

b) Lawyers Want It Documented in the Record

The fact that an error or medical misadventure happened is often not evident from the record. If what happened on a given day must be guessed at, most lawyers will not take the case. While this may sound like it argues for not charting findings, that is clearly not the import of the message.

Instead, what lawyers do is they look at the records not only with an eye toward how they will make their claim, but also what the likely defense will be. Is the clinician going to claim that he performed a task or did a check he didn't document? Is the case going to be about documentation, or about something else?

Generally speaking, the better your documentation, particularly the situation the patient was in before coming to see you, the better.

One thing that makes lawyers salivate is to see something that should be documented missing from the record. If the patient should have received their medications, but did not receive them according to the records, the lawyers will argue that if it wasn't charted, it wasn't done. This may not be true, but it makes the plaintiff's job easier.

c) Plaintiffs Want Large Damages

In almost every state, damages for non-economic injury are now capped at a figure between $150,000 and $500,000. These caps make cases that are about pain and suffering less viable for attorneys. For this reason, a malpractice claim where the injured party is a 35-year-old family breadwinner working two jobs to save for his children's college, is better than the same claim for a retired teacher. The teacher will not have lost any income. The teacher will not have lost any fringe benefits. The young man will have lost all of those things.

Generally, elderly patients who have recently retired will not command large judgments or settlements of their malpractice claims. Thus, lawyers look for young men and women with serious, life-changing injuries like paralysis. Injury cases are always better than death cases because injury cases always carry with them the increased costs of medical care into the future.

H. KEY POINTS

- Medical error is not always medical negligence.
- Medical negligence is always medical error.
- Not all error produces a negative outcome.
- Medical error should be disclosed to patients.
- It is possible to disclose medical error without admitting fault or liability.
- The cost of medical error is very high.
- Systems should be analyzed to determine if they are at fault, rather than individual clinicians.
- Plaintiff has the burden of proof in a medical negligence case.
- The defendant doesn't have to prove anything, unless he asserts an affirmative defense.
- Statutes of limitations, statutes of repose, assumption of the risk, contributory fault, and professional judgment are the most commonly asserted affirmative defenses.
- Negligence is a deviation from the standard of care.
- Causation means that the negligent act caused or contributed to cause the injury or damages.
- Damages are economic, non-economic, or punitive in nature.
- Plaintiff usually proves the standard of care through an expert.
- Plaintiff usually proves causation through an expert.
- Therapists can commit other torts, like fraud, slander, libel, breach of fiduciary duty, and assault against patients.
- The best way to protect yourself against malpractice claims is good documentation.
- Documentation should be simple, clear, accurate, legible, and promptly done.
- Documentation should not contain the five "I"s: inaccurate, illegible, improper, irrelevant, and inflammatory.
- Communication is important.
- Good communication prevents lawsuits.
- Therapist-to-nurse and nurse-to-therapist communication should occur in private to reduce misunderstandings by visitors and patients.
- Lawyers want cases easily made from the documentation.

- A lawyer wants a case he can get multiple experts to say "they blew it" and one that is easily understood by a jury.
- Bad documentation is better for lawyers, bad for clinicians.
- Lawyers want cases with very large damages.

I. SUMMARY

Medical negligence and liability are hot button topics in today's world. The issues are complex and the cases are varied. But in the end, every malpractice case comes down to an allegation that something could have been done better, and should have been.

These cases are very difficult for plaintiffs to bring, and very expensive for defendants to defend. They are emotionally draining, and not every case ends with a plaintiff's verdict. But every case changes those who go through it. If you follow the ideas in this book, it should minimize your chances of being sued.

CHAPTER 9

What Every Therapist Should Know About Risk Management

It is easier to perceive error than to find truth, for the former lies on the surface and is easily seen, while the latter lies in the depth, where few are willing to search for it.

Johann Wolfgang von Goethe
18th Century German Literary Giant

A. INTRODUCTION

Every hospital of any size has a risk management department. The primary goal of the Risk Manager in a hospital is to protect the hospital from liability—to constantly look for areas that put the hospital at risk, and to take corrective action when those areas are found. Unfortunately, too many hospitals have a person who considers it her job to "answer complaints." These institutions "don't get it." While complaining patients is one aspect of risk management, the larger purpose of the department is to give life and vitality to the idea that vigilance results in safer patient care. Risk management is part quality assurance, part medical error prevention, and part customer satisfaction. It is also the department that has the greatest impact on how the facility is perceived by angry or upset patients and visitors.

Smaller health care organizations, like durable medical equipment or home care companies, those which are often run by therapists, can't recruit a full-time Risk Manager because it would be prohibitively expensive.

And some group medical practices employing therapists as patient care-givers have risk management departments in name only. But risk management should be a defined job (even if the job is handled by a person whose primary job is something else) in any health care environment. Even if there is no dedicated person or department, risk management should be a major part of every employee's job. Every employee should be trained to look for liability and safety risks and report them to those who can fix the problems.

The job of preventing medical error, improving quality, avoiding litigation, and enhancing patient satisfaction with the organization ultimately rests with each and every employee. Every hospital employee should do exactly what the Risk Manager does: look for hazards, report them, and fix them. Unfortunately, even in good organizations, too little emphasis is placed on risk management. The job is not well-funded. Few resources are given to that department, and very few of the hospital's employees are trained in risk management techniques.

B. WHAT DOES A RISK MANAGER DO?

The first goal of the Risk Manager is to help everyone in the organization avoid medical error. In the hospital environment, this is normally accomplished through aggressive vigilance with respect to patient complaints, incident reports, and employee morale. It includes being notified and involved in the investigation whenever there is a credible allegation (by the physician, the family, or staff) that there has been a medical error. It includes developing systems and methods that allow for the identification of problem areas and problem employees and independent contractors.

It also requires an approach that brings everyone into the tent, so to speak, to make sure that everyone who has a piece of the problem participates in its resolution. Often patients think they have a problem with the hospital, because that is where they were when the problem arose. When careful listening and problem-solving skills are brought to bear on the problem, the issue is really one of dissatisfaction with the physician or a failure of understanding about the disease process itself.

It can't be repeated often enough that while there may be a "Risk Management" department in most hospitals, the **job** of risk management—preventing medical error, managing known risks, and investigating and negating unknown risks—is the job of every employee in the hospital.

1. What Is Systems Analysis?

Systems analysis is the careful and systematic evaluation of a problem, with an eye toward preventing similar errors in the future.

When Robert Courtney began diluting chemotherapy intended for the Kansas City–based physicians he serviced, he never believed he would be caught. Courtney had looked at the system and found a loophole. Cancer drugs are the most expensive drugs available. Chemotherapy is frequently no more than a life-extending process; very few patients obtain a cure from chemotherapy. All but a few patients with cancer were expected to die anyway.

Courtney knew that the individual clinicians who bought their chemotherapy from him (a group of physicians and a gynecological oncologist in the same building) were not doing intensive or focused quality review, improvement, or assurance. So he simply altered the doses that were ordered. When a drug costs $2,000 per dose, and when you give multiple doses, cutting 50% of the dose results in a $1,000 profit per patient. Courtney diluted the drugs and began to pocket the difference.

But for every action there is a reaction, and the reaction to the diluted drugs was that people who should have been experiencing side effects from their chemotherapy—nausea, vomiting, loss of hair—did not experience the side effects. Everyone thought their chemotherapy treatments were incredibly easy to tolerate.

When attorneys interviewed the physicians, their staff, and the patients after the scandal broke, all the patients said the same thing: "I never got sick, I never lost my hair, I thought chemotherapy was the easiest thing I'd ever been through." To a one, the patients treated with outpatient chemotherapy purchased from Courtney didn't suffer symptoms as severe (if they suffered any at all), and almost none of them improved with treatment. The nurses and the clinicians did not pick up on the lack of side effects. Every single clinician—except one—failed to put two and two together.

The physician who did put the pieces together, a courageous and honorable gynecologic oncologist named Verda Hunter, broke the story to the FBI when the sales representative for Eli Lilly continued to ask for proof that she had purchased Gemzar from Courtney. For some reason the drug representative wasn't getting credit. He had asked his company to investigate, and they couldn't give him an answer.

Hunter, an oncologist who specialized in very tough cancer cases, suddenly started putting the pieces together. Continued requests for confirmation of drug purchases, lack of side effects, failures of therapy, patients expiring faster than they would have been expected to die.

Hunter contacted the drug company to find out if it could test a sample of its own drug for potency. The drug company was not able to help her. She finally found an independent laboratory and sent off a sample of the drugs. The laboratory found what should have been a 70% solution of the drug was a 1% solution of the drug.

Hunter contacted the FBI, who had a broader sample of chemotherapy tested. They found that some of the drugs tested were no more than sterile saline solutions. Courtney was investigated, arrested, prosecuted, and ultimately convicted on a guilty plea. He received a 30-year sentence.

The critical piece of the story, however, is that until someone provided a missing scrap of information, the puzzle wasn't pieced together. If the physicians had been doing routine quality analysis, comparing their treatment results with national averages, and their side effects with national statistics, they might have realized much more quickly what Courtney was up to in his pharmacy.

The physicians in the case were not sued for medical negligence even though a credible claim could have been made that they had not picked up on the fact that Courtney's chemotherapy (1) didn't make patients sick, and (2) didn't reverse their disease processes. Simply put, no one was looking for adverse symptoms that did not appear! The main reason that none of Verda Hunter's patients wanted to sue her is the way Hunter handled things.

She did not shrink from her duty and begin buying chemotherapy from someone else. She did not quietly walk away, recognizing that there might be liability. Instead she confronted the problem head on, calling each patient individually, telling that patient what she had learned, and starting a new plan of care. Hunter's attitude and honor won her the respect not only of the patients and their families, but also of the lawyers investigating the case. Hunter was as much a victim as the patients—you could see that in her eyes at her deposition. Her approach to the problem prevented her from being sued.

From a systems point of view, however, if the patients' adverse reactions, including their response to the chemotherapy drugs, had simply been statistically tracked and compared with those of other patients, Courtney's illicit scheme would have been uncovered much sooner.

One of the main reasons that hospitals and health care organizations should track this kind of clinical information (for example, heart rate increases with bronchoactive drugs), is to ensure than when there is a problem with a drug, it can be detected and fixed before patient harm results.

2. Would Systems Analysis Have Stopped Efren Saldivar?

No one may ever know, but it might have, if it had been conducted scientifically, by a Risk Manager instead of by an interested department head who wanted to believe that he ran a department with competent and caring therapists.

When Efren Saldivar was reported to have a "magic syringe" that frequently resulted in patient deaths, the supervisory staff at Glendale Adventist Hospital quickly tallied up deaths on his shift and didn't see any patterns. Oddly no one put together the fact that when Saldivar's patients died, he drew a face with "X" eyes and a protruding tongue on the treatment board. This bit of blindness may have been due to three things: First, the natural tendency to think you work with competent and caring individuals; second, a belief on the part of the supervisors that the individual filing the report had an axe to grind with Saldivar; and third, a desire to protect Saldivar's supervisors from a report to the California Board for Respiratory Care.

When the therapist who initially reported to supervisors that Saldivar might be killing patients discovered Succinylcholine chloride in Saldivar's wall locker, he didn't take further action. The therapist remembered that his original report to his supervisor went uninvestigated (or so he had thought). Since he had entered the locker unlawfully, and knew he could get in trouble for it, he didn't make a report of finding the drugs in the locker.

Only when an ex-convict trying to make a buck through a "reward" scheme told the hospital about Saldivar's acts did the hospital call in the police—more than a year after Saldivar had first been brought to the attention of the hospital. In fact, when Efren Saldivar came in for his police interview, the police had pretty much written off the incident because everyone at the hospital (except the person who originally reported him) denied the story.

The managers in the department and the Risk Managers at the hospital were not looking for any patterns in patient deaths, even though Saldivar was certainly not the first (and not even the last) to use paralytics to cause patient deaths. The circumstances of numerous deaths in the facility, all occurring in roughly the same manner, should have put the facility on notice if they had been conducting proper quality assurance and undertaking a systems analysis of the problems.

3. Why Is Systems Analysis the First Line of Defense?

Nobody wants a problem. Everyone expects not to find a problem. Everyone is happy when everything is okay. That is what social scientists call a "comfortable assumption." For these reasons, and several others related to the practice of cognitive dissonance, most hospitals don't thoroughly analyze the problems that occur. This "stick your head in the sand" attitude leads to liability problems, and lets hospitals get blindsided when the truth finally comes out.

The first line of defense in a hospital is a systems analysis approach to data gathering that looks at quality indicators from the same perspective as a detective investigating suspicious events. If statistical information changes, there must be a reason. Identifying the reason is important. There can be no unexplained variances if a hospital is to avoid liability issues.

In the Saldivar case what the hospital did was leave a wonderful trail of negligence for the civil attorneys to follow. The employee who heard rumors discharged his duty by reporting, but failed to discharge his duty when he found evidence of diverted drugs and drugs that a therapist never uses. His negligence, under the doctrine of *respondeat superior,* would be imputed to the hospital. Similarly, a therapist who was sleeping with Saldivar admitted to the Grand Jury that she had supplied Succinylcholine Chloride to Saldivar for use in his "magic syringe." She was present and did not object to his euthanizing patients. Her active participation shows a willful and wanton disregard for the health and safety of the patients at the medical center, and probably subjects the hospital to punitive damages.[2]

Hopefully, Glendale Adventist has learned from its failures. According to testimony before the Grand Jury, Saldivar (and the therapist who assisted him by getting drugs for him), obtained the medications when they were left sitting on a windowsill in a patient's room. Simple adherence to basic ac-

---

[2]In an odd twist, Saldivar's conduct probably does not subject the hospital to liability. The hospital did not assign him duties where he would normally have used Succinylcholine chloride, and his actions were so far outside the scope of practice of a therapist that the facility could not be charged with liability under *respondeat superior.* The negligence of the supervisory staff and the staff therapists, in failing to detect Saldivar's mercy killing, however, could be (and would be) imputed to the hospital.

countability procedures for dangerous drugs would have prevented Saldivar's access to the medications. More importantly, hopefully Glendale has imposed some mechanism for tracking adverse events.

Every department in a hospital should have means of tracking adverse events and should have a mechanism for the reporting of dangerous and unlawful conduct. Designing systems that encourage the investigation of patient harms is central to a good risk management system.

4. Is This a Search for a Scapegoat?

While a good system is helpful, it must be married with a fair yet rigorous process for finding answers to problems that, more often than not, are **system** problems, not people problems. The quick and easy answer to a therapist turning off the wrong mechanical ventilator is to fire that therapist. However, if the system is also to blame, it should be modified to prevent a recurrence. Any time a therapist discontinues life support or extubates a patient, there should be a two-person check to ensure that it is the correct patient and the correct orders are being followed. Procedures that result in mortality cannot be undone, and must be perfect.

The Duke University Hospital learned this lesson the hard way with transplant recipient Jesica Santillan. Santillan was O positive, and received organs that were A positive. CNN reported, "They told us there had been a mistake and there had been a clerical error and Jesica had received type-A organs. The doctor took full responsibility. He said that it was his mistake; he should've typed the organs, but he failed to do so."

Her body immediately began rejecting the organs, and Santillan fought for her life. They counted on a system that matched organs to donors, and never expected that their system would fail. But personnel had forgotten the basis for the system. While they later blamed the error on a clerical mistake, the real problem was the attitude of the caregivers. The system seemed so certain to avoid error that the staff forgot to question their basic assumptions. When the transplant team requested organs, the transplant donor agency just assumed they had requested the right blood type. They never checked.

Making matters worse in the Santillan case, her surgery had been funded in part by a local donor who brought the child from Mexico. After the first error, the donor complained that the hospital administration had been very hard to deal with. He claimed they did not want unflattering publicity. So the donor hired a medical malpractice attorney.

The hospital countered by trying to block the donor from seeing the child in the hospital. This petty, stupid, and useless tactic resulted in an intervention by Senator Elizabeth Dole. In the end, Jesica died and the hospital suffered a horrible public relations catastrophe. Basic risk management checks could have avoided the entire debacle.

5. How Should Investigations Be Handled?

Once a medical error occurs, it should be promptly investigated. This is not something that should wait weeks for action. People have better memories of events closer to the time something happens, and nothing good comes of waiting. It also sends a bad message to the public: the institution doesn't really care. Investigations must begin promptly.

Investigations must be conducted fairly and impartially, with an eye toward patient safety. Therapists whose care is suspect should be suspended when there is any doubt as to the safety of patients, and the doubt issue should be resolved with a wide margin for error on the part of patient safety. Put another way, there is never a reasonable way to explain how an employee suspected of causing patient harm was allowed to continue to have access to patients.

Scapegoating is never an effective way to deal with a quality issue, or with a risk management issue. While assigning of blame makes those who didn't have any fault feel better, it doesn't solve the problem. The system problem that allowed the error in the first place is completely unaffected by parceling out blame.

Consider a situation, drawn from my personal experience. A therapist changes out a Cascade humidifier and dumps Dakin's solution into the device instead of sterile water. This happens on the evening shift in the middle of a busy night, and isn't discovered right away. Although no patient harm is documented, the patient's family is very badly upset that their mother was exposed to chemical fumes from the Dakin's solution.

In investigating, we found that the cause of the accident was two-fold. First, the therapist did not ascertain that she was using a clean and new bottle of sterile water, one that had not been previously mixed with bleach. Similarly, the nurse had used the top of the ventilator as her own personal work space, and had left the bottle, with but a very small label, capped and available.

Both the therapist and the nurse shared fault for the error; although the primary fault was with the therapist who had the ultimate responsibility to ensure that she was delivering proper care. Neither was officially disciplined by the hospital. Coordination between nursing and the respiratory care department developed several ideas to prevent a recurrence. First, bottles of solutions used by nursing would be kept on the nursing cart, and no place else. Second, a closed-system filler device would be purchased for refilling the Cascade humidifiers.

By implementing two simple but effective system changes, repetition of the error could be easily avoided. Interestingly enough, the incident revealed a problem with the teamwork between the therapists and the nurses. Nurses and therapists were asked to brainstorm ways that teamwork could be improved. The result: improved teamwork between the therapists and the nurses led to several other recommendations that ultimately improved care in the ICU.

As mentioned earlier, searching for someone to blame is a natural human tendency, but it should be avoided. The goal is to find the real culprit, which often is in the system, not the people.

6. How Important Is Identifying Individual Error-Makers?

The best thing an institution can do is maintain what experts call a "blame-free" environment in its organization.[3] It is important to communicate to staff that individuals are not going to be <u>unduly</u> punished for mistakes.[4] It is also important to communicate to staff that the institution realizes that many problems are not individual personnel problems but systems problems, as discussed above. A blame-free environment is essentially a promise to staff to be fair when conducting an investigation.

Adopting the idea that placing blame doesn't solve the problem instills a culture of safety in the organization. Errors and mistakes in patient care are inevitable because people are human, and what is important is to learn from those mistakes and not to cover them up. If an institution encourages reporting of error, it also encourages an investigation so that the root cause is

---

[3]This is because in a hospital where there is a "find a scapegoat" approach to problem solving, the "problem" is considered fixed when someone is identified as responsible and fired. This clearly doesn't fix a system problem.

[4]Blame-free doesn't mean punishment free. If the result of the investigation reveals incompetence, abuse, neglect, or lack of attention to detail, these personal faults should be addressed through appropriate discipline.

found, and so that people who report problems are not the messengers who get shot for delivering the bad news.

7. How Should Investigations into Abuse and Neglect Proceed?

Patient care investigations that involve serious allegations of abuse and neglect must be handled swiftly and conducted so as to protect the privacy of both the patient and the caregiver. They must also be conducted with an eye toward "rumor control" because human nature says that stories that are just too good not to repeat will be repeated, and usually inaccurately. When patients and visitors hear these stories, it impairs their confidence in the hospital, and it also increases the chances that the patient or his family will hear the most incorrect version of what happened to them or to their loved one.

When there is an allegation of abuse or neglect, the first thing that must happen is a prompt and thorough inquiry conducted by someone who speaks for the hospital and has the full authority of the administration to conduct the investigation. The approach should be consistent, and should make sure that individuals and departments inside the facility who ought to know about an investigation and its results are informed.

For example, an investigation into the case of a therapist accused of abuse should include the Risk Manager, the Respiratory Care Director, the Director of Nursing, the Medical Director of Respiratory Care, and the patient and her family. In many situations, it may be necessary to involve the Corporate Compliance Officer, particularly if there is any claim that the therapist engaged in any improper care or delivered care that can't be reimbursed.[5] In some instances, it is a good idea to involve the Public Relations staff (the earlier the better) if the media will eventually learn of the purported wrongdoing.

Early involvement of counsel is also important in situations where there may be liability issues. The debacle of Jesica Santillan and her care at Duke University was made much worse by the attempts of the hospital to thwart an investigation and to shut out Santillan's benefactor from the process. This, more than the error, created the public relations crisis because it made the hospital look like it had something to hide.

---

[5]For example, suppose a hospital learns that a therapist's license lapsed three months earlier. The care delivered by that therapist during that three-month time cannot be compensated by Medicare because it was not given by a licensed provider in accordance with government regulations.

C. HOW DO WE FIND OUT WHAT WENT WRONG?

A good systems approach looks at several different potential areas of inquiry and fully investigates each. The first factor to be investigated is the human factor. Human factors look at the caregiver and what he or she did.

1. What Human Factors Should Be Investigated?

The first human factor is intent. The investigator should determine whether this is a situation where the caregiver who made the error or mistake did so with the intent to cause deliberate harm. In analyzing this issue, the first question is very brief: "Was the action intended?" (e.g., Did the therapist intend to turn off the alarms?). And the next question is, "Did the therapist intend the adverse consequences of this action?" (that the patient would become hypoxemic and die). If either is admitted (as in Saldivar) or discovered (as in Swango), it should be immediately dealt with through suspension and termination of the employee, and reporting of the individual to police for arrest and prosecution.

It is important, however, not to conflate the analysis into one question. We are not trying to determine guilt or innocence. We are trying to determine intention, which is a state of mind. The issue of whether the action was intended is different, and must be determined first. The issue of the result of the action is saved for last.

Let's examine a hypothetical situation where a therapist turns off the alarms on a ventilator and the patient suffers a disconnect and dies. If the therapist turned off the ventilator alarms, he or she may not have understood the consequences that would have resulted from the action. This would be reasonable in a therapist fresh out of school working with a ventilator he or she did not know well. It would not be reasonable in a therapist who had worked for 12 years in the same facility with the same ventilators and the same type of patients.

The first question, however, is "Did the therapist turn off the alarms?" Recently, in a Kansas City hospital, a careful systems analysis resulted in murder charges being brought against a husband who visited his wife in the ICU. The hospital personnel believed that the husband had purposefully turned off the alarms and let his wife (a victim of domestic violence) die. Police personnel were involved quickly, and the prosecutor brought murder charges.[6]

---

[6]The jury acquitted the man of the charges because there was insufficient evidence.

If the therapist turned off the alarms, the next question is whether that act was intentionally done. In other words, did the therapist intend the result? Any therapist who has spent more than ten minutes in an ICU environment has turned off ventilator alarms, or rendered them ineffective on the patient who simply alarms all the time. But usually those patients are one-on-one patients who receive more careful monitoring. Sometimes, however, a therapist will silence alarms and perform an intervention with the idea that as soon as the intervention is completed he or she will turn the alarms back on. A failure to do that is sometimes not discovered until the next ventilator check. Thus, while the act itself was purposeful and intended (shutting off the alarms), the result (patient death) was not intended because the therapist had an intention of restoring the alarms once he was finished. A choking emergency in the next room may have caused him to leave the patient, and forget to restore the alarms. This is negligence, not an intentional act.

Intentional acts do occur, however, and when they do, they must be carefully investigated. Where there is any suspicion that the act may have been intentional, trained criminalists and forensics investigators should be involved.

Many facilities fail to report deliberate harm to authorities for fear of what that might do to their reputations. However, if deliberate harm is disclosed and the media finds out about the conduct through a wrongful death suit or through some other means, the media firestorm will be worse. It is always better to discharge the duty to report to authorities whenever a patient has been deliberately harmed.

2. What About Mere Negligence?

Negligence doesn't get reported to the police, but a good systems analysis looks at the root cause. For example, is the root cause a lack of education or experience in the caregiver? Did the therapist not understand that a patient with epiglottitis cannot be visually examined, or was the therapist just not skilled in pediatrics? Had the therapist who silenced the alarms just forgotten that alarms could be silenced for one minute at a time?

In analyzing the negligence aspect, the investigator looks to determine whether the therapist departed from the protocol or procedures. If there were no protocols, why were no protocols available? If there were protocols and the therapist departed from them, was there a valid scientific reason to do so, or did the therapist lack a complete understanding of the basic disease processes involved? Does the therapist need remedial training on the life support equipment?

Negligence is best addressed through improved training and supervision followed by monitoring of performance through quality improvement. If the therapist continues to make errors, the therapist should be considered for increasingly proportional discipline including suspension or termination.

3. What About Impaired Mental Function?

Another factor to consider is whether the therapist who committed the error is impaired by a mental or physical disability. Sometimes therapists get sick, and no one knows about their medical condition. For example, a therapist might have an eating disorder or undiagnosed medical condition that may impair her judgment. She may handle things well until at some point she becomes incapable of dealing with the stresses of her job. A person with a health problem should be treated and re-evaluated for duty.

Even a therapist with a sprain or a muscle pull might create a negligence problem. The therapist with a sprained ankle can't move as fast and doesn't want to walk as much, so he takes shortcuts. He stops doing full ventilator checks every two hours and instead abbreviates his ventilator checks so he can get off his feet.

Incapacity comes in other forms too. Was the therapist impaired chemically? Does she have a substance abuse problem? Often these therapists don't mean to commit error or induce harm, but they lack the ability to control their addictions. These personnel should be dealt with through employee assistance as the first step, and suspension or termination if repeated.

Hospitals should keep in mind, however, that where a patient death results from the actions of an impaired caregiver, police and prosecutorial agencies may be much less forgiving, and may consider the action of a therapist who works with life support equipment while impaired to be tantamount to intentional wrongdoing in much the same way as the alcoholic who drives while he is drunk. Colorado authorities recently prosecuted an anesthesiologist who fell asleep during a pediatric surgery where the patient died.

4. What Is the Substitution Test?

A key factor in sorting through the human factor issues in an investigation is to examine things through the substitution test. In the substitution test the question is, "Would a similarly trained person, under the same or similar circumstances, have made the same error?" If so, then the problem is most likely a systems problem, not necessarily a human factors problem.

For example, in the case of the patient exposed to Dakin's solution, would another therapist coming into the ICU likely have made the same mistake the night shift person made? If the answer is yes, then the system, not the individual, is the problem. That was what the investigation found because the bottle was improperly marked and placed where the therapist would have assumed it was her supply of sterile water. This pointed out a systems problem.

In another instance, drawn from my personal experience as a manager, a therapist was assigned to provide care in the NICU. When a patient there required resuscitation, he could not get the ambu bag to function properly. An investigation showed that he may have panicked, did not have sufficient training to work with the ambu bag, and was unprofessional in his conduct toward other staff. This <u>was</u> a human factors problem. If you put another therapist in the same situation, almost any of them could have avoided the problem, or taken other corrective action (such as getting another ambu bag).

Only a few months earlier, during a code, an adult resuscitation bag failed to function because it had been incorrectly assembled by a new unlicensed assistant. This person, whose job was to wash and reassemble equipment before sterilization, had not been taught to test resuscitation bags by occluding the end and squeezing the bag. For that reason, when she assembled one incorrectly, she had no way of discovering it. A similar worker of her training level and experience would have made the same error. That error pointed out training and supervision issues, as well as quality control issues.

If the above methodology involving systems analysis seems particularly well thought out, the author can take no credit. It was developed by the National Patient Safety Agency in the United Kingdom for analysis of critical patient incidents there. A copy of the decision-tree setting out the basics of this methodology can be found at http://81.144.177.110/web/display?contentId=3020.

D. IS QUALITY IMPROVEMENT A PART OF EFFECTIVE RISK MANAGEMENT?

Done properly, quality improvement—which looks at improving the quality of care and quality of decisions affecting care—is a part of an overall risk reduction program. Unfortunately, too many hospitals give lip service to Quality Improvement, or maintain such an office only because the Joint Commission requires them to have one.

Ideally, QI is a forward-looking process that tries to identify ways to improve outcomes and procedures. Unfortunately, for many therapists, it becomes no more than a statistical tracking exercise looking at numbers that have no "real world" meaning.

E. HOW DOES TRACKING ERRORS IMPROVE CARE?

Tracking errors improves care by refining failed systems that lead to errors.

Tracking errors, including medication errors, is an important part of quality improvement, but it should never be the only part of the process. All negative quality indicators should be tracked (missed treatments, medication errors, etc.), but in addition, certain proactive screens should be done.

For example, supervisors and managers should go talk to patients and learn what they think about the care they are receiving from staff therapists. Therapist charting and compliance should be assessed for missed therapy, but also for what they do right. The hospital or health care organization should spend some time finding out whom patients identify as the best and most caring therapists, and why. They should then use this information to teach new therapists and re-train employees to improve overall quality.

1. Should Therapists Be Tracking Side Effects of Medications?

Yes, both their existence and, if it happens, their absence, should be recorded.

As mentioned earlier, tracking side effects of medications is a good way to know whether medical supplies are becoming stale or out-of-date. If bronchoactive medications are not causing heart rate increases, or are causing increases only for certain therapists, there may well be an issue with respect to patient teaching or personnel performance. Are certain therapists just "assuming" that there is a heart rate increase? Are the drugs fresh? Is patient care being delivered according to policy and procedure?

Periodically all therapists should be evaluated for what could best be termed "institutional laziness." The process of copying data from one prior reading to the next, without actually assessing the patient, is more common than most department heads would want to believe.

While no one wants to feel as if "big brother" is watching, some effort should be made to actively supervise employees on all shifts. No one paid much mind to the night shift at Glendale Adventist until patients started showing up with Succinylcholine chloride in their veins and respirations absent. Active supervision and follow-up is the best way to avoid an "Efren Saldivar" situation.

2. How Do We Encourage Error Analysis?

When errors are uncovered, thorough analysis of what went wrong, and how it was discovered, should be examined. The "lessons learned" from the experience should be written into the policies and procedures of the institution. There should be a great deal of investigation into ways to avoid similar problems, and research should be conducted at other institutions. How does another hospital handle the same problem? That information could be very useful to therapists in developing systems that prevent these errors from recurring.

3. What Is the Golden Rule of Avoiding Litigation?

In countless presentations to therapists and other health care providers across the country, I have shared my experience with patient litigation. I have told clinicians what I consider to be the golden rule of health care law: people do not sue medical providers whom they like. They do not sue hospitals that they believe are generally good places with generally good management. Put another way, no one sues a friend.

Whom do they sue? They sue that uncaring person who didn't listen to them. They sue that large, faceless corporation that sent them a $15,000 bill for six hours in the emergency room, where they were not even able to save the patient's life. They sue the nurses who were rude. They sue the physicians who were uncaring and would not answer their questions. And most importantly, they sue people who they believe tried to cover up wrongdoing.

Consider the instance where a patient has a very bad outcome from surgery. The bone in her arm develops avascular necrosis, and she loses a sizable amount of length from the arm. She endures two very painful restorative procedures. She is upset at the hospital.

She brought her case to me. She explained that she wanted to sue the hospital. After a thorough review of the medical records, the conversation went something like this:

> *Me:* *We've analyzed the hospital records, and we have determined that the surgeon made a horrible error when he did your surgery. You have a cause of action against the surgeon.*
>
> *Her:* *I don't want to sue the surgeon. The surgeon plays golf with my husband. I want to sue the hospital.*

Me.   But the hospital didn't do anything wrong.

Her: What? They brought me the wrong food tray. They gave me the wrong medications. And the nursing staff was very rude to me.

This lovely lady then launched into a ten-minute recitation of everything the hospital had done wrong. After examining each one, we analyzed the error or omission from the standpoint of causation: did the error cause her arm problem and the loss of use of the arm? The answer was always no.

Our law firm declined her case, but another attorney might have felt differently about it. It is important to remember that patients don't sue people they like, but they have no problem suing those they don't like, even when there may be no basis for doing so.

4. How Does This Affect Patient Incidents?

It has been my experience that patients will frequently talk to their respiratory therapist about the nurse, to the nurse about the therapist, and to anyone who will listen about their doctor. If they like their doctor, they will sing his praises. If they do not, they will tell you how he bills $115 to see them in the hospital, and spends less than ten minutes with them. The point is, when a patient gets upset about something that has happened, they tell someone, and that's a good thing.

Sometimes it is tempting to write off what a patient tells you as a "silly" concern. The family notes something different about Cousin Earl sitting there in the bed, and a few hours later he is in ICU from respiratory failure. The family complains "we tried to tell the respiratory therapist he was doing badly, but she wouldn't listen."

Of course, at the time, the therapist had seven other treatments to give, she had medications that were due to be delivered, and it was a weekend when she was working with insufficient staff and supervision. She was busy, and she didn't understand or care about the family's view that Cousin Earl didn't look quite right. From the therapist's perspective, Earl didn't look right when she came on—she didn't notice any change.

These are the kinds of incidents that lead to malpractice claims. When you hear a family member say something about what a bad job the floor nurse did in a particular case, that information should be reported to the Risk Manager as quickly as possible, not because it is true, but because it must be investigated. If the family complains about another therapist, that should be reported to the department head even if you know the therapist and believe that therapist delivers excellent care.[7]

The reason for the report is not to give the therapist, nurse (or heaven forbid, the physician) a hard time. The reason is to give the Risk Manager a chance to evaluate the patient's complaint while the Risk Manager can still do something about it. If the Risk Manager can talk to the patient and investigate, that is often all the family member wants.

Many times, if a patient thinks they have been listened to, and if they believe that negative feedback will be acted on, they will talk to the hospital personnel. If the hospital gives no indication that it cares one way or the other what the patient thinks, then the feedback will come in the form of a lawsuit filed against the hospital.

5. When Should I File an Incident Report?

Every time a therapist knows of an adverse event, bad outcome, or medical error, that information should be reported directly to Risk Management. This is equally true when the person making the error is a physician, because the hospital is just as apt to be blamed for the doctor's error as it is an error on the part of the staff.

Although most physicians are caring, competent, diligent perfectionists, everyone has a bad day now and then, and there are a few physicians who simply do not care if they make an error. Many simply refuse to recognize an error. But if the patient or family is upset by what they perceive as an error, that should be reported to the Risk Manager, to allow him to deal with the problem.

This is especially important to the health care organization. Frequently the hospital is blamed for "not providing information" to the physician, and the physician for not acting on information provided. The hospital is always in the stronger position when it has provided the information. The hospital is also in a stronger position when it cares about the quality of care that its patients are receiving. This allows it to gather information that can be used to defend it, and its personnel, from a lawsuit.

---

[7]Once a complaint like that is lodged, it is a good idea to assign the patient to another therapist to prevent an allegation of "retaliation" later. Therapists should also not take the complaining personally. A therapist who has never been the subject of a patient complaint likely is not doing his or her job.

6. Can You Admit Error Without Admitting Liability?

One of the most important things a Risk Manager can do is admit error without admitting liability. If that sounds somewhat contradictory, it is because when we make a mistake, we traditionally think in terms of "my fault." Fault, however, is similar to liability, and admitting fault is the same, in many jurisdictions, as admitting liability.

But error and liability, as established earlier, do not always go hand in hand.

C. H., a 40-year-old single woman, 60 inches tall, 320 pounds, is admitted to Big N Mighty Hospital with a potential colloid cyst in her uterus. She is supposed to get some diagnostic testing, including radiographic imaging and CT scanning, but this is delayed by a series of trauma patients. Her family continues to ask when she will be seen.

On her third hospital day, her temperature spikes to 104 and her blood pressure starts to drop. Emergency surgery is scheduled. Due to problems with the surgical field, the surgeon is not able to get all the infected material. The patient becomes septic and dies.

How does the Risk Manager handle the situation when the family says "if you guys had done your CT scan on time, my daughter would still be alive?"

First, again, it is important to isolate the medical error in the case (failure to diagnose peritonitis, failure to complete surgical removal of necrotic tissue, sepsis, and death) with the issue of liability. Admitting liability would mean admitting that the hospital caused the patient's death.

The Risk Manager here listens to the family. He asks questions. "Are you saying you believe, or you've been told, that if we had gotten a CT scan earlier this event might have been avoided?"

This is the most important part of the process. Sometimes the family is just upset that their loved one died. All they really want is some compassion and someone to understand the loss they feel. A Risk Manager who is an active listener helps achieve this goal.

When the family responds to that question with a definitive "yes," the Risk Manager says, "well I understand completely how you could feel that way." Validating the family's right to feel angry and upset is an important part of making the family feel that their complaints have been heard, and not ignored.

When the family is finished grieving and complaining, the Risk Manager says "I am truly sorry for your loss. I know how upset I would be if my sister died under these circumstances, and I understand you're upset because we didn't get a CT done. A hospital has a duty to serve all patients, and under the rule of "triage" certain critically ill patients must come before others."

"Let me see if I can explain this," the Risk Manager continues. "If we have a patient with a traumatic injury to the abdomen, he is going to get bumped in front of someone like your daughter because he is a known emergency. At the time your daughter's procedure was rescheduled, we didn't know she was an emergency. Nothing in her vital signs told us that. When she got sick all of a sudden, the decision was made to take her to surgery right away, without a CT scan. That was the best thing we could do under the circumstances. But even with a CT, there is no guarantee that surgery would have been a success. I can assure you that triage was handled appropriately. But we are very sorry that she died."

"Now, as you know, your daughter died from sepsis, which is from an infection. She obviously came in with that infection. The doctor did everything he could to find and clean out the infection. Now, I don't speak for him, but I know he is very upset that he wasn't able to save your daughter. Would you like me to set up an appointment for you to visit with him about this?"

In our example here, the Risk Manager has expressed his regret over the outcome, and has explained the choices the hospital made. He has effectively apologized with the explanation, and has offered an opportunity for the family to be heard by the doctor.

In most situations this will end the claim of malpractice right here. The family understands that the trauma patient was an emergency. The family understands that the hospital tried its best. In 99% of the cases, this explanation will satisfy the family and will permit them to achieve some closure without the necessity of bringing a malpractice lawsuit.

This happens because the patient's family knows that they have been heard.

But what about the situation where the error is entirely on the part of the hospital? Suppose we have a situation where the therapist, as noted earlier, puts Dakin's solution into a ventilator Cascade?

Here, the Risk Manager explains the error, explains why it happened, and what the hospital's investigation revealed. The Risk Manager apologizes for the outcome: "we're sorry your mom had to breathe those fumes for so long." Then the Risk Manager says, "we've identified a system problem here, and we've studied why it happened and have worked out a system to prevent this error from ever occurring again."

Again, the Risk Manager has carefully avoided accepting fault for the error, but instead, simply expressed his remorse for the outcome.

Sometimes family members want more. "I don't think we should have to pay for the two extra days that dad was in the ICU!"

In those situations it is frequently a good idea to make an economic concession, but when the hospital makes that concession, it may be an unofficial admission of liability. When a discount or cost savings is given to the family for what happened, some courts interpret that as an admission of liability. Those courts may reason that if the hospital had not been at fault, it would not have made the concession.[8]

For this reason, when a therapist makes an error and decides to "just not charge you for the treatment," he may be making a binding admission on his part and his employer's part. This is not something that should be done without the concurrence of Risk Management and hospital counsel.

7. When Should a Mediator Be Considered?

Sometimes in smaller health care operations, for example, the home health care company owned and managed by a therapist, there is simply no way to have a separate Risk Manager, and therefore, no way to effectively deal with situations where there is a potential for liability.

In this situation either an attorney should be hired or a mediator should be retained. Suppose the issue is whether a particular piece of equipment was functioning properly and may have contributed to a patient being re-admitted to the hospital. Since the DME business is a small company, it is possible that the owner may be the one who set up and inspected the equipment. Because he is simply "too close" to the situation, he is not the ideal person to deal with the risk management problem because he cannot be objective.

Although hiring an attorney may send the wrong message to some people (i.e., "sue me") it may be the smartest course of action. An attorney can explain things to the patient's family, and can take steps to protect the small business owner from liability.

A mediator is similarly a good choice. An individual who specializes in mediating disputes is ideally equipped to approach the family on behalf of the business owner, and this is something that should be considered, depending on the nature and severity of the situation.

---

[8]Conversely, courts do not generally permit evidence of corrective measures taken after such an incident (for example, changing to a closed humidification system) because public policy supports the idea that hospitals should improve care, and an improvement in care is not necessarily related to negligence.

Any patient death or serious injury that is credibly linked to human or product error presents a liability risk. Irrespective of whether the business owner ultimately uses the services of a mediator or attorney to contact and deal with the family, malpractice carriers should be notified and an attorney should be retained. That attorney should be asked to provide guidance on what can be said and what should not be said to the family.

8. Why Is It Necessary to Protect the Medical Record?

Another key task of the Risk Manager is protecting the medical record from alteration or destruction. There is a rule of evidence that allows a jury to assume that altered or missing records would have supported the patient's case against the provider. The Risk Manager's first task on learning that there is a claim of medical error is to flag the record and impose a copying control on the record.[9] That is necessary because, unfortunately, there are people (including physicians) who will try to change things in the medical record after the case is filed. This is neither smart, nor helpful.

9. What's the Problem with Record Alteration?

The worst problem with altering, amending, or destroying a medical record is the impression it leaves in the jury's mind. You, the health care provider, have something to hide, or you didn't do something you should have.

If a medical record is lost or destroyed, that is almost a prima facie admission that the record contains information that hurts, rather than helps, the therapist's case. There is no way, in most jurisdictions, to escape an instruction from the judge that the jury may consider this in determining fault.

The other major problem is that if records are altered or changed after the fact, that alteration or change will most likely be detected. Inks can be dated. Handwriting can be compared at the microscopic level. Forgeries, where someone scrawls the name of another provider in order to cover their own tracks, are almost always the easiest of cases for an attorney to have.

While some alterations might go unnoticed, the damage to the case if it happens is simply too great. That's why, good or bad, the Risk Manager seizes the record the minute there is lawyer involvement, and isolates it from

---

[9]Any request for medical records from an attorney should be referred first to the Risk Manager for evaluation. Counsel may need to be involved at this stage to determine whether there is a reason to report the matter to the facility's insurance carrier.

any other provider, including the physician. A log is kept of the record's storage, and who had access to that record on what dates. If a physician or therapist needs to review the record, that should be done under the watchful supervision of a Risk Manager to prevent any alterations from being made.

10. Do Late Entries Create a Problem?

Yes, but not as much as record alteration or destruction. As mentioned earlier, getting a record admitted into evidence relies on the fact that the annotations were made at or near the time of the events recorded. If an entry is made a month or more after the event, the altered part of the record will most likely not be admissible because it will not fit within the exception to the hearsay evidence rule. For this reason, late entries should be kept to an absolute minimum.

11. Why Index the Medical Record?

Any time there is a lawsuit, the medical record should be indexed. Every page should be stamped with a unique number, and care should be taken to get the front and back of every page in the medical record. A chronology should be prepared for each provider who administered care, setting forth which entries are their entries, what dates and times they provided care, and whether or not they figure into the liability issues in the case.

Even when a therapist doesn't provide care that is directly related to the liability issues, she may still be subpoenaed to provide testimony about the patient. For this reason, it is important to know how many times a therapist saw a patient, where she saw him, and what she did to him when she saw him. An index to the medical record prevents the therapist from having to browse the entire record to see the care she provided.

Many therapists and nurses review medical records for plaintiffs' attorneys. They examine patient care records looking for deviations from the standard of care as well as indexing the caregivers, physicians, and medications given. Therapists are frequently paid from $50 to $125 an hour for such work, depending on the quality of their end product.

12. What About Departmental Records Not in Medical Records?

Some records in the hospital are not routinely made a part of the medical record, but are still subject to discovery. While the blood gas report may be easily rewritten after the fact to conceal a hypoxemia situation, the computerized record of blood gas results maintained in the instrument, or the paper record maintained by the instrument, are still subject to review and subpoena.

Likewise, quality control records showing that the blood gas instrument was out of control, or was not functioning properly at the time of a critical event, can be subpoenaed even though they are not part of the medical record. Therapists should be careful about mentioning such records when they are deposed, unless they are asked directly about them. It might appear to a juror that the therapist or facility had something to hide by maintaining what amounts to two separate sets of records of test results, with only one of those going on the chart. Remember, what may be innocent to you, may make you look guilty to a jury.

13. What Is an Incident Report?

An incident report is a privileged communication[10] from a hospital employee to a Risk Manager, attorney, and insurance company. It sets out the facts of what happened in a place and manner separate from the medical record, so that there will be an alternate record of what went on.

The rationale for an incident report seems to be that when care is delivered, that is recorded in the chart. When errors external to the patient are made (for example, a therapist leaves the bed rails down on a patient with dementia, and the dementia patient falls and breaks a hip). The error should be documented in something other than the chart because while the outcome of the error is important in treating the patient, the error itself is not. The patient record contains the statements: "Patient found on floor. Assessment shows left leg externally rotated and shorter than right. Patient transported to Radiology. . . ."

The incident report, however, contains the information that the therapist saw the patient at 1:00 a.m., left the room, and the nurse found the bed rails down and the patient on the floor at 1:33 a.m.

From day one, hospital employees are wrongly taught to fear the incident reporting system. An "incident report," to most employees, is the same thing as a disciplinary incident. (Although incident reports cannot be used, in most hospitals, as the basis for a disciplinary action, the facts and circumstances brought to light by an incident report can be.) For this reason, no one wants

---

[10]In most states, a "work product" privilege attaches because the document is prepared on advice of and for the use of counsel.

an incident report written on them, and no one wants to write one because he or she doesn't want to get a fellow therapist or employee in trouble.

14. How Important Are Incident Reports?

They are vital because memories fail. In fact, incident reports are the most vital part of the risk management process because these are documents that are, in **most** jurisdictions, privileged, and more than likely contain information not in the medical record.[11] That means that the hospital can document the facts and circumstances of what happened without worrying about the incident report falling into the hands of a plaintiff's attorney.

15. What if My Small Company Doesn't Have Incident Reports?

Most hospitals, nursing homes, and health care facilities of any size have an incident reporting system. Some smaller businesses, like home care and DME companies, do not. When a therapist does not have an incident report form to fill out, he can accomplish the same goals by taking a clean sheet of paper and writing at the top of the sheet "NOTES PREPARED FOR MY AT-TORNEY IN ANTICIPATION OF LITIGATION" and, at the bottom of the page, "ATTORNEY-CLIENT and/or WORK PRODUCT PRIVILEGE." The therapist can then write out the facts and circumstances of the event. The notes should be placed in a sealed envelope with the same instructions on the outside, and held for the therapist's attorney if a lawsuit is filed. Documents should be maintained for at least one year past the statute of repose date.[12]

16. Is an Incident Report a "Gotcha!"?

It should never be used as a gotcha. Some hospitals and department directors use it that way, but it should not be used that way.

---

[11]Some states do not recognize a privilege for incident reports, and do not shield them unless they are prepared by or on behalf of an attorney or an insurance company. Check with your attorney in your jurisdiction to find out whether incident reports are privileged.

[12]An attorney should advise you on how long to maintain these documents. The attorney should be retained to provide the advice and, if he won't charge you additionally for the service, should receive a copy of the original document for his records and retention. Therapists should remember that when an event involves a minor or an incompetent patient, statutes of limitation do not apply, and only a statute of repose would terminate the rights of the patient to sue. Every therapist should know what the applicable statutes are in his or her state.

Because there is a universal feeling among employees that an incident report is a "gotcha" report, Risk Managers and department heads need to instill confidence in the process by writing reports themselves. The idea that an employee can be fired for an incident report is universally accepted in most hospitals and is also universally untrue in most hospitals.

The purpose of the incident report is not "gotcha" but "don't let the lawyer getcha." An incident report takes the employee's best recollection of the events and circumstances that occurred at the time, and records them so that if a lawsuit is filed, the lawyers representing the therapist or hospital have a factual record made at or near the time of the incident, which they can use to refresh the memory of the therapist about important facts and circumstances.

Sometimes a nurse will write an incident report, and the therapist might think that satisfies the requirement. The problem is, the nurse will write down what is important to her, and not what is important to the therapist. She may gloss over breath sounds, pulse oximetry readings, and other clinical data that the therapist feels is important and justifies the actions taken.

Sometimes nurses write incident reports as "gotchas" aimed at a particular therapist. In some hospitals, if an incident report is written by one party, no one else may write an incident report on the same incident.[13] Moreover, for administrative reasons, once an incident report is written, all copies must be controlled and accounted for.[14] This is one reason why a therapist must also keep separate records if there is conflict about what happened and who did what. The form just described with the attorney-client privilege information properly placed at the top and bottom is one way to keep a record for your own personal files.

Of great importance in the incident reporting process is the admonition not to place any record or reference to the incident report in the medical record:

> *8:20 p.m. Found ventilator oxygen setting at 100%. Reset oxygen to 50% as ordered. See Incident Report. Sally Smith, RRT*

A notation of the preceding variety is the kind of thing that will remove the privilege from the document because the medical record now refers to, and

---

[13]This kind of muddle-headed thinking is what makes plaintiffs' lawyers wealthy.

[14]A document is only privileged if it is designed to be privileged. If everyone gets a copy of the incident report, there may be no way to maintain the privilege.

incorporates by reference, an external document. This removes the shield of privilege because by referencing the incident report document, the writer is intending for a reader of the medical record, in order to get the full story, to look up and read the incident report. This should never be done.

17. How Do I Write a Good Incident Report?

In the 1950s and 1960s, Jack Webb portrayed the television detective Sergeant Joe Friday in the crime series Dragnet. Webb's signature line in the series was "just the facts ma'am." Friday viewed detective work as "a glamourless, thankless job that's gotta be done."[15] He was never interested in the emotions or the "why" of what went down, just the "what" of it. It made him a good TV detective, and a bit of an icon.

Friday's Rule, as lawyers know it, is to just get the facts. In interviews, that is rarely easy. An interview with a new client often takes 30 to 45 minutes because people want to talk about the why of what happened rather than the facts of the incident.

Do not fall into this trap when writing incident reports. Incident reports are not a place where you, as therapist, should attempt to even the score by including every invective known to man about the clueless, hapless LPN who extubated your patient:

8:23 p.m. Called stat to the ICU where Donita had extubated Mr. Jones. She claimed she was trying to move him up in bed and left his hand untied for a minute and he extubated himself. But really what I am pretty sure happened is the idiot just forgot to move the tubing holder when she pulled him up, and the tube just came right out. I had told her three times this shift that I needed her help in retaping the tube, but no, she couldn't help me because she had to sit on her fat butt and jawbone with Clarice and Monica at the nurses station. And because she is lazy, I wound up having to try to stick a tube in this guy who has a fat neck and is a PIA to intubate. Shelly Smith, RRT	"she claimed" "what really happened?" "idiot" "sit on her fat butt and jawbone..." All of these statements are emotional and would not help an attorney defend a claim of negligence against the therapist.

Figure 9-1 Example Incident Report

---

[15]In this respect, police work and respiratory care share similar aspects. The role of the therapist is rarely filled with glamour.

Rather, an incident report should be a short retelling of what you saw, what you heard, what you did, and what is important to the defense of any claim:

8:23 p.m. Called to ICU to reintubate Mr. Jones. Patient found with labored respirations, pulse oximetry reading 90%. Preoxygenated with 100% oxygen. Sprayed with Cetacaine in two small bursts. Two attempts made to intubate, complicated by patient's thick neck. Used a Miller #4 to intubate because I could not get visualization with a macintosh blade. No trauma to teeth. Pulse oximeter never went below 90% during attempts. Intubated on third attempt. Placed on 100% oxygen for five minutes, and then returned to previous 50% setting. Heart rate did not go above 120. Respiratory rate 28–30. Patient anxious but cooperative. Stayed with patient for 10 minutes after event to hold his hand and calm him down. I did not see extubation. I heard a nurse say that Mr. Jone's hands were not tied down. His hands were tied when I entered the room. Shelly Smith, RRT	Factual account of incident. No emotion. All relevant clinical data. Lawyer would take from this report the fact that patient was not harmed. Ideally much of this same documentation would go in the medical record as well, but without the last paragraph.

Figure 9-2 Example of Better Incident Report

Incident reports should not include suppositions about what happened, what a person thinks might have happened, who might be at fault, and especially, it should never point out blame as to any party, especially a physician. Record the facts. An incident report, in some instances (and through lawyer error) can sometimes be discovered. When that happens, you don't want to appear to a jury to be a loose cannon who was blaming everyone else without accepting any responsibility. The way around that is to record the facts, not your suppositions, beliefs, and emotions.

18. How Important Is Guest Relations?

Guest Relations is the second pillar of the temple of risk management because good guest relations keep patients, visitors, and family members happy. It may not appear obvious that a portion of this chapter is aimed at guest relations, but the keystone of any good risk management plan is an excellent guest relations plan.

19. Do Guest Relations Affect Lawsuits?

Yes, absolutely! The golden rule of litigation is that people don't sue people they like. They go to those people and work out their differences. Being liked is seldom at the top of the therapist's list. We have to poke people with needles, give them treatments that make them cough when they have large abdominal incisions, and we have to do unpleasant things to people on ventilators. So being liked is seldom at the top of the list because we care about the person, not what they think of us.

But it is vital to the therapist and the facility to build a rapport and relationship with each patient and his or her family in order to prevent litigation later on.

A good guest relations program begins with an analysis of the facility (or, in the case of a physician's office or home care company, the business). Ideally, this is done by a professional facilitator who can find out what the facility does well, what it does poorly, and where it can most improve.

A site survey is conducted where patients who are out of the hospital one week or less are interviewed. A second survey is done of patients one month out of the hospital (always a different group). A third survey is done on patients and their family members who last went to the hospital six months ago. The first group has the experience fresh in their minds and may be able to highlight subtle areas of improvement that won't come out in the later interviews.

The one-month and six-month interviews will highlight the most important flaws in the hospital guest relations program because they will be looking at things that patients remembered long after they were discharged.

The information from this survey is placed into a matrix, and a wide range of issues evaluated. Is the hospital properly signed? Can patients find Radiology when they need to, and can they distinguish between Radiology and Radiation Oncology? Do outpatients have to wait too long? Do patients coming to the hospital for stat care get appropriate service?

Several months ago I was evaluated for a potential blood clot in my left leg. I was sent to our local hospital with orders for a STAT EKG, Stat D-Dimer, and an ultrasound of both legs. On arrival at the hospital, which is not the hospital I routinely use, I was asked to wait for 20 minutes while they found an Admissions person, and then the Admissions person had me wait another 15 minutes in her office while she tried to figure out which test should be done first.

"Don't you think maybe those stat tests should be done first," I prompted.

"No, doctors write 'stat' all the time," the Admissions person confided, hooking the first two fingers on both hands over her head as she said the word "stat."

If stat means "do it when you feel like it" at that particular facility, it is no wonder that doctors write it all the time. Admitted with a diagnosis of "rule out DVT," I didn't feel very important when it took three hours to get the stat EKG. The message to the patient was clear: we don't care.

Doubtless the hospital administration is completely clueless about the message they are sending to the community through their Admitting department. A good guest relations program would help to remedy that by identifying the areas for improvement.

Once areas are identified, those that are easy to fix (like signage) are addressed first. Then all hospital personnel, and especially all the physicians admitting at that facility, are required (as a condition of continued privileges at the facility) to participate in a two-hour guest relations training program.

Guest Relations is everyone's job at the hospital. If a patient's family member is lost, it's the job of the respiratory therapist who finds them wandering the halls to get that family member back to the patient, unless, of course, they have a stat call that takes precedence.

20. Why Is a Patient's Perception Important?

A patient's perception is his or her reality. From a litigation-avoidance perspective, that is the only perception that matters.

You see, there is an interesting bonus that comes from understanding and applying guest relations principles. A therapist who makes sure that Mildred finds her husband, John, in the Radiology Department is thought of not so much as another faceless worker, but as "that lovely man from Respiratory who made sure I got back here." As a result of this one act of kindness, every therapist is thought of as competent and professional (unless he or she demonstrate otherwise). The housekeeping person who waters the patient's plant is not thought of as just another housekeeper, but a friend who looked after a sick person's plants. The hospital is thought of as a "caring and respectful" facility. The hospital may in fact be a bona fide "Three Stooges" operation. They may not be capable of finding the patient in the bed, but patient perception is reality because most patients cannot objectively evaluate quality of care.

Post-program evaluations at the one-week, one-month, and six-month time frames are conducted after training to document the improvement. Almost universally, the thing that people say is "what a change I have noted here." Patients believe the hospital has more caring and attentive staff, and the community believes that the hospital is a good place to go when sick.

The perception of the community changes, but not the reality. The hospital's therapists are no more competent than they were before the training. They are no more professional. But they are viewed that way because the patient associates courtesy, caring, and attention with professionalism and competence, even though the two may not be related at all.

In short, every employee wins, but especially the Risk Management department. The reason is simple and bears repeating yet again: people don't sue hospitals, health care providers, and therapists that they like.

F. KEY POINTS

- Risk Management is the science of avoiding litigation through management of known risks and identification of unknown risks.
- Risk Management may be assigned to one department, but it is every person's job.
- Good Risk Management focuses on systems, not individuals.
- Every bad outcome should be investigated to determine what could be improved.
- Systems Analysis is the first line of defense of a hospital.
- Quality Improvement is an integral part of risk management.
- Quality Improvement pays attention to errors and omissions as well as normal routine factors.
- Quality Improvement should be aimed at detecting both the presence of error and absence of expected outcomes (e.g., detecting that patients are not having heart rate increases with bronchoactive drugs).
- Every bad outcome should be investigated with an eye toward systems analysis, not scapegoating.
- While individuals may be the cause of problems, they are frequently not the only cause of problems.
- An investigation examines:
  - Was the action deliberate?
  - Was the harm intended?
  - Was there a lack of knowledge, skill, or training?
  - Was there negligence?
  - Was there an issue with health or substance abuse?
  - Would a similar therapist under the same circumstances make the same error (if so, it's a system problem)?
- The Golden Rule of Litigation is that people do not sue people they like.

- The therapist should be the eyes and ears of the Risk Manager and report when patients are unhappy with care.
- Incident reports should be routinely written whenever there is an error.
- Incident reports should not place blame, but should record what happened, limited to just the facts of the incident.
- When an incident report form is not available, you can prepare confidential notes for your attorney.
- The best malpractice insurance is good guest relations.
- Guest Relations is important because it promotes a good community image.

G. SUMMARY

Risk management is not just a department in the hospital; it is a way of life in today's health care environment. For this reason it is important for every therapist to be cognizant of what Risk Managers do, and how they can help therapists.

CHAPTER 10

Protecting Yourself and Your Employer

Litigation: A machine which you go into
as a pig and come out of as a sausage.

Ambrose Bierce
20th Century American Author and Satirist

A. INTRODUCTION

Because therapists have a limited scope of practice, they normally work in the hospital environment, and not in home care, physicians' offices, or other settings. While there are some notable exceptions, and some therapists have blazed the trail in these other venues, for the most part, the majority of therapists continue to practice in the hospital environment.

Therapists tend to think of their employers as entities that provide a job and paycheck. While for some therapists the issue of "loyalty" to the institution is founded on the next paycheck, and does not arise out of some deep-seated love for the institution, it nonetheless inures to the benefit of the therapist to actively protect his facility's interests in doing his job.

This chapter highlights the duties that therapists have in protecting their facility from five different types of claims related to special health care statutes. It examines the clinician's duty to report abuse, and the clinician's duties with regard to the state licensure system. It examines Antitrust, Consumer Fraud, and Class Action litigation as it applies to hospitals, and ends with a discussion of Corporate Compliance in the health care industry.

B. WHAT ARE A CLINICIAN'S DUTIES IN REPORTING ABUSE AND NEGLECT?

Simply put, if you have reason to suspect abuse of a minor or an elder, you are obligated to report it.

State laws and local ordinances may require that a respiratory therapist who becomes aware of violence directed at senior citizens, children, and spouses report that abuse to law enforcement or other authorities. These statutes normally contain a criminal penalty clause for failure to report.

1. What About Elder Abuse?

In Missouri, as one example, a health care worker is required to report abuse of an elder, defined as a person 60 years of age or older. The statute says:

> *565.188. 1. When any* . . . **home health agency** *or* **home health agency employee; hospital and clinic personnel** *engaged in examination, care, or treatment of persons;* . . . **other health practitioner;** . . . **or other person with responsibility for the care of a person sixty years of age or older** *has reasonable cause to suspect that such a person has been subjected to abuse or neglect or observes such a person being subjected to conditions or circumstances which would reasonably result in abuse or neglect, he or she shall immediately report or cause a report to be made to the department in accordance with the provisions of sections 660.250 to 660.295, RSMo.* . . .
>
> *2. Any person who knowingly fails to make a report as required in subsection 1 of this section is guilty of a class A misdemeanor.*

The highlighted terms in the statute comprise most of the places where therapists work, and most of their duties. Some states name respiratory therapists by name, while others lump them in under "other health care workers."

The statute is important. A therapist who knows of "reasonable cause to suspect" abuse must report it, and that duty is not discharged by telling a physician or nurse to report it, or relying on those professionals to do it. The only way you discharge your duty to report is to pick up the phone and make the report. Simply put, there are no exceptions.

Should a therapist be directed not to report something that he has a legal duty to report, his adherence to hospital policy on this issue will not be a defense in the criminal action brought against him. The therapist cannot say "my boss told me not to report" and defend a criminal charge. It will not matter because no one may command you to disobey the criminal law.

What Happens When You Don't Report?

In 1999, nursing home executive Charles Kaiser had implemented a policy that prohibited nurses and administrators from reporting abuse and neglect in his nursing homes. In 2003, he was convicted for failure to report because he did not alert proper authorities to the abuse a patient suffered while his company was managing the nursing home.

It may not appear obvious, but one reason why the statute regarding reporting abuse is a land mine for therapists is that failure to report and protect an elder creates the situation where a therapist breaches a mandatory state-imposed duty to protect the elder. This breach of duty can be the basis for a tort lawsuit against the therapist and his or her employer for damages. The theory of that lawsuit will be *negligence per se*, that the therapist knew of the law, and consciously chose not to obey it. This also becomes a basis for punitive damages!

Every therapist should be cognizant of the duty to protect elders and report abuse so as to prevent a claim that the therapist or hospital breached a duty and caused the patient to receive further damages.

3. What About Child Abuse?

Like elder abuse, most states require the reporting of injuries to children that a clinician "reasonably suspects" of being inflicted through abuse. When should a clinician report abuse? Whenever there is any reasonable suspicion. Failure to report can be tragic not only for the child, but for the clinician. In 2004, nurse Leslie Ann Brown was accused of a misdemeanor count of failure to report child abuse when a small child, Dominic Foster, died after abuse by foster parents. Although the charges were later dismissed by the prosecutor in a plea agreement, Brown fought her case all the way to the Supreme Court. You can find the case at Appendix C-2.

Like the requirement to report elder abuse, the duty to report child abuse is statutorily imposed, and breach of that duty not only subjects a therapist to potential criminal liability, but may subject the organization or entity to both criminal liability and civil liability in tort.

Therapists must always ensure that the duty to report has been fulfilled in order to fully protect themselves and their organizations.

4. Do the Same Rules Apply to Spousal Abuse?

Not in most states. Spousal abuse has not been elevated to a level consistent with child or elder abuse, and most states do not have mandatory reporter laws. However, that does not rule out a duty to report facts and circumstances to appropriate authorities. Under *Tarasoff v. Regents of the University of California,* 17 Cal.3d 425, 551 P.2d 334, 131 Cal.Rptr. 14 (1976), the California case that placed a requirement on psychotherapists to reveal threats of harm directed at particular individuals, therapists should be aware that the duty to report may be applied by analogy to a situation where a therapist or clinician knows that a patient is being abused by a spouse, and lets the abuser take that patient home knowing that the abuse will be repeated.

C. DO LICENSURE LAWS CREATE PROBLEMS FOR HOSPITALS?

Another area where hospitals and clinicians can come onto hard times is by failure to abide by hospital and therapist licensure laws. At this writing, 48 states in the country have either licensure or legal credentialing laws for respiratory care. Notably, Hawaii has no therapist licensure laws, and as such has wound up as a kind of "dumping ground" for therapists whose licenses have been suspended or revoked in other jurisdictions.

Compliance with licensure laws is mandatory, and a hospital can lose the confidence of the community if patients are treated by an unlicensed therapist. Department heads can face fines, jail, and loss of credentials if they knowingly employ unlicensed persons. In addition, care given by unlicensed individuals would not be eligible for Medicare or Medicaid reimbursement. For this reason, hospitals and employers must have a means to verify licensure and must do background checks on all hires to ensure that their licenses are valid.

Another problem is that hospitals may not be able to seek reimbursement from commercial insurers for therapy performed by unlicensed providers, and the facility may have to pay back funds wrongfully paid. Because most inpatient bills are DRG related, and are a "one price" bill for the total service, there is a possibility that any patient who received therapy might well have his or her entire payment refunded to the government because the hospital failed to comply with the Conditions of Participation.

D. HOW SHOULD A THERAPIST APPROACH A PROBLEM WITH A LICENSURE BOARD?

Carefully, and never without an attorney.

The public's view of a licensure board is that it is a friendly forum for the health care professional unlucky enough to come up for review. Populated by similar professionals, the board should be willing to look at therapists with a sensitive eye. Rather than demanding blind adherence to regulations, certainly a board would understand how a therapist might have to deviate now and then.

This is what the public thinks. It is not, for the most part, how the board behaves.

The board's mission is to protect the public from dangerous and incompetent practitioners. In most cases, that means people who break the law and get caught; it doesn't mean people who make honest mistakes. Honest mistakes might be malpractice, but they are not normally thought of as grounds for discipline. But every board has different standards, and for that reason, every therapist should be wary of the state board.

1. When Should I Seek Counsel?

If you are unlucky enough to receive a formal accusation by the Board of Respiratory Care in your state, or a "Statement of Issues" (if you are applying for licensure and are denied), you should immediately contact an attorney specializing in regulatory defense to handle your case.

This is not an area of the law that your average general practitioner can handle. The attorney needs expertise in dealing with agencies, and not simply a general understanding of the law. The rules that govern licensure procedures are different from the laws and rules applied in most other areas of the law. For this reason, you need a specialist.

It is tempting to think that you can meet with investigators, explain your side of it, and walk away free and clear. That is tempting because you want to believe it. It is, for the most part, untrue. The investigator has your license as his target, and he may not feel he is doing his job if you retain your license at the end.

For that reason, any time you have any interaction with the Board or its investigators, you should immediately retain counsel. Again, this is not just another lawyer, but someone who has defended professional discipline cases previously.

Sometimes investigators show up at work, having been summoned by hospital administrators or supervisors, and demand an immediate interview. You are guaranteed a right to counsel by the Constitution, and if you do not take advantage of it, your license may well be lost. Do not be bullied into talking to anyone until you have talked to a lawyer.

Politely but firmly inform the investigator that under no circumstances will you meet with him and discuss anything unless and until you have an attorney at your side.

"But if you have nothing to hide, why do you need a lawyer?"

That is often a question investigators, who want to prevent you from knowing your rights, use to get you to waive a lawyer. The proper answer to that question is "I want to make sure that my rights are fully protected from overzealous or bad faith enforcement." Terminate the interview politely. Contact an attorney immediately. Direct the Board to communicate solely with your attorney.

It is never—repeat never—in your best interest to talk to a board investigator without counsel, even if you are not the person being investigated. Do not waive that right. If you say something inappropriate, you might wind up a target of the investigation too.

You also have the right to schedule the interview for a time when you are rested, relaxed, and have had time to review the medical records of the patient that complained or whose care is implicated in the board enforcement action.

An analysis of disciplinary documents from cases in California shows clearly why it is necessary to obtain counsel.

One therapist, whom we'll identify by her initials, UA, gave material assistance to Efren Saldivar by providing him with a bottle of Succinylcholine chloride. She was interviewed by police and by investigators and ultimately confessed to having given him the materials he needed to kill patients. Her grand jury testimony was as follows:

Q. Can you tell me how it came about that you gave Efren Saldivar Succinylcholine chloride?
A. I just handed it to him
Q. Where did you get it from?
A. The rooms in the Surgical Intensive Care, they have windows dividing each room. There is like a windowsill. I just saw it sitting on the windowsill . . .
Q. Now, did you know what Succinylcholine chloride was at the time.

A.   Yes.
Q.   What is it?
A.   It's a paralyzing agent . . .
Q.   And why did you give it to Mr. Saldivar?
A.   I don't know.
Q.   Had he asked you to get him some Succinylcholine chloride?
A.   No.
Q.   Were you aware that Mr. Saldivar was injecting people and killing them?
A.   Yes.
Q.   When did you find that out?
A.   Early months of '97.

***

Q.   What was your relationship like with Mr. Salidivar?
A.   We were close friends.
Q.   Were you having sex with him?
A.   Yes.

2. When Should I Report Someone to the Board?

You should follow the dictates of the state licensure statute and regulations promulgated under that statute.

Most state statutes require that a professional who is aware of another professional's misdeeds must report that professional. California arguably has the strongest stand on this issue. Its state statute says:

§ 3758. Report on suspension or termination for cause

(a) Any employer of a respiratory care practitioner shall report to the Respiratory Care Board the suspension or termination for cause of any practitioner in their employ. The reporting required herein shall not act as a waiver of confidentiality of medical records. The information reported or disclosed shall be kept confidential except as provided in subdivision (c) of Section 800, and shall not be subject to discovery in civil cases.

(b) For purposes of the section, "suspension or termination for cause" is defined to mean suspension or termination from employment for any of the following reasons:

(1) Use of controlled substances or alcohol to such an extent that it impairs the ability to safely practice respiratory care.

(2) Unlawful sale of controlled substances or other prescription items.

(3) Patient neglect, physical harm to a patient, or sexual contact with a patient.

(4) Falsification of medical records.

(5) Gross incompetence or negligence.

(6) Theft from patients, other employees, or the employer.

(c) Failure of an employer to make a report required by this section is punishable by an administrative fine not to exceed ten thousand dollars ($10,000) per violation.

§ 3758.5. Reporting violations

If a licensee has knowledge that another person may be in violation of, or has violated, any of the statutes or regulations administered by the board, the licensee shall report this information to the board in writing and shall cooperate with the board in furnishing information or assistance as may be required.

The California statute requires an employer to report any employee whom it discharges for cause, defined to include gross incompetence, negligence, patient abuse or neglect, sexual contact, or use of controlled substances. Arguably someone who is discharged because they fail to come in to work after having had too much to drink the night before would be reported to the Board since the cause of the termination was the use of alcohol. Additionally, the statute requires that any licensee who has knowledge of violations must make a report in writing.

Interestingly enough, the California statute has an added twist. It requires that if an employer discharges an employee for cause, a report is made not only on the employee, but also on the supervisor of that employee. Thus, a department director has an incentive to discharge an employee for almost any other reason than one listed above so as to prevent a report being made on her. The statute says:

§ 3758.6. Report on supervisor

(a) In addition to the reporting required under Section 3758, an employer shall also report to the board the name, professional licensure type and number, and title of the person supervising the licensee who has been suspended or terminated for cause, as defined in subdivision (b) of Section 3758. If the supervisor is a licensee under this chapter, the board shall investigate whether due care

was exercised by that supervisor in accordance with this chapter. If the supervisor is a health professional, licensed by another licensing board under this division, the employer shall report the name of that supervisor and any and all information pertaining to the suspension or termination for cause of the person licensed under this chapter to the appropriate licensing board.

(b) The failure of an employer to make a report required by this section is punishable by an administrative fine not to exceed ten thousand dollars ($10,000) per violation.

Missouri does not codify its requirement to report misconduct in the statute itself, reserving this for the code of state regulations. The code governing the Board of Respiratory Care states:

4 CSR 255-5.010 Code of Ethics

(N) Within the limits of the law, a respiratory care practitioner or permit holder shall report to the board all knowledge of suspected violations of the laws and rules governing the practice of a respiratory care practitioner as defined in section 334.810, RSMo, and any other applicable laws and rules.

(2) Failure of a respiratory care practitioner or permit holder to adhere to the code of ethics constitutes grounds for discipline of the license or permit.

Thus, in Missouri, a practitioner is required to report all knowledge of suspected violations of the law and rules to the board, and failure to do so constitutes grounds for discipline.

3. Can You Survive the Disciplinary Process?

In most states, once the state board is involved, it becomes the prosecutor, judge, and jury, mixing its roles in a constitutionally precarious way. In Missouri, for example, the hearing is set before the Administrative Hearing Commission and the Board acts as prosecutor. If the Administrative Hearing Commission determines that there is cause to discipline the licensee, the Board then has the power to impose discipline as it sees fit. Any challenge to the board's action must be brought in the local circuit court, and can be appealed to the State Court of Appeals or the Missouri Supreme Court. Other states have similar procedures.

During the pendency of a charge, the state has the ability to take depositions of witnesses, as does the licensee. The case can be disposed of by motion or by hearing on the merits.

Several years ago, a physician asked me to represent him before the State Board for the Registration of the Healing Arts. The experience convinced me that no licensee should be without an attorney.

At one point the board served on my client a subpoena that required him to bring all his records on all of his patients 210 miles to Jefferson City, Missouri, for the purpose of a disciplinary interview. In addition to summoning him for an interview, the subpoena commanded that if he failed to honor the subpoena, this would be grounds for discipline. The physician was looking at having to hire a Ryder Truck to bring all his records to the Board Office. Obviously this created some serious privacy issues for the records.

Fortunately the Attorney General agreed to reduce the request to six separate records, which we produced at an interview where the Board ultimately agreed it did not have a case.

4. Isn't It Better to Cooperate and Be Nice?

Honestly, no. It is almost never a good idea to cooperate fully with the board without involving an attorney, because the board's view and your view of cooperation could be two different things. For some state boards, cooperation means voluntarily placing your head on the chopping block after sharpening the axe first.

Boards frequently abuse their authority. Not because the people on the board are bad people, and not because the board is not trying to perform its public protective function. But often the professionals on the board are unskilled in the legal analysis required. They have access to counsel through the Attorney General, but frequently fail to use it. As such, they tend to overstep their authority.

The problem is that, without an attorney, this physician would have complied with the request and wound up guessing wrong. The Board was interested in two discrete incidents, which it later found not to be valid causes for discipline.

Strong legal representation by someone who knows the process is vital to ensuring that a practitioner's rights are fully protected. This is because frequently the licensee doesn't know what rights the law provides.

E. WHERE IS THE GOVERNMENT HEADING IN HOSPITAL REGULATION?

The government is interested in several significant areas. They are: violations of the Antikickback statute, violations of the Stark laws, Antitrust, and false claims. These three areas present the greatest threat to a hospital's financial viability. The government frequently pursues all these issues as criminal law issues, and frequently goes after managers and administrators for prison time.

F. WHAT ARE ANTIKICKBACK VIOLATIONS?

It is the payment of anything, in cash or in kind, in order to induce someone to either recommend a provider's services to a federal medical beneficiary, or as payment for referrals. Not only can hospitals be sued by the government for such violations, violations can carry civil and criminal penalties. More importantly, even insubstantial activities may result in liability.

At Our Lady of Perpetual Billing Hospital, Rufus Drager, the owner of Medicare Pays Home Care, comes to see the Department Head. He tells the Department Head that they are looking for someone to do monthly in-service education for their staff on Respiratory Care issues. They'd like to hire the Department Head, strictly as a sideline business venture, to provide that service. They agree to pay him $200 for every monthly in-service.

The Department Head agrees. He makes several trips to the Home Care company and finds the staff to be very caring and compassionate. As a result, he starts recommending to nurses and to the discharge planners to contact MPHC for services. Several months in a row, he is unable to make the trip and do an in-service, and the company pays him anyway. But every third or fourth month he gets in an in-service.

1. Is There a Problem with This Arrangement?

42 U.S.C. § 1320A-76(B) provides the following definition of what violates the antikickback statute:

*The knowing and willful solicitation, offer or payment of any remuneration (broadly defined to encompass **anything** of value), whether direct or indirect, overt or covert, in cash or in kind, in return for:*

> *referring an individual for the furnishing of any item or service; or purchasing, leasing or arranging or recommending or arranging for the purchase, lease or ordering, of any item or service paid in whole or in part under any Federal Health Care Program. (The Health Insurance Portability and Accountability Act of 1996 ("HIPAA") defines Federal Health Care Program to include "any plan or program that provides health benefits, whether directly, through insurance, or otherwise, which is funded directly, in whole or in part, by the United States Government" other than the Federal Employees Health Benefit Program (42 U.S.C. § 1320a-7b).)*

In *United States v. Anderson,* 261 F.3d 993 (10th Cir. 2001) *cert. denied* 122 S. Ct. 818 (2002), the Tenth Circuit Court of Appeals adopted the Third Circuit "one purpose" test, holding that if *any* purpose of a payment is to induce referrals, the statute is violated. Under the facts stated above, the department head is in serious civil and potentially criminal trouble. He is taking money, and at least one purpose of the money is to induce referrals because the director is being paid every month whether he provides a service or not. This looks less like a payment for in-service than a payment for referrals.

2. What Are the Penalties?

Civil monetary penalties of up to $50,000 and damages of up to three times the total amount of remuneration offered, paid, solicited, or received may be assessed for violation of the antikickback statute (42 U.S.C. § 1320a-7a(a)) This means our director is being subjected to a $600 payback every month that the scheme goes on, and that he might be assessed a civil penalty of $50,000. And that is not the worst of the director's problems. Criminal penalties and exclusion from Medicare's payment system remain penalties for violations of the antikickback statute.

If our director is excluded from Medicare, it is possible the hospital will be excluded. If he is excluded from the Medicare program, it is doubtful that he will ever be able to work in health care again in any kind of productive role (except, perhaps, as a bad example).

3. How Do Courts Interpret the "Knowing and Willful" Intent Standard?

The *Hanlester* Standard (adopted in the Ninth U.S. Circuit Court of Appeals) is the least stringent standard for measuring criminal conduct under the antikickback statute. It says that "knowing and willful" conduct requires knowledge that the statute prohibits offering or paying remuneration to induce referrals, and prohibited conduct taken with the specific intent to disobey the law. The court, in that case, found that neither of the defendant entities met both standards; they believed the physician joint venture arrangements were lawful. *Hanlester Network v. Shalala* (51 F.3d 1390 (9th Cir. 1995) Applying that standard, our Director may escape criminal liability. However, other circuits use other standards. For example, in *United States v. Jain* (93 F.3d 436 (8th Cir. 1996)), the Court held that the antikickback statute "only requires proof that [defendant] knew that his conduct was wrongful, rather than proof that he knew it violated 'a legal duty.'" Our Director could be in really hot water if a court determined that he knew he shouldn't have been paid for the in-service presentations he did not give.

4. How Is a Hospital Department Head to Know?

Ask the Office of Inspector General of the Health and Human Services Department. Recently, that department offered "supplemental compliance guidance" (government talk for "what you will do") on the subject of anti-kickback laws. It said that the government views compliance with the anti-kickback statute as a condition of participation under Medicare and the other federal health care programs, and that a violation can lead to further sanctions under the False Claims Act. The OIG offers the following analytical tool to help hospital department director avoid trouble in this area:

- Does the hospital have any remunerative relationship between itself (or its affiliates or agents) and persons or entities capable of generating federal business, directly or indirectly, for the hospital? If so:
- Could one purpose (not just the sole purpose) of the remuneration be to induce or reward the referral or recommendation of business reimbursable under federal health care programs? If the answer is yes, the antikickback statute may be implicated.

If an arrangement implicates the statute, the Supplemental Guidance lists four aggravating circumstances that are likely to place the hospital at greater risk of prosecution. If the arrangement: (i) has the potential to interfere with clinical decision-making; (ii) includes the potential to increase costs to the government, beneficiaries, or enrollees; (iii) contains the potential for over-utilization or inappropriate utilization; or (iv) presents increased risks to patient safety or quality of care, then the arrangement should be scrutinized carefully.

The statutes and the federal guidance make it clear that anything a hospital does to influence persons to send them business must be carefully scrutinized. The same goes for anyone outside the hospital looking for referrals from inside the hospital. This is not always easy to see. If a drug store offers to provide free unit-dose medications for the pulmonary rehabilitation program, with an eye toward obtaining the medication business of these patients, it might well be soliciting referrals. Therapists would be wise to seek a legal opinion before agreeing to any contract that might be seen by the government as violating this statute.

G. CAN HOSPITALS BE SUED FOR ANTITRUST?

The federal antitrust statute says:

Every contract, combination in the form of trust or otherwise, or conspiracy, in restraint of trade or commerce among the several States, or with foreign nations, is declared to be illegal. Every person who shall make any contract or engage in any combination or conspiracy hereby declared to be illegal shall be deemed guilty of a felony, and, on conviction thereof, shall be punished by fine not exceeding $10,000,000 if a corporation, or, if any other person, $350,000, or by imprisonment not exceeding three years, or by both said punishments, in the discretion of the court.

15 USC § 1

The idea behind the antitrust statute is to prevent too few people from controlling a market and thereby setting prices without competition. This is the conduct that Microsoft was alleged to have engaged in by monopolizing the market for its internet browser (Internet Explorer).

Trusts and monopolies have traditionally been defined as "concentrations of wealth in the hands of a few." This is thought to be injurious to the public and individuals because such arrangements minimize, if not eliminate, normal competition over goods and services in the marketplace and produce undesirable price controls.

To prevent restraints on trade or commerce from reducing competition, Congress passed the Sherman Antitrust Act in 1890, at a time when railroads and large banking trusts were having a ruinous effect on the economy. The Sherman Act was designed to promote freedom of contract, and to eliminate restraints on trade and competition. The Sherman Act is the main source of federal Antitrust law.

Almost all states also have some similar statute prohibiting antitrust activities. Massachusetts' statute, for example, says:

Chapter 93: Section 6 Discouraging competition

Section 6. It shall be unlawful for any person engaged in trade or commerce, in the course thereof, to lease or make a sale or contract for sale of goods, wares, merchandise, machinery, supplies or other commodities, patented or unpatented, for use, consumption or resale in the commonwealth, or fix a price charged therefor, or discount from, or rebate upon, such price on the condition, agreement or understanding that the lessee or purchaser thereof shall not use or

deal in the goods, wares, merchandise, machinery, supplies or other commodi-
ties of a competitor or competitors of the lessor or seller, where the effect of such
lease, sale or contract for sale or such condition, agreement or understanding
may be to lessen substantially competition or tend to create a monopoly in any
line of trade or commerce in the commonwealth.

Antitrust law simply prohibits any agreement to fix prices or limit competition for customers. It has application in the health care world in that, frequently hospitals compare prices for services that they charge, and use that comparison to adjust their prices. If Hospital A charges $560 for a complete pulmonary function test, and Hospital B charges $650, Hospital A is likely to raise its charges to keep pace in revenue production. The act of getting together and comparing prices can sometimes be construed as price fixing.

Therapists should be careful about engaging in conduct that treads closely to an agreement in restraint of trade. Suppose Hospital A suggests that since it is adding a new outpatient surgery suite, it will do bronchoscopies for physicians. In order to get Hospital B to give up the bronchoscopies, it suggests that it will not do any more pulmonary function testing. Arranging with another hospital not to offer one service, and refusing to schedule some similar service as a concession, is an agreement in restraint of trade. It is presumptively unlawful.

A patient, a physician, a competitor, or anyone damaged by the arrangement can sue for treble damages under the Sherman Act. For this reason, therapists should be very careful when making agreements between hospitals, even for purposes of sharing equipment, because such an agreement might be seen in the big picture as an agreement in restraint of trade.

Antitrust at the heart of the dispute between two major respiratory care product suppliers, Tyco's Nellcor business unit and Masimo. The dispute is over pulse oximetry sales, and how Nellcor pressured group purchasing organizations (GPOs) into sole-source supplier contracts. In March, 2005, a California jury placed some serious brakes on GPOs and vendors who engage in anticompetitive marketing practices. They awarded $140 million in damages to Masimo because they found that Tyco's Nellcor unit engaged in "anticompetitive" market manipulation through group purchasing arrangements. Under the Sherman Act, that $140 was then trebled (tripled) to a whopping $420 million, and Masimo will have its attorneys fees (amounting to as much as another million, potentially) paid by Tyco.

In determining that Tyco Healthcare violated antitrust laws related to the sales of its pulse oximetry technology, a federal jury found that Tyco had utilized various anticompetitive practices, including sole-source and high compliance agreements, bundled rebates, and co-marketing agreements, to exclude Masimo from the marketplace.

The exclusionary contracting practices of GPOs have also been the subject of three Senate Judiciary Antitrust Subcommittee hearings led by Senators Herb Kohl (D-Wis.) and Mike DeWine (R-Ohio). Last October, Senators Kohl and DeWine introduced the Medical Device Competition Act of 2004, which would ensure open and fair access to innovative, cost-effective medical technologies. Several federal and state agencies, including the U.S. Department of Justice, are also investigating these practices.

Joe E. Kiani, Founder and CEO of Masimo, in a prepared statement, said, "We sued Tyco to seek relief from Tyco's actions that prevented purchasing decisions from being made based on merits of the products. We are gratified that the jury found in our favor. We hope this verdict will benefit patients and our nation's health care system by fostering vigorous competition, thereby promoting innovative, cost-effective technologies."

Tyco has already announced that it will appeal the verdict. "We are confident that we will ultimately prevail when the legal process is completed," Nellcor President David Sell said.

What does this mean for therapists? "It should probably be seen as a victory for patients and clinicians," Masimo Vice-President Brad Langdale said. "The big companies with market share have no incentive to innovate, and if they tie up the market by bundling and tie their discounts to those bundles, the sole purpose is to shut out the smaller competitors from the market. That means less competition. Less competition means less innovation, and higher prices. It's simple Economics 101."

It may also mean hospitals will want to think long and hard before getting into GPO contracts that contains the types of agreements that the federal jury found suspect. Hospitals will ultimately benefit from the verdict if the appeals court sides with Masimo.

The verdict also calls into question the manner and methods that many larger vendors in the health care marketplace (not just Tyco, but vendors like Hill-Rom and Becton-Dickinson) use to market their big-ticket items to hospitals. KCI, the bed company, sued Hillenbrand Industries for anticompetitive practices based on the same theories as Masimo (after a jury verdict in favor of KCI, Hillenbrand paid $250,000,000 to settle the case). The same can be said of Retractable Technologies, who has sued Becton-Dickinson, and included in that suit are several GPOs. In short, the verdict in the KCI and

Masimo cases should give hope to the therapist-manager who may be locked into a contract for equipment she does not believe presents the best clinical options for her patients. The fact is, free competition benefits everyone.

H. DO HOSPITALS FACE CLASS ACTIONS?

Class action lawsuits are brought on behalf of a large number of plaintiffs for essentially small amounts of damage. The theory is that when a merchant overcharges a client by $1.50 for 10 months, and has more than five million customers, the overcharge quickly adds up to big profits, and absent a class action, no consumer would sue to get relief for the unlawful acts. Class Actions are the legal vehicle meant to redress this wrong. They are permitted in state and federal court throughout the country.

In order to be resolved by a class action lawsuit there must be numerous claims. Exactly how many claims is not well settled. In the Courtney chemotherapy dilution case discussed earlier, more than 60 plaintiffs sued in the first few weeks, and at least three law firms filed class action cases on behalf of all the plaintiffs. The court never ruled on the class action allegations. Instead it consolidated the cases under one senior judge who was in charge of the cases for the next three years. When the cases finally settled, the Court simply converted the first case into a class action complaint and ignored the previously-filed ones. By this time, however, more than three thousand patients had been affected by what Courtney's pharmacy had done.

The court's next concern is whether the claims involve common questions of law. In other words, in deciding the case, will the questions of law (regarding the admissibility of evidence, what body of law applies, etc.) be common so that the court can rule on an issue once and have that ruling apply throughout the case?

If the court finds that there are numerous and common claims, the next step the court takes is to see if the claims brought in the case are typical of the claims others could bring. For example, in the Fen-Phen Diet Drug Litigation cases, the claims were for product liability (a dangerous and defective product) and for failure to warn (of the adverse effects). These claims were typical of the claims patients were bringing all over the country, and so the case was suitable for resolution as a class action.

Finally, the court examines the question of whether the parties who are designated as class representatives will fairly and properly represent the class members. This may sound odd, but collusive class action lawsuits do occur.

Sometimes when a company discovers that it has created a defective product, or has engaged in conduct that might be seen as fraudulent, it finds itself facing multiple class action lawsuits.

Some of those lawsuits are brought by law firms that specialize in that litigation, and the company knows that if that case is certified as a class action, it will be held to account fully for what happened. Unfortunately, there will also be companion or "copy cat" cases that have many of the same claims, but are brought by law firms and plaintiffs who are more apt to see things the way the defendant sees things. Instead of requiring payment of money directly to the plaintiff class, for example, the "friendly law suit" will work out a settlement with the defendant early on to provide for relief in the form of coupons. Since the coupons will rarely, if ever, be used, the defendant doesn't have to worry about a large cash payout. The defendant is happy, the class plaintiffs are paid significant sums of money, and the lawyers representing this friendly class are well compensated. These lawsuits are closely examined by the state and federal courts because they result not from arms-length litigation over the issues, but from a desire from a law firm to make a quick profit at the expense of several thousand consumers, and the desire of the corporation to minimize its liability.

If all the claims are numerous, typical, common, and provide for fair representation the court can "certify" the class action, which means that the result of the trial will ultimately bind all the members in the class action. Since jurors are apt to award large damages in class action cases, defendants settle most class action lawsuits before trial.

Class Actions are typically settled for large amounts of money that are paid back in very small ways, and depending on the difficulty of the case, it may sometimes be to the consumer's best interests to have a "coupon" settlement. For example, consider this class action settlement notice at Appendix H. In this case the damages would have been very difficult to establish, and the class action worked out an arrangement beneficial to class members and the company too. Although there were objections, the class was eventually approved by the court.

I. CAN HOSPITALS COMMIT CONSUMER FRAUD?

Most states have laws that protect consumers from consumer fraud. A consumer fraud is a fraud perpetrated against an entire class of consumers. As with class actions, in consumer fraud cases the injury may be small in amount, but massive in scope.

When the tobacco cases were brought by the State Attorney Generals' offices in 1997 and 1998, those cases were filed primarily under the doctrine of consumer fraud. The theory advanced by the Attorneys General in almost every state was the consumers had been promised one thing (that cigarettes would not hurt them) and given something completely different (a dangerous and defective product).

State consumer fraud statutes not only permit class action litigation against defendants, but they also can provide for enhanced remedies including double and, in some cases, triple damages.

Recently, these statutes have been turned against corporate not-for-profit hospitals. Although it is too early to say at this point whether the cases will be successful, the incident underscores why it is important to fully disclose the facts to patients.

In these not-for-profit hospital cases, the theory is that the hospital bills itself in the community as a "charity" hospital where the uninsured and underinsured can come and receive compassionate care. These same hospitals, however, frequently charge the full rack rate for their rooms and care to the very people who can least afford it (the indigent). The net effect is that an indigent person who comes to a charity hospital may wind up losing his house or his assets to the hospital in a lawsuit where the indigent person may wind up being billed two to three times what Medicare or a private insurance company would pay for the same care. This, the plaintiffs allege, amounts to fraud.

Although there is no law specifically on point that says a hospital cannot do this, the consumer fraud statutes, which prohibit deceptive conduct in trade or commerce (defined as something that has the capacity to mislead the average person) are the closest to providng a remedy.

Almost all of these cases resulted from the hospital's lawsuits against the uninsured persons, and illustrate the importance of getting good legal advice before pursuing collection actions against patients.

1. Is Corporate Compliance Important?

Every hospital should have an active and engaged Corporate Compliance Officer who is empowered to cross divisional lines and investigate any hint of wrongdoing in the hospital environment. Having a compliance officer in name only is more dangerous than not having one.

As mentioned earlier, the Chief Compliance Officer is the administrative person in the hospital who oversees the Corporate Compliance Program. He or she is in charge of functioning as an independent and objective body that reviews and evaluates compliance issues/concerns within the organization. The compliance officer has two bosses: the CEO and the Board of Directors, and must be completely free to interact with both without the permission or approbation of the other.

The position ensures that the Board of Directors, management, and employees are in compliance with all the rules and regulations of various state and federal regulatory agencies. He or she makes sure that company policies and procedures are in accordance with federal and state law, and are being followed to the letter. Finally, the CCO makes sure that behavior in the organization meets the company's Standards of Conduct as set out in its Compliance Program.

The Corporate Compliance Officer, and those under his or her control, serve:

- As a fair and impartial person who will receive complaints in absolute confidence and then direct a fair and appropriate investigation aimed at resolving the compliance problem; and
- As the final internal check and balance for resolving problems in the organization. When a therapist or clinician cannot resolve a clinical issue with physicians, other departments, or some other internal entity, the CCO deals with the concerned parties and may communicate after other formal channels and resources have been exhausted.

The Chief Compliance Officer directs all compliance/ethics efforts of the hospital and provides guidance for the Board of Directors and senior administrators on matters relating to compliance. The Chief Compliance Officer, together with the Corporate Compliance Committee, is authorized to implement all necessary actions to effective compliance.

J. DOES HIPAA RAISE CONCERNS FOR HOSPITALS?

Of all the laws recently passed by Congress, the HIPAA statute has created more work for health industry lawyers than that created by malpractice lawyers. HIPAA created a new regulatory framework for analyzing privacy issues in medically-confidential material, and the disclosure of information outside the ranks of the health care worker can create serious problems.

"HIPAA" stands for the "Health Insurance Portability and Accountability Act of 1996."[1] Most of this act concerns reforms to the insurance market and

---

[1]The Health Insurance Portability and Accountability Act of 1996, Public Law 104-191, 110 Statutes 1936 (August 21, 1996) ("HIPAA"), codified in portions of the Social Security Act.

fraud and abuse prosecution issues. Over the past few years however, HIPAA has emerged as a large area of concern for all hospitals, and a source of confusion for individual clinicians and physicians.

HIPAA itself did not set standards for privacy. Instead it authorized the Department of Health and Human Services to promulgate detailed regulations for its implementation. It has taken some time for these regulations to be developed and published.

Subtitle F of HIPAA required the adoption of privacy regulations only if certain conditions weren't met. Legislation was not enacted, and so, in 1999, HHS began to issue rules regarding privacy.

Under HIPAA, state law regarding patient privacy controls if it imposes "requirements, standards, or implementation specifications that are more strict than the requirements, standards, or implementation specifications imposed under [HIPAA]."[2] A state law is considered "more stringent" when:[3]

- It provides for greater limitations on uses or disclosures of protected information, in terms of numbers of potential recipients, amount of information that may be disclosed, or circumstances in which information may be disclosed;
- It gives individuals greater rights of access to or amendment of protected information, except to the extent that it pertains to the disclosure of Protected Health Information regarding a minor to parents, guardians, and others acting in loco parentis;
- It provides for greater penalties;
- It provides for more information to be disclosed to individuals upon request;
- It makes it more difficult to get, or otherwise provides more restrictions on, the form individual authorizations for use or disclosure of protected information.
- It requires more detailed or more lengthy record retention.
- It otherwise provides greater privacy protection for individuals.

The statute says HIPAA applies only to "individually identifiable health information," defined as:

any information, including demographic information, collected from an individual that . . . is created or received by a health care provider, health plan,

---

[2]HIPAA § 264(b)(2).
 [3]See Privacy Rule, 45 CFR §§ 160.201—205.

employer, or health care clearinghouse; and . . . relates to the past, present, or future physical or mental health or condition of an individual, the provision of health care to an individual, or the past, present, or future payment for the provision of health care to an individual, and . . . identifies the individual; or . . . with respect to which there is a reasonable basis to believe that the information can be used to identify the individual.[4]

Based on the government's initial reading of HIPAA's intent, the draft Privacy Rule limited its application to a category called "protected health information" ("PHI"), which was "individually identifiable health information" that "is or has been electronically transmitted or maintained."[5] This did not hold up, and PHI now includes information in any medium, written, oral or electronic.[6]

HIPAA provides criminal penalties for using health information that is unlawfully obtained. HIPAA also provides civil remedies against hospitals and individuals who violate its provisions. It is a far-reaching statute that will continue to create problems in the near future until health care organizations adopt policies and procedures to meet its mandates.

HIPAA provides for civil and criminal penalties for violations.[7] Of the two, civil penalties are likely to be much more common, while criminal penalties are likely to be much more severe. What determines whether a civil or criminal penalty attaches is generally whether the United States Attorney is interested in punishment or collections.

HIPAA civil money penalties may be assessed at the rate of no more than $100 per violation, to an annual cap of $25,000 per violation of each "identical requirement or prohibition."[8] Most of the "requirements and prohibitions" appear to be things a hospital could only do once; however, others might be violated each time a routine activity (like releasing medical records to lawyers) is conducted. It might be possible to reach the maximum penalty quickly.[9]

The Privacy Rule is enforced by the Office of Civil Rights ("OCR") at the Department of Health and Human Services.[10] No one knows how enforce-

---

[4]HIPAA § 1171(6).

[5]See Draft Privacy Rule, 64 Fed.Reg. at 59928, 60053 (proposed section 45 CFR § 164.504).

[6]See 45 CFR §§ 160.103 (definition of "health information") and 164.501 (definition of "protected health information").

[7]See HIPAA §§ 1176, 1177.

[8]See HIPAA § 1176(a)(1).

[9]E.g., routine transmission of unencrypted email including ePHI would violate 45 CFR §164.312(e)(2)(ii) in the absence of proper justification, and many organizations might very quickly exceed the 250 transmissions necessary to reach the annual maximum.

[10]See generally the CMP Rule.

ment will be handled, although it appears that The Centers for Medicare and Medicaid and the Office of Civil Rights will be primarily involved in coordinating certain investigations.[11]

It appears that, so far at least, enforcement is principally through "voluntary compliance." Hospitals and health care organizations are given "technical assistance" from the Office of Civil Rights on how to cooperate.[12] In this context, a good faith attempt to comply should likely provide a credible defense to civil money penalties and criminal prosecution.

In short, HIPAA requires that confidential information about patients be kept confidential. This not only means that information can't be given to persons outside the hospital without a need to know, it means that information cannot be given inside the hospital unless there is a need to know.

The key area where therapists are at risk is that of diagnostic testing and in patient care areas whenever visitors are present. A therapist cannot simply assume that because someone else is in the room, it must be okay to talk about medically-private information. The patient should always be consulted. "Mr. Jones, do you mind if I ask you some questions about your health while your wife is in the room?" Most of the time the patient will say he doesn't mind. But, when there is a problem, that should be respected.

Similarly, when a patient comes by to pick up a copy of a pulmonary function test, a test that might not be in the medical records department, that test should be handed over only when you are satisfied that the patient is the person whose test is being requested (and that is normally done by checking identification) or when you have a valid, notarized authorization permitting you to turn the documents over.

K. FALSE CLAIMS ACT LIABILITY

As mentioned earlier in this book, the government likes to pursue recipients of federal money for refunds when it is clear that the hospital should not have received the funds. If a hospital issues false billings to Medicare or Medicaid, if it performs unnecessary services, if it hires and routinely uses unlicensed professionals to deliver care, it can create liability under the False Claims Act. See Chapter Four on Whistleblower Statutes for more information on this topic.

---

[11]See U.S. Department of Health and Human Services, *CMS Named to Enforce HIPAA Transactions and Code Set Standards,* HHS Office for Civil Rights To Continue To Enforce Privacy Standards (October 15, 2002), available at http://www.hhs.gov/news/press/2002pres/20021015a.html (visited July 18, 2003).

[12]See the preamble to the CMP Rule, 68 Fed.Reg. at 18897.

L. KEY POINTS

- In protecting your employer, you must pay attention to mandatory reporting laws.
- Most states have mandatory reporting laws for elder abuse and child abuse.
- Failure to report can be a felony if you have information from which you can derive a reasonable suspicion of abuse or neglect.
- Hospitals must follow licensure laws.
- Licensure laws are designed to protect the public.
- The licensure agency has a duty to investigate and prosecute wrongdoing.
- Sometimes Licensure Boards handle their duties poorly.
- Therapists should always get an attorney to help them if they are called before the Board for Respiratory Care.
- Hospitals should ensure that licenses are kept current because failure to do so might invalidate multiple patient care charges.
- Hospitals can face lawsuits if they engage in anticompetitive practices.
- Hospitals can face lawsuits if they engage in consumer fraud.
- Hospitals can face lawsuits if their employees violate the antikickback provisions.
- Individual employees can face federal criminal and civil penalties if they violate the Antikickback Act.
- Hospitals and individuals can face False Claims Act lawsuits if they violate the federal antikickback laws.
- One particularly bad form of lawsuit is the lawsuit filed as a class action.
- Hospitals should have corporate compliance programs.
- Hospitals should be careful to fully implement HIPAA.

M. SUMMARY

Protecting the health care organization requires attention to the issues that get hospitals sued, including paying attention to mandatory duties imposed by law. Although neither a risk management department nor a corporate compliance department are required by law, they are both exceptionally important departments in the hospital in terms of keeping the organization out of the courtroom.

CHAPTER 11

Business Law—Protecting Your Own Business

Discourage litigation. Persuade your neighbors to compromise whenever you can. As a peacemaker the lawyer has superior opportunity of being a good man. There will still be business enough.

Abraham Lincoln

A. INTRODUCTION

Respiratory therapists are smart, innovative persons who frequently think of better, faster, and more clinically efficient ways to do things. Therapists have frequently parlayed their knowledge of medical issues into sideline businesses that have turned out to be massively successful. There are thousands of durable medical equipment, home health care, and other life science companies that got their start in the minds of respiratory therapists passing time on the night shift.

Unfortunately, it isn't easy being a therapist who wants to take a great idea and make money with it. Around nearly every corner, there is a potential legal pothole for the unwary. A therapist's idea stolen by a big corporation can quickly become a huge nightmare. Failure to protect an idea with a patent could result in loss of the idea. Failure to obtain business insurance could mean that a very profitable year winds up being a corporate bankruptcy. Instead of riding your ideas to profit and success, it is completely possible to lose your house, your car, and your means of making a living.

This chapter highlights the things you can do to protect yourself and any business you set up to capitalize on your respiratory knowledge.

B. WHAT IS THE BEST WAY TO SET UP A BUSINESS?

The most common form of business is called the "sole proprietorship." A sole proprietorship is the quintessential "mom and pop" operation. Pop owns the company along with his wife. When he has a child or two, he passes the company to them. If all goes well the company winds up listed on the New York Stock Exchange after 50 years of excellent business. Unfortunately, too many simply churn their profits back into the family and coast along until disaster strikes.

Suppose Derrick invents a new method of securing an endotracheal tube. The ET tube holder Derrick invents works well, and he obtains a patent. He secures business insurance for $2,000,000. He starts small, marketing the device locally, and before long he is selling his device all over the U.S. After 11 years, his sales reach $450,000, and he is bringing home a handsome profit of $250,000 per year.

Then one day in Wyoming, a state without caps on liability limits, his device cracks, an ET tube slips out of position, and the patient dies. The hospital blames the device, and the lawyer sues Derrick's unincorporated sole proprietorship for damages. Derrick's insurance company fights the action, but the defendant will not accept a policy-limits offer of $2,000,000 and takes the case to trial. At trial, a jury awards $6,000,000. The insurance company pays its $2,000,000, and the plaintiff comes after Derrick for the rest. Derrick sells his company for $150,000 to a competitor. The plaintiff gets this money, and forces Derrick into bankruptcy, stripping him of his house, his car, and all his savings.

Not a very pretty picture, is it?

But let's back up a bit. Instead of electing a sole proprietorship, Derrick, after getting his patent, forms Tube Derrick LLC, a limited liability company, or Tube Holder, Inc., a corporation.

Now, when sued, the corporation must defend, not Derrick personally. When the judgment is rendered, Derrick's company may be bankrupt, but Derrick doesn't lose his house or his car.

There are many different forms of business that allow a therapist to engage in business without exposing the therapist's personal assets. They include corporations, limited liability companies, limited liability partnerships, limited partnerships, and foreign corporations. We will examine the different types of business forms and determine which make the most professional sense for the therapist.

1. What Are Corporations?

There are three types of corporations: general, close, and non-profit. Most therapists entering into business want to form either a close corporation or a general business corporation, depending in large part on whether the company will have a few closely-held owners, or will be a large company that issues stock.

a) What Is a General Business Corporation?

When most people think in terms of a corporation, they think of a company like General Motors Corporation, a company that has offices in numerous states, employs tens of thousands of workers in countries all over the world, and has stockholders who receive dividend payments. The number of shareholders of a company like General Motors is huge. Individual shareholders who own 1000 to 5000 shares have little practical power with their stock, other than to sell it. General Motors is operated by a board of directors, and those officers are directed by the groups of people who hold tens of thousands of shares of stock and who vote blocks of stock together.

General Motors is a general business corporation.

A general business corporation is a company with numerous stockholders. In most states, a company with more than 50 shareholders is considered to be a general business corporation.

Of course, companies like General Motors are different from the large number of general business corporations with multiple stockholders in that General Motors stock is "publicly traded." That means you can buy and sell your shares of GM stock on the New York Stock Exchange. Just because a business is a general corporation doesn't mean that the stock is traded publicly. Publicly traded stock is governed by rules relating to securities and investing, which are beyond the scope of this book. Suffice it to say that the guidance in this book is aimed at helping therapists determine what corporate form may be best for them.

Corporations must follow certain rules. In order to be set up, they have to file articles of incorporation, usually with the Secretary of State of the state where they are incorporated. Some larger companies incorporate in Delaware because Delaware has the most liberal corporation law in the United States. There are companies that specialize in helping the small business owner form and manage a Delaware Corporation. A clinician can set up a corporation in any state, and do business in any state, but is usually required to register in the state where they do business. Registration normally requires payment of a foreign corporation registration fee in addition to the fees paid to the state of Delaware. For this reason, unless your attorney insists on Delaware for some business reason, it is almost always smart to incorporate in your home state.

Beware of corporation companies that promise to set up your corporation in "tax free Nevada." Most states have tax statutes that require money earned in that state to be taxed in that state, and attempting to shield assets from taxation through a Nevada corporation is rarely a good idea.

In addition to filing articles of incorporation with the Secretary of State, the corporation must appoint a registered agent for service of process. This is someone who will receive the lawsuit papers if the corporation is sued. If John Doe is sued, the sheriff can find his house or work address and serve him personally. But the Sheriff might not be able to find John Doe Corporation, particularly if it was a small company. So the law requires the incorporators to appoint someone to receive the process. If this isn't done correctly, the secretary of state may wind up receiving notice of the lawsuit for the corporation, and a default judgment may be taken against the company.

Another "corporate formality" is a minute book and a corporate seal. A corporate seal is an embosser that formalizes the acts of the company like a signature. The "minute book" is the place where the minutes of the corporate meetings are held. At least one meeting every year is required.

Sometimes, particularly in smaller corporations, it is tempting not to adhere to these formalities and have annual meetings. Failure to have annual meetings and failure to keep a corporate minute book can be disastrous. In some states, if you do not adhere to the formalities, you lose the benefits (including the liability protections) of a corporation.

If a corporation enters into an agreement to buy or sell something, and then defaults, the corporation, not the individual who owns or manages it, is liable. Thus if the Doe Corporation wants to borrow $400,000 from the local bank, and cannot pay it back, John Doe is not personally on the hook, and the bank has to seize the assets of the corporation if it wants its money back.

Because of the liability protection afforded corporations, banks, credit unions, larger companies, insurance companies, and others may well require what is called a "personal guarantee."

A personal guarantee is a document signed by a corporate officer or director that pledges their personal credit, and their personal assets, in the event the corporation defaults on its obligations. That way when the corporation gets sued, and cannot pay its debts, the bank or the other business that has extended credit has someone to go to in order to have the obligation satisfied.

In short, a general corporation, like any corporation, is a company that provides liability protection for its owners. The corporate personnel must meet certain guidelines and must adhere to certain formalities, and the company can have unlimited shareholders.

b) What Are Close Corporations?

The close corporation is much like the general corporation, except that in most states the number of shareholders is kept to less than 50. A close corporation is usually a family-owned business. When Beard's Painting and Art Gallery incorporates, the corporate shares are owned by three people: Papa Beard, Ben Beard, and Brad Beard. Papa Beard owns 51% of the stock of the company, and is entitled to 51% of the distributions from the company. Ben and Brad each have 24.5% of the stock. Set up this way, Papa Beard can always control what happens in the corporation.

On the death of the elder family member, the shares can be passed through a last will and testament to Mama Beard, or distributed to Ben and Brad in equal shares. However, normally a smart attorney handling such a transaction will insist that one person have at least 51% of the stock so that there is no issue with respect to who controls the corporation.

Sometimes close corporations are set up with 50% interest for two people, in much the same way as a partnership. But if a business disagreement erupts later on, then neither of the two owners can conduct business without the other, and neither may want to conduct business if it helps the other. Thus the company may fall apart.

For this reason, shareholder agreements and articles of incorporation are usually drafted so as to provide for some form of dispute resolution. Business break ups are particularly well suited to mediation and arbitration, and these mechanisms are frequently inserted into business documents.

Like the general corporation, ownership is by shares of stock, and the number of shares is unlimited. But, the number of shareholders is not unlimited, and in most cases can be no more than 50.

c) What Are Not-for-Profit Corporations?

Not-for-profit corporations are set up as regular corporations under the business law of the state in which they operate. They file separate paperwork with the Internal Revenue Service for exemption under Section 501(c)(3) of the

Internal Revenue Code. This section provides that a corporation set up for charitable or beneficial purposes is not required to pay federal income taxes.

The law of not-for-profit corporations is too detailed to explain in this book. If you desire to set up this kind of corporation, you'll need expert tax advice from an accountant, and expert legal advice from a seasoned attorney.

2. What Are the Benefits of Incorporation?

In addition to liability protection, corporations are viewed as serious businesses, more so than simple partnerships or proprietorships. Corporations are registered with the Secretary of State and tend to get noticed by banks and lending organizations, which frequently make credit proposals to these entities. It is almost always easier to secure business insurance for a corporation than for a sole proprietorship.

The main benefit, however, is protection from personal liability for the corporation's owners. If General Motors gets sued for a defective car, the owners of GM stock do not have to pay if the judgment bankrupts the company (which is somewhat unlikely). If a sole proprietorship gets sued, and the judgment is more than insurance, the owner can be forced to pay the difference.

Keep in mind that in most situations the corporate form will not relieve the corporation's officers of any duties to pay the corporation's debts. Most banks and loan companies want a "personal guarantee" of any loan. So if the corporation goes bankrupt, the individual is still on the hook to pay back the money.

The benefit comes entirely from protecting the owner of the business from personal liability for the acts of his employees. If the owner of the company commits a tort, the corporation and the individual may both be liable.

3. Are There Duties of Corporate Record-keeping?

In addition to keeping minute books and other corporate records, there are always accounting issues that occur in both general and close corporations. These accounting issues include whether to be viewed as a General Corporation for tax purposes or an S or C corporation.

Tax advice is beyond the scope of this book. Anyone thinking of forming a corporation (or any other business association for profit) should secure tax advice from an accountant or from an attorney who limits his practice to tax issues.

Unlike other areas of the law, making a bad choice with respect to how a corporation or business entity is taxed can frequently have long-lasting and dreadful consequences. Secure an opinion from your tax adviser before you secure your business organization.

4. How Are Corporate Names Protected?

Suppose you want to form a company that lays sod, and you want to form that company in Missouri. Suppose you want to call that company Ground Concepts Incorporated. A quick check of the Missouri Secretary of State website will show that the name is taken. What do you do?

One thing you can do is go to a different state and incorporate there; however, if Ground Concepts has registered its name and service mark with the United States Trademark and Patent Office you may be violating the law by appropriating a name that is already taken.

Instead, your best bet is to find a name that is not taken and pay the proper amount to the Secretary of State to reserve that name. The reservation lasts only for 30 days or so, and for that reason it is important to find a good business attorney and work with her before reserving your name. It may take your attorney several weeks to draw up the papers necessary to form your corporation.

5. How Does One Go About Filing the Papers?

In recent years, hundreds of companies have sprung up that promise to file all the paperwork to get you your corporation. "Why pay an attorney $500 to $1000 to form your company," they ask, "when we can do it for $75 and filing fees?"

It is also possible, of course, to lance a painful lesion on your tongue using a mirror and tools designed for that purpose. But the process is painful and the results are uncertain. It is always better to go to a doctor and have the job done, simply because if you screw it up you have to pay the doctor to fix it, and it is less painful to have it done right than to have it done wrong and then fixed later.

The same advice applies to filing the paperwork for corporations. It is far less expensive to hire an attorney to represent you in the process of setting up your business than it is to set up a business on your own without professional help, and then have to rely on an attorney to unwind things later.

Charlie is an inventor. He develops a new laryngoscope that has the capacity to make intubation easier. He sets up a partnership with his son. He will continue his life as a respiratory therapist working in the hospital while his son Brad sells and markets the device. One year later, the two are squared off in court because they did not have an attorney draw up an agreement between them. Father says the son isn't behaving right. The son says he is doing all the work and the dad is getting all the money. Without a written agreement governing their relationship, the entire situation is a mess for the lawyers and the courts.

Charlie saved $500 by not going to a lawyer. He paid his attorney six times that just to get a "corporate divorce" from his son.

C. WHAT ARE PROFESSIONAL CORPORATIONS?

A professional corporation is a corporation set up for a degreed professional (doctor, lawyer, therapist, accountant, etc.) who practices as a corporation more for tax purposes than for liability purposes. Professional Corporations are business forms that allow a professional to shield some assets, but do not relieve the professional of his duty of care. In other words, even though a physician may be a professional corporation (Dr. John Smith, PC), Dr. Smith is still responsible if he commits malpractice. He cannot simply avoid liability by saying that the professional corporation is at fault.

For this reason, it is not always a good idea to form a PC unless an attorney or tax advisor suggests it is the most effective way to avoid taxation. For the professional, it does not provide malpractice liability protection.

D. What Are Limited Partnerships?

Another form of limited liability business organization is the limited partnership. In a limited partnership, there is a general partner (almost always a corporation) and a series of limited partners who, for the purpose of sharing their investments, maintain an ownership interest in the company.

In a limited partnership, only the general partner is liable in tort and contract for the debts and wrongdoing of the company. Physicians often set up small group practices this way.

A general partner is formed as a corporation. That entity is in charge of the day-to-day activities of the organization. The limited partners are investors who share in the profits, but who do not routinely share in the day-to-day operations of the company. If there is a lawsuit in contract or tort that arises out of the company, the most the limited partner can be liable for is his or her "contribution" to the partnership.

Suppose Doctors A, B, C, and D want to form a limited partnership. Together, they form Docinthebox Corporation to be their "general partner." The general partner is a corporation, so the liability of that corporation is already limited by state law. Now Doctors A, B, C, and D all pool their money by putting $15,000 together to get an office lease, lease equipment, obtain insurance, and hire employees.

If the limited partnership is sued, the most the doctors can lose is their $15,000 investment; they cannot be held personally responsible for more because they are limited partners.[1] However, as noted earlier, the liability shield applies only to the activities of the corporation. Since corporations cannot practice medicine (only doctors can) the liability protection does not attach to the professional activities of the professional, only to the business activities of the partnership.

Each state has different laws with regard to limited partnerships, and this is not a business organization that can be set up without legal help because making the wrong determination under state law could result in losing liability protection. But it is one option when a small number of investors want to form a business.

Like corporations, limited partnerships must adhere to strict rules on formation, and must engage in minute- and record-keeping in order to retain their liability shield.

E. WHAT ARE LIMITED LIABILITY PARTNERSHIPS?

Law partnerships are often set up as Limited Liability Partnerships. Like a Limited Liability Company (LLC) below, the LLP is a closely-held partnership where each partner has limited liability, and where there are no general partners. LLPs can be set up with differential ownership; for example, one partner can have 50% ownership, and two other partners could have 25% ownership.

Like the LLP and the Professional Corporation, the liability protection for professionals in an LLP is scant since the professional can still be

---

[1]They can be liable individually if their actions are at issue. In other words, if they performed a negligent intubation while working at their company, the corporate form doesn't protect them any more than a professional corporation protects a professional.

independently liable for malpractice. But, on the positive side, in an LLP the record-keeping requirements are greatly reduced. Limited liability is not lost if the professional does not keep good minutes of annual meetings in most states.

Like limited liability partnerships and professional corporations, forming an LLP is not something for an off-the-shelf software kit or a $75 corporation service. Again, the key in forming a corporate entity is not in filing the papers, but in determining which form of business makes the most sense.

F. WHAT ARE LIMITED LIABILITY COMPANIES?

A relatively new form of business, the Limited Liability Company, like the LLP, is a company organized for the purpose of minimizing the liability of the owners. Just as with an LLP or a Professional Corporation, a professional who practices through an LLC is not insulated from professional liability by virtue of the LLC. But like an LLP, there is almost no requirement for corporate formalities, and LLCs can have an unlimited life span in most states.

LLCs also offer the ability to be taxed as either a sole proprietorship or a partnership. Thus, tax liability is minimized depending on which form is chosen. Normally, for a sole proprietorship, the most sensible approach is to tax the company as a sole proprietorship so as to avoid double taxation. If taxed as a partnership, the partners must pay taxes on company earnings (the first tax), and then pay regular income taxes on income they derive from the LLC (the second tax). For obvious reasons, it makes good sense to have an LLC for tax purposes over almost any other form of sole proprietorship.

LLCs are formed, like corporations, by filing "Articles of Organization" with the state, and appointing a registered agent for service of process. When multiple individuals will be partners or shareholders in the venture, an internal operating agreement is usually drawn up in order to settle potential issues among the partners. A good operating agreement provides for what happens on dissolution of the LLC, and who gets what back from the organization.

In some states, LLCs have eclipsed corporate filings because they offer such tremendous benefits for the small businessperson. However, as with any corporate form, the real trick in setting one up is not the paperwork, but the advice received. Getting a good operating agreement drafted at the inception of an LLC can often spell the difference between success and failure.

G. ARE THERE ISSUES COMMON TO ALL CORPORATE FORMS?

In every business organization, three common issues arise, which anyone thinking of forming a business should think about and prepare for before forming the business. Those are the requirements of record-keeping and annual reporting, the need for officers, directors, and shareholders, and the rights of the shareholders or partners on dissolution of the business.

1. Does Record-keeping Matter?

In most states, corporations, professional corporations, limited partnerships, and general partnerships are required to file an annual report with the Secretary of State or Corporations Commission. This annual report normally lists the officers and directors, the number of shares outstanding, and the names of the senior beneficial owners. Some corporation laws require annual financial reporting.

Failure to file an annual report usually results in a fine or penalty, and, if the annual report is not remedied quickly, the corporate form can be lost or declared not in good standing. Compliance with the annual reporting requirement is one reason for selecting certain corporate forms (LLC, LLP) over others (corporation, limited partnership).

2. Who Appoints Officers, Directors, Shareholders?

Each corporate entity, whether a close corporation, general business corporation, LLC, LLP, or otherwise, will have someone in charge. Corporations usually appoint officers and directors of the company to oversee the business affairs. In every corporation there must be a President, a Secretary, and a Treasurer; although, in most states one or more roles can be performed by one person. So, a President might also be Treasurer or Secretary.

Directors are elected by shareholders and represent the shareholders' interests in the management of the company. Certain companies have different shares of stock with different voting rights. Holders of preferred shares may get to vote for more candidates or may have extra votes, while holders of common stock may not enjoy such preferences. How a company organizes its shares, its management, and its corporate officers is normally a matter requiring sound legal advice. In a close corporation, such matters may not be terribly important if it is widely understood that the person owning the majority of the stock owns the majority of the company and makes the decisions. In larger companies, and in some partnerships where partners have an equal say in the management of the company, how those senior management positions are allocated can be a source of severe internal friction.

3. What Happens on Dissolution?

Prenuptial agreements are designed to make things easier if the marriage doesn't work out. Operating agreements for corporations, LLCs, and similar business organizations are essentially business prenuptial agreements. When the great idea is in hand and everyone wants a piece of the pie, that's the time to decide who gets to have what say in the organization. That time is not 16 months later when the original investments have run dry, when the product is not being delivered, and when creditors are knocking on the door.

When businesses break up, the most common dispute is over money, and who is or who is not getting theirs. The second most common reason is ego. Everyone wants to be president; no one wants to be the janitor. How officers and directors are elected, as well as how they are compensated, is a source of internal friction and can ruin a company if not spelled out in advance.

In close corporations especially, where there may be two or three primary investors, how disputes get resolved is tremendously important. Simple "majority rules" procedures may be woefully inadequate to protect individual members of the company, and there are certain methods that attorneys use to set up and advise clients to avoid these kinds of problems.

But the rights of each individual on the breakup of the corporation, as well as their responsibilities, should be clearly spelled out. If a guarantee is executed by the president, making him or her personally liable for the corporation's debt, it is vitally important that other officers and directors execute similar documents and have similar responsibilities so that the "majority rules" process doesn't leave one person holding the bag.

4. Do Businesses Need Insurance?

Insurance is the one thing no business can afford to be without. Even if the company has very small revenues and insufficient customers to justify a hefty salary for its officers, there should be no scrimping on insurance. Insurance is what keeps the wolves away from the door, and there are plenty of wolves out there.

a) What Is Comprehensive General Liability Insurance?

A Comprehensive General Liability policy, or CGL, is necessary to protect the business from accidents and injuries occurring on the business premises. It also provides general liability protection from torts like negligence, advertising injury, and similar harms. It is designed to protect the business from everything except professional negligence, motor vehicle accidents, and intentional acts.

b) What Is Professional Negligence Coverage?

If any part of the corporate duties for any employee involve the rendering of professional services (for example, a durable medical equipment company that allows therapists to set up equipment and deliver in-home instruction), that employee should have professional liability insurance, and the company should have a policy covering the company for any acts or omissions by the professional.

c) Are Automobile Policies Necessary?

Usually, yes. If an employee will drive his own vehicle or a company car to see patients, deliver equipment, or otherwise engage in acts on behalf of the employer, a corporate automobile policy is mandatory. The employee's policy may cover him for his personal car when not on company business, but most personal liability policies issued to individuals do not cover the use of the car in any business pursuit. An employee can cause a business to be sued for negligent acts engaged in while driving on behalf of his company.

d) Does a Business Need Workers' Compensation Insurance?

If the business employs anyone other than the proprietor, including children, nieces, nephews, aunts, uncles, cousins, or brothers-in-law, those individual employees should be protected by a Worker's Compensation program.

In most states, if a small business does not purchase a Worker's Compensation plan, and an employee is injured while performing tasks for the employer, the state pays the employee and files an action against the business to recover its costs. Worker's Compensation insurance, while not inexpensive, is vital to protect the company's assets. Also, some corporate forms

do not protect a business owner from liability if the state goes after the officers and directors of an insolvent or defunct corporation.

e) What Are "Umbrella" Policies?

A good umbrella policy is an excellent investment if any portion of the corporate entity is involved in the delivery of patient care. Even though the policy may never be used, if there is a catastrophic injury, the protection it provides will be very much worthwhile.

5. Must Businesses Keep Tax Records?

Depending on which internet shyster you listen to, you can legally avoid
all taxes with the right corporate form. Do not believe this, even for an instant. In a battle between you and the IRS, the IRS always wins. The IRS can
take your home, your car, your bank accounts, and it can attach your earnings. The IRS is not an agency to be trifled with.

The first investment any business person should make is a good attorney,
and behind that, a good accountant to provide good tax advice. Taxes are not
easy or simple for businesses, and even relatively successful entrepreneurs
get caught up in the IRS rules and regulations and wind up bankrupt.

Most states have similar corporate taxes. It seems that everyone wants a
piece of a small and successful business. It is tempting to cheat the tax man.
It is never wise. You may get by with it once or twice, but never in the long
run. It is better to pay your taxes with your income than to pay for your
crimes with a jail sentence.

Unless your attorney is also an expert in taxation, do not rely on your attorney for tax advice. Accountants make their living manipulating the tax
system, and hence are usually better prepared to advise you in this regard.

H. SHOULD OWNERS PLAN FOR SUCCESSION?

While any good attorney plans for dissolution in an operating agreement
used to form a corporation, not all plan for succession. While you may be operating the business today, ten years from now you may wish to retire. You
might want your son, daughter, co-worker, or someone else to take on the
corporate logo and continue doing business.

Good business advice on this subject is vital to preserving what you want
for your business.

1. Should Your Lawyer Act as Advisor?

While lawyers are usually terrible tax advisors (unless that is their specialty), they are relatively good business advisors. If a personal guarantee sought by the bank is the right way to approach a loan, they can tell you. Every important contract signed by your business should be run by the attorney, not only to be sure it is proper and legal, but also to ensure you do not make a bad business judgment.

One of the things lawyers see is what happens when business agreements go bad. Knowing how they go bad, they are usually well suited to advising on how to keep a business out of hot water.

Most people have a family physician who knows the family members and who is there to provide medical care when something goes wrong. A business attorney is much like a family doctor in that regard. If the business attorney helps put the business together, and knows the parties, he can help to advise the business so as to avoid the major pitfalls. This lawyer is not a litigator, but a consultant. His job is to advise the business on how it can operate more profitably and more efficiently. He owes a duty of loyalty to that business.

There is one caveat, however. The lawyer, when hired by the corporation, LLC, LLP, or other corporate-type entity, represents the business or the corporation, not the individuals. So if John and Joan go together to form a business, and become involved in a dispute that will require litigation of the issues, the lawyer cannot represent either one of them. Since he represents the business, he is a witness and cannot get involved by taking sides. Similarly, it is important to understand that a business attorney hired by and paid by the corporation owes a duty to that corporation over his duty to any one individual, even if that individual is his primary contact. There won't be a privilege between John and the lawyer, or Joan and the lawyer with respect to personal things they may tell the lawyer. There will be a privilege as to anything they tell him related to the business. This is important to understand because it has the potential for real problems. If it appears that litigation will be necessary, a litigator, not a consultant is needed, and should be hired.

2. Should You Plan for Business Disputes?

No matter how hard you try, it may still be necessary to go to court to solve problems. If that happens, in most cases you do not need an attorney who specializes in tort law, but rather, an attorney who specializes is business litigation.

Business litigation is different from medical malpractice. In a business lawsuit, the issues are economic; in a medical malpractice lawsuit, they are often personal. And while some business breakups can mirror a bad divorce (this is especially true when there is a divorce at the center of the business dispute), most can be mediated out of court if the parties are properly advised and reasonable.

3. Is It Possible to Avoid Litigation?

Obviously, the best approach is to avoid litigation. That means getting good business advice up front from a seasoned attorney and tax advisor, and it means following that advice.

If an attorney wasn't used to set up the business, or if the business is a partnership or sole proprietorship that has no corporate form, time is of the essence. Every day the business operates without corporate protection, liability issues arise. The first step in avoiding litigation of all types is to make sure that all the corporate forms are properly filed, and all the corporate formalities attended to.

4. How Do I Structure Agreements Properly?

Involve a lawyer who is loyal to you.

If one party or another wants to put together a corporation with someone else, then in some cases it is wise to get independent legal advice. It may sound silly to pay two lawyers to form a corporation, but it is often in the best interests of the parties if there are significant differences in terms of what individuals are bringing to the table.

Consider the situation where one person has a patent for a medical device, and another person is an expert in sales and marketing. The sales person can add value to the medical device by properly advertising and marketing it. He possesses skills and abilities that the inventor does not.

The inventor holds the patent. Instead of placing the patent into the company as a business asset, the inventor wants to issue a "license" to the company and draw royalties from the use of the patent. In addition, he wants to split the profits 50% with the marketing and sales person.

At first blush this might sound like a good idea, until you recognize that the inventor is being compensated twice: first for the use of his patent, and second for his status as a shareholder in the company.

So, if the company sells $500,000 in goods, and pays a 10% royalty to the patent-holding shareholder ($50,000), and the profits, after the cost of goods sold are deducted are $100,000, then the patent holder gets $100,000 for his role in the company, and the marketing person gets $50,000. This may or may not be fair depending on how much work and effort the marketing person put into selling the product. Since a patent holder may revoke a license, the marketing person could be in the position of working very hard to make a profit, only to have the patent license revoked once the product becomes profitable. Under the situation described, the inventor could simply license the patent to a competitor and derive additional income on which the marketing person would have no claim. A good business lawyer could have foreseen this and prevented it.

A business attorney might well agree to set up a company in any manner he was asked, although he should probably advise the parties as to the effect of their agreement. But, if the inventor hired the lawyer to put the corporation together, the lawyer owes a duty of loyalty to the inventor, not the marketing person. He must do what the inventor wants him to do. He does not become the lawyer for the corporation until the corporation is formed (if at all).

Here, the marketing person should have a separate lawyer review the documents and corporate form to make sure that his rights are protected.

I. KEY POINTS

- If you are going to conduct business, you should do so in a form that minimizes your personal liability.
- You need legal advice to determine what form of business to use.
- Companies that do the paperwork without providing legal advice do you a disservice.
- All businesses involving more than one person should plan for dispute resolution.
- All businesses should plan for succession.
- All businesses should maintain some form of insurance to protect the assets of the company.
- Record-keeping is an important part of any business.
- Businesses need a retained lawyer as an advisor in order to comply with the law.

J. SUMMARY

Filling out the proper papers is essential to forming a corporate entity, but it isn't the filling out of papers that makes a lawyer necessary. It is the knowledge of what happens inside corporations; how corporations, partnerships, and limited liability companies are governed; and the methods by which business disputes can be avoided that allow the attorney to earn his money.

If you are thinking of forming a business to protect your assets or to improve your profitability on a product or service you offer, you do not save money by doing the paperwork yourself. All you really do is make it more likely that you'll need a more expensive lawyer down the road.

CHAPTER 12

The Civil Law—Protecting Yourself and Family

Avoid lawsuits beyond all things; they pervert your conscience, impair your health, and dissipate your property.

Jean de la Bruyere (French Satirist)

A. INTRODUCTION

Of the hundreds of people who came to my office to see me about suing someone, none of them ever wanted to be there in the first place. None of them knew the first thing about lawsuits or litigation, and very few of them had any serious idea about what to expect. Those who did know something usually knew something wrong.

Most people form their opinions (and obtain their information) about the legal system from television or the media. From television, we learn that every case can be wrapped up in an hour (two if it's a movie), and that the good guy always wins. Unfortunately, that is not always true. Frequently, justice is blind, not just. People do not always get an even break, and the guilty do get away with murder.

Yet, from politicians we learn that lawsuits are lotteries for the injured and disabled, a way of making a killing from a misfortune. As Don Henley and Glenn Frey put it:

You haven't been the same since you had your little crash,
But you might feel better if they paid you some cash . . .

The fact is, most people who come to see a lawyer aren't thinking about getting wealthy from a lawsuit. Most of them come because they know they've been wronged, and they want accountability for that wrong. This is after dealing with the person who committed the wrong, and sometimes, after dealing with the insurance company.

As I have said elsewhere, it is not so much what happens that drives a person to see a lawyer, but rather, how a person is made to feel by the experience. For example, a person in an automobile accident who suffers a back injury and who receives timely treatment from a good physician will likely be unwilling to hassle with a lawsuit if the insurance company treats her right, and pays her medical bills. Most people do not view misfortune as their ticket to better economic times. If she owes the doctor $5,000, and gets $7,000 for her claim, in most cases she is happy.

But what happens when the insurance company wants her to see their doctor, and that doctor essentially tells her that in spite of her sciatic pain and stiffness, she isn't hurt? When the insurance company refuses to pay for an MRI because it considers it "frivolous medical testing," it angers the patient. And when the insurance company tells the client that they've paid all the medical bills they intend to pay, and that they've determined that they aren't liable anyway, the injured person goes ballistic.

A good friend of mine, an experienced and highly successful personal injury attorney in Kansas City, says that he has never gotten a multimillion-dollar verdict from the defendant, that it has always been the defendant's insurance company that has given it to him. In essence, when people act unreasonably—when they refuse to become accountable—they increase their chances of being sued, and they increase their chances of getting hit with a big verdict.

The fact is that most people who are injured never sue. Those who do, sue because of one of several factors. They are either lied to, treated badly, or treated as if they do not matter by someone who ought to know better. This is the honesty factor. The other reason is the misfortune factor. Their lives have changed; they cannot continue to work; they miss payments; they lose possessions; they begin to spiral toward bankruptcy. In fact, the number of personal injury claims referred from bankruptcy attorneys would probably be surprising to most people.

Over the years, some of my best clients have been former respiratory therapists who came to my firm because of me. They came with stories of medical negligence, nursing home negligence, and products liability. Most, when they walked through my door, didn't understand the process of the law, and most didn't grasp the idea that when they are injured through no fault of their own, and because of someone else's negligence, that they are owed compensation. None of them came seeking wealth—and any attorney who promises you wealth is promising you the wrong thing. Each came expecting to get back what they were out of pocket and were likely to be out of pocket over time. In most cases, we were able to recover something for them. In none of the cases did the compensation match, in any credible terms, to the loss they had suffered. The law is far from perfect.

Therefore, in this chapter we'll start with some basic legal protections available to consumers, including statutes that protect credit and identity. We'll discuss bankruptcy law, and the different kinds of things about which people bring lawsuits. Much about the elements of these lawsuits has already been discussed in the Torts chapter, and this is but a brief review of those causes of action. Finally, we'll discuss the thorny issue of domestic relations and divorce law.

B. SHOULD I HAVE PRIVACY CONCERNS?

In short, yes. Everything you do in any economic sense of the word is linked, one way or another, to your social security number. Every person's social security number is a key piece of information sought by businesses wishing to sell to or buy from you. They want that information because everything in this country is indexed by that number.

If you were to go to www.freecreditreport.com and select your credit report, you would most likely be amazed at what is reported on you. You would find that, for the last seven to ten years, the business world has been keeping close track of what you've been up to. Not only will every instance where you have requested credit appear, but so will every instance where someone checked on your credit.

"Wait a minute," I can hear you saying. "How could someone check my credit without my asking them to?"

The answer is devastatingly simple, and unfortunately, transparent to most people in the United States. Anyone can check your credit if they have your social security number, and almost anyone can get your social security number if they have your name and you have an address or driver's license.

Once someone accesses your social security number, they can, if they have a "legitimate business purpose"—which includes pre-qualifying you for a credit offer, even if such a credit offer is never extended—find out all about your credit. Private detectives can use your SSN to gather "location information" and find out what entity employs you.

But, of course, far worse than these insidious uses is the use that everyone fears—identity theft. If a criminal knows your social security number and your address, he can file a change of address form with your credit card company and begin receiving your credit card statement. Then he files a notice of a lost or stolen card, gets the card issuer to re-issue the card to the new address, and before you know it you've just paid for Jerry and six of his closest friends to spend a week on Maui.[1]

For this reason, you should guard your credit and your SSN very carefully. You should check your credit report every six months at a minimum, and should follow the guidelines to dispute invalid entries as soon as possible (see following). You should not print your social security number on correspondence or other information unless you are certain that the number won't be disclosed. You should insist on your driver's license number being changed to a number that is not your social security number, and you should offer your new driver's license number (and not your SSN) on documents that are liable to be seen by others (for example, you have no guarantee that the clerk at the grocery store who writes down your social security number isn't also using that number to steal you blind).

Guard your identity and your privacy jealously—once they are invaded, getting back your safety and security is a little like un-ringing a bell.

If you do suffer identity theft, the Fair Credit Reporting Act provides procedures to let others know you've had this problem. Credit issuing agencies can be alerted via a "fraud alert" in your file. You can also take steps with each of the credit reporting agencies to help prevent or reduce your exposure.

If someone does clone your identity, however, you must immediately alert law enforcement personnel. The United States Attorney prosecutes identity theft cases, and federal prison terms for this crime are stiff and mandatory.

C. WHAT IS CONSUMER PROTECTION LEGISLATION?

Consumer Protection Legislation, generally speaking, is legislation that is aimed at protecting you from the unscrupulous in the world. And, in some ways, it is designed to protect you from yourself. Charles Ponzi, the architect of the "Ponzi scheme"—a self-pepetuating pyramid scheme he used to steal millions from investors—said he never cheated an honest man. What made Ponzi rich (and ultimately, what sent him to jail) was the desire most people

---

[1]Of course, federal law limits your liability on this, and identity theft is a federal crime. But it goes on every day.

have to make lots of money without doing a lot of work. Ponzi took people's greed and made it work for him. Hundreds of enterprising entrepreneurs do the same thing every day.

Ponzi was caught, convicted, and ultimately imprisoned. But he was a pioneer, and since his time, thousands of people have taken his work and copied and adapted it to their own particular situation.

Most of the Consumer Protection legislation in America is aimed at preventing this kind of fraud.

1. Is *Caveat Emptor* the Law?

There is a Latin phrase called *caveat emptor,* which means "let the buyer beware." For many years in this country, that was the rule in business transactions. If the rental company could convince you that you could get a 42-inch television for $28 a week, and you were silly enough to rent your television, you pretty much got taken for a ride.

In the late 1950s and early 1960s, a group of predatory business people began to set up companies that could gouge consumers. Television was becoming a big thing, and everyone wanted one. "Easy credit" made that possible. All a consumer had to do was buy the television and agree to pay over time. Revolving credit, with rates of interest at 15% or more, began to become a drain on working people. Slowly, state legislatures and Congress began to address the problems in two ways. First, they addressed the quality of the goods through "lemon laws," and second, they addressed the merchandising schemes through merchandising practice statutes.

2. What Is a "Lemon Law"?

One of the first laws of the era of consumer protection was the automobile lemon law. First passed in California and New York, these statutes required new car dealers to honor their warranty, and provided for a means of relief if the dealer didn't.

Other states passed similar laws, and since those early laws the statutes have been amended to dilute most of the consumer protections.

A listing of the lemon laws (www.yourlemonlawrights.com) in all 50 states is found at a website owned by the law firm of Krohn & Moss, Ltd.[2] If you have a complaint with your new automobile, check out the law in

---

[2]The author does not imply any endorsement of the law firm.

your state before going to the dealer and complaining. Sometimes knowing what your rights are before you walk into the dealership pays off.

Lawyers are rarely mean or abusive. They have the law on their side, and they don't care if the dealer makes a concession or not. The dealer can either pay the money now, or pay the money later, and so they don't get angry and raise their voices. They simply make simple clear demands and follow them up in writing. You can do the same:

Ima Tiredathis
101 E. 19th St.
Clemson, MO

Dear Mr. Bigg:

I bought my new 2005 Toyota from Bigg Ole Toyota on January 5, 2005. Within a week I had to have the seat belt replaced, and a week after that I had to have the brakes repaired. On February 11, 2005, I had an electrical failure where all the lights went out on my car. Your dealership examined the car on February 12, 2005, and could not find anything wrong with it.

The blackout reoccurred on February 19, 2005, while taking my son to soccer practice. My son missed his game, and we were nearly rear-ended at twilight when we could not get the lights to work. On February 21, 2005, your dealership again examined the Toyota, and this time decided it must be the fuses. You ordered parts, which were replaced on February 28, 2005. In spite of this, on March 11, 2005, while going to a wedding, the electrical system failed and the car had to be towed back to my home from St. Louis.

The lemon law provides you four opportunities to fix the problem. You have had your opportunities, and you continue to fail in fixing the problem. I demand a replacement vehicle. Please contact me when you have a similar vehicle for me to examine.

Sincerely,

Ima Tiredathis

D. WHAT DOES THE FEDERAL TRADE COMMISSION DO?

Although it sounds like one of those federal agencies that simply works in the area of foreign trade, the Federal Trade Commission (FTC) is the main consumer watchdog agency. They work hard at protecting citizens from unscrupulous merchants.

At the federal level, the FTC is charged with regulating unfair and deceptive merchandising practices in interstate commerce. The FTC is charged with enforcing numerous federal statutes including:

- **Federal Cigarette Labeling and Advertising Act of 1966** (15 U.S.C. §§ 1331-1340, as amended)
- **Truth in Lending Act** (15 U.S.C. §§ 1601-1667f, as amended)
- **Fair Credit Billing Act** (15 U.S.C. 1666-1666j)
- **Fair Credit Reporting Act** (15 U.S.C. §§ 1681-1681(u), as amended)
- **Fair Credit and Charge Card Disclosure Act** (codified in scattered sections of the U.S. Code, particularly 15 U.S.C. 1637(c)-(g))
- **Equal Credit Opportunity Act** (15 U.S.C. §§ 1691-1691f, as amended)
- **Fair Debt Collection Practices Act** (15 U.S.C. §§ 1692-1692o, as amended)
- **Electronic Fund Transfer Act** (15 U.S.C. §§ 1693-1693r)
- **Comprehensive Smokeless Tobacco Health Education Act of 1986** (15 U.S.C. §§ 4401-4408)
- **Telephone Disclosure and Dispute Resolution Act of 1992** (codified in relevant part at 15 U.S.C. §§ 5701 et seq.)
- **Telemarketing and Consumer Fraud and Abuse Prevention Act** (codified in relevant part at 15 U.S.C. §§ 6101-6108)
- **Credit Repair Organizations Act** (15 U.S.C. §§ 1679-1679j)
- **The Children's Online Privacy Protection Act** (15 U.S.C. §§ 6501-6506)
- **Identity Theft Assumption and Deterrence Act of 1998** (codified in relevant part at 18 U.S.C. § 1028 note)

Federal law (15 USC § 57) gives the authority of the FTC to issue rules and regulations that prohibit certain unfair or deceptive conduct in interstate competition. The statute also provides for civil lawsuits by victims of consumer fraud.

The FTC regulates fraud in the area of pay-per-call (900 number) charges, telemarketing, and in the area of credit reporting and debt collecting. In general, if a consumer has a complaint against a company from another state that attempted to sell something through the mail or over the telephone or internet, the FTC is often the first stop in making a complaint and bringing a lawsuit.

The FTC offers consumers advice through its website at www.ftc.gov. There, a consumer can find information about buying automobiles, credit, diet, health and fitness, the internet, franchise and business opportunities, identity theft, investments, telemarketing, and travel.

1. What Does the FTC Do About Scams?

The FTC works for the consumer to prevent fraudulent, deceptive, and unfair business practices in the marketplace and to provide information to help consumers spot, stop, and avoid them. To file a complaint, or to get free information on consumer issues, visit www.ftc.gov, or call toll-free, 1-877-FTC-HELP (1-877-382-4357); TTY: 1-866-653-4261. The FTC enters internet, telemarketing, identity theft, and other fraud-related complaints into *Consumer Sentinel*, a secure, online database available to hundreds of civil and criminal law enforcement agencies in the United States and abroad. For this reason, the FTC should be one of the first stops consumers make when they suspect that they've been scammed.

2. What Are "Little FTC" Statutes?

These statutes are special laws passed in almost all the states, which make consumer fraud both a target of the Attorney General, and a vehicle to get compensation when a consumer is defrauded. Taking the lead of the federal government, most states enacted consumer protection laws to protect their citizens from the exact type of fraud that the FTC statutes cannot reach. If a business operates inside a state, and sells only to people within the state, the FTC statute may not be an effective deterrent to the fraud. States developed their own consumer protection statutes to give the Attorney General and citizens a weapon to combat fraud.

There is no comprehensive listing of state consumer protection statutes available on the internet; however, a Google search with "deceptive trade practice" and the name of your state will most likely yield a link to your state's law.

Under a state consumer protection statute, you can bring an action if you are defrauded while purchasing goods or services. Some states do not allow actions for "services" claims, but others, like Missouri, allow a person to proceed against someone who sells a service that turns out to be worthless.

If you've been sold a bill of worthless goods, you should either contact an attorney or log on to your Attorney General's website to learn whether the state has an active consumer fraud section. State consumer protection statutes are meant to protect consumers from unscrupulous merchants who prey on those who do not know their rights. In some states, the Attorney General will pursue the wrongdoer for you.

E. WHAT IS THE TRUTH IN LENDING ACT?

The Truth in Lending Act was designed to remedy certain practices by lenders, which hid the amount of money a person taking out a loan was required to pay back. Regulation Z, as promulgated by the Federal Trade Commission, makes lenders comply with a number of disclosure requirements including disclosures as to whether there is a pre-payment penalty.

Most people barely read the documents presented to them with a new car loan or a home loan. To many they are long, confusing, and don't tell them what they really want to know, which is how many payments, and how much the payment is. If they have to pay $20,000 in interest on a $40,000 loan, many people don't give it a second thought if they can afford the monthly payment.

Very few lenders violate the Truth in Lending Act, and where there have been violations they have, for the most part, been technical or mathematical errors that have been fixed once they were brought to the attention of the lender.

The Truth in Lending Act, however, is an important part of providing consumers with a good education about the cost of the credit they obtain.

Recently, a group of predatory lenders have come into existence called the payday loan lenders. Payday loans are small ($50–$500) but exceptionally high cost loans. A person can borrow $50 and pay back $65 to clear his or her debt. The payday loan companies obtain "security" in the form of a post-dated check. Essentially, the loan agreement calls for automatic payment of the debt on a certain date.

If, for any reason, the payday loan customer cannot or will not make good on the check when it is sent through, the loan company has a very big "strong arm" collector it can use—the county prosecutor—who files criminal bad check charges against those unfortunate enough to default on their payday loan obligations.

This has prompted a number of lawsuits against these lenders, and almost every lender now requires a borrower to make an express pledge not to act as a class representative in any class action litigation. The pledge enables the litigant to file an action in small claims court, but not to file a big class action case against the lender. At present, none of those agreements has been challenged, but there is good public policy, which, in many states, will hold those agreements null and void.

Recently, I helped a young woman pay off her payday loans. A $500 loan for two weeks exacted an annual percentage rate of 469% interest. In other words, if the $500 loan went unpaid for a full year the interest alone would be $2,345, requiring the payday loan recipient to pay back $2,845 to the lender. In many states, such a high interest rate would violate usury laws, but the payday loan industry has obtained exemptions from legislatures enabling them to continue to charge such egregiously high rates.

Under no circumstances should a therapist ever obtain a payday loan, or the cousin of the payday loan, the car title loan. These organizations are no more than legalized loan sharking operations, and the therapist who does business with them will soon be broke, or bankrupt, or both.

Worse, if the payday loan company retains your "post-dated check" and runs it through your bank when you don't pay off the loan, you could wind up with charges from your bank. If the lender sends your check to the county prosecutor for action, you could wind up being charged with passing a bad check.[3] In essence, these payday loan sharks don't need a 300-pound "leg breaker" to do their collection work; they let the long arm of the law do it for them. Lives, careers, and families have been ruined dealing with these lenders.

1. What Is the Fair Debt Collection Practices Act?

Another act enforced by the Federal Trade Commission, it is designed to keep collectors (but not creditors) off the backs of working people. In the 1960s and 1970s, unscrupulous debt collectors would call debtors at work, at home, in the middle of the night, and on weekends and holidays in order to harass them into paying debts that often were incorrect or exaggerated. Congress passed the Fair Debt Collection Practices Act to put an end to this kind of abuse.

The Fair Debt Collection Practices Act protects "debtors." If you use credit cards, owe money on a personal loan, or are paying on a home mortgage, you

---

[3]In most cases, since the check was given as security for a loan, and not with an intent to defraud, the criminal charge would not stick if the debtor were represented by competent counsel. However, hundreds of people have gone to jail dealing with payday loan companies.

are a "debtor." If you fall behind in repaying your creditors, or an error is made on your accounts, you may be contacted by a "debt collector." The act applies to debt collectors (normally collection agencies and lawyers collecting debts), but it does not apply to creditors. For that reason the Act can be used to prevent phone calls from ABC Collection Agency, but can't stop phone calls by Acme Mastercard. The creditor (the person to whom you owe money) can avoid the terms of the act (although most honorable credit card companies comply with it).

a) Does the Act Reduce a Person's Debt?

The Fair Debt Collection Practices Act requires that debt collectors treat you fairly and prohibits certain methods of debt collection. Of course, the law does not erase any legitimate debt you owe. It simply prevents the creditor from collecting it in an improper way.

The FDCPA covers personal, family, and household debts. This includes money owed for the purchase of an automobile, for medical care, for charge accounts, for lines of revolving credit, or for gasoline and travel credit cards. Again, it is important to remember that the actual creditor (Shell Oil Company, for example) is not subject to the FDCPA unless, for example, Shell has a subsidiary (Shell Collections, LLC) that does its collecting using the Shell name.

b) Who Is a "Debt Collector" Under the FDCPA?

A debt collector is any person, agency, or entity who regularly collects debts owed to others. This includes collection agencies and attorneys who collect debts on a regular basis.

Because there is a history of abuse by debt collectors, the Act limits how a collector can contact you. A collector may contact you in person, by mail, telephone, telegram, or fax. However, a debt collector may not contact you at inconvenient times or places, such as before 8 a.m. or after 9 p.m., unless you agree. A debt collector also may not contact you at work if the collector knows that your employer disapproves of such contacts.

c) How Can I Stop Collector Harassment?

Like calls from the IRS, calls from collectors (or visits or letters) are annoying and sometimes downright harassing. You can stop a debt collector from contacting you by writing a letter to the collector telling them to stop. It is never enough to simply tell them over the telephone to stop calling. You must send a letter, and in most cases, the best way to send it is by certified mail, and if possible, by facsimile. If you use a return receipt, you can prove the collector received your letter telling them to stop contact. If you have a fax receipt, you can prove they got the correspondence that way.

Once the collector receives your letter, they may not contact you again except to say there will be no further contact or to notify you that the debt collector or the creditor intends to take some specific action. Please note, however, that sending such a letter to a collector does not make the debt go away if you actually owe it. You could still be sued by the debt collector or your original creditor. Sometimes, debt collectors like to deal directly with the debtor, and sometimes they apply pressure by calling friends and family and implying that you owe money and are going to be sued. They will often use this method to extract payment from parents and others.

d) Why Might I Need an Attorney?

If you have an attorney, the debt collector must contact the attorney, rather than you. If you do not have an attorney, a collector may contact other people, but only to find out where you live, what your phone number is, and where you work. Collectors usually are prohibited from contacting such third parties more than once. In most cases, the collector may not tell anyone other than you and your attorney that you owe money.

e) What Are Predatory Collectors?

Predatory collectors are companies that buy the bad debt of a company or business and then attempt to collect it using high pressure and the threat of litigation. These speculators will buy a Mastercard account with $5,000 in charges for $150, and then attempt to collect the debt from the person who had the account.[4] Often, computers do not get updated, and payments do not get posted. Frequently, the debt collector has the amount wrong, or has the wrong person's name associated with the account. For that reason, the law provides some safeguards against predatory collection tactics.

---

[4]And sometimes, they get the wrong person. When an identity criminal runs up charges in your name, you may face multiple collection actions from creditors who will try to claim the debt is yours.

f) What Protections Exist to Ensure That Only Valid Debts Are Collected?

Within five days after you are first contacted, the collector must send you a written notice telling you the amount of money you allegedly owe, the name of the creditor to whom you owe the money (if it is different than their name), and what action to take if you believe you do not owe the money. A collector may not contact you if, within 30 days after you receive the written notice, you send the collection agency a letter stating you do not owe money. However, a collector can renew collection activities if you are sent proof of the debt, such as a copy of a bill for the amount owed.

The FDCPA prohibits certain conduct on the part of collectors. That conduct includes:

Harassment. Debt collectors may not harass, oppress, or abuse you or any third parties they contact.

For example, debt collectors may not:

- use threats of violence or harm;
- publish a list of consumers who refuse to pay their debts (except to a credit bureau);
- use obscene or profane language; or
- repeatedly use the telephone to annoy someone.

False statements. Debt collectors may not use any false or misleading statements when collecting a debt. For example, debt collectors may not:

- falsely imply that they are attorneys or government representatives;
- falsely imply that you have committed a crime;
- falsely represent that they operate or work for a credit bureau;
- misrepresent the amount of your debt;
- indicate that papers being sent to you are legal forms when they are not; or
- indicate that papers being sent to you are not legal forms when they are.

Debt collectors also may not state that:

- you will be arrested if you do not pay your debt;
- they will seize, garnish, attach, or sell your property or wages, unless the collection agency or creditor intends to do so, and it is legal to do so; or
- actions, such as a lawsuit, will be taken against you, when such action legally may not be taken, or when they do not intend to take such action.

Debt collectors may not:

- give false credit information about you to anyone, including a credit bureau;
- send you anything that looks like an official document from a court or government agency when it is not; or
- use a false name.

Unfair practices. Debt collectors may not engage in unfair practices when they try to collect a debt. For example, collectors may not:

- collect any amount greater than your debt, unless your state law permits such a charge;
- deposit a post-dated check prematurely;
- use deception to make you accept collect calls or pay for telegrams;
- take or threaten to take your property unless this can be done legally; or
- contact you by postcard.

g) Do I Have a Say in How My Debts Are Paid Off?

Debtors do have some say over how debts are paid off. If you owe more than one debt, any payment you make must be applied to the debt you indicate. A debt collector may not apply a payment to any debt you believe you do not owe.

Of course, some collectors simply refuse to be bound by the law. They are operated by shady characters who prey on the uninformed. They assume that debtors cannot afford legal representation, and as a result, go after them with a vengeance. You have the right to sue a collector in a state or federal court within one year from the date the law was violated. If you win, you may recover money for the damages you suffered plus an additional amount up to $1,000. Court costs and attorney's fees also can be recovered. A group of people also may sue a debt collector and recover money for damages up to $500,000, or one percent of the collector's net worth, whichever is less.

Debtors can report any problems with a debt collector to their state Attorney General's office and the Federal Trade Commission. Many states have their own debt collection laws, and your Attorney General's office can help you determine your rights.

Sometimes, however, the State Attorney General is not a helpful resource, and an attorney is needed. To help your attorney you should:

- Keep a copy of everything the collector sends you.
- Keep a copy of everything you send to the collector.

- Make notes about what the collector said at or near the time the collector talked to you.
- Record the telephone conversation (if legal in your state) if the collector repeatedly calls back or uses harassing and abusive or profane language.
- Never lose your temper with the collector.

An attorney can often take blatant evidence of violation of the FDCPA and use it to negotiate an end to collection activities, and sometimes a settlement of all claims.

h) A Word About Student Loan Debt

Student loan debt is unlike most other forms of debt. Although the protections against abusive collection apply with equal vigor to the collectors hired by the Department of Education, student loan debt is unique in several respects.

If you borrow money from Acme Lending, and you don't pay that loan back, the statute of limitations makes it impossible to sue on that debt after five to ten years, depending on the state. In some states there are statutes of repose. But those statutes, by virtue of federal law, do not apply to student loan debt.

In fact, just the opposite is true. There is no statute of limitations on a federally guaranteed student loan. A loan can be reduced to judgment after 20 to 30 years of not being paid—something that could never happen to a commercial debt.

Also of importance, the federal government can employ other remedies, including the suspension or revocation of professional licenses, to enforce payment.[5] If you are working and are in default on a student loan, the Department of Education doesn't need a court order to garnish your wages.

The bottom line: do not default on student loan debt.

F. WHAT IS THE FAIR CREDIT REPORTING ACT?

The Federal Trade Commission also enforces credit laws that protect your right to obtain, use, and maintain credit. These laws do not guarantee that everyone will receive credit, only that everyone will have an equal opportunity to do so. The credit laws protect your rights by requiring businesses to give all consumers a fair and equal opportunity to receive credit and to resolve disputes over credit errors.

---

[5]This is also true with respect to delinquent child support obligations.

Your credit payment history is recorded in a file or report called a credit report. These files or reports are maintained and sold by "consumer reporting agencies" (CRAs). One type of CRA is commonly known as a credit bureau. You have a credit record on file at a credit bureau if you have ever applied for a credit or charge account, a personal loan, insurance, or a job. Your credit record contains information about your income, debts, and credit payment history. It also indicates whether you have been sued, arrested, or have filed for bankruptcy. The information in your credit report is considered by businesses granting credit to be accurate unless you dispute it.

The Fair Credit Reporting Act (FCRA) is designed to help ensure that CRAs furnish correct and complete information to businesses to use when evaluating your application.

Your rights under the Fair Credit Reporting Act include the following:

- You have the right to receive a copy of your credit report. The copy of your report must contain all of the information in your file at the time of your request.
- You have the right to know the name of anyone who received your credit report in the last year for most purposes or in the last two years for employment purposes.
- Any company that denies your application must supply the name and address of the CRA they contacted, provided the denial was based on information given by the CRA.
- You have the right to a free copy of your credit report when your application is denied because of information supplied by the CRA. Your request must be made within 60 days of receiving your denial notice.
- If you contest the completeness or accuracy of information in your report, you should file a dispute with the CRA and with the company that furnished the information to the CRA. Both the CRA and the furnisher of information are legally obligated to reinvestigate your dispute.
- You have a right to add a summary explanation to your credit report if your dispute is not resolved to your satisfaction.

When you apply for credit, you fill out a credit application. When creditors evaluate a credit application, they cannot lawfully engage in any discriminatory practices including discriminating on the basis of race, color, national origin, or where your money comes from.

1. How Does the Equal Credit Opportunity Act Affect Credit Reporting?

The Equal Credit Opportunity Act (ECOA) prohibits credit discrimination on the basis of sex, race, marital status, religion, national origin, age, or receipt of public assistance. Creditors may ask for this information (except religion) in certain situations, but may not use it to discriminate when deciding whether to grant you credit.

The ECOA protects consumers who deal with companies that regularly extend credit, including banks, small loan and finance companies, retail and department stores, credit card companies, and credit unions. Everyone who participates in the decision to grant credit, including real estate brokers who arrange financing, must follow this law. Businesses applying for credit also are protected by this law.

Your rights under the Equal Credit Opportunity Act include the following:

- You cannot be denied credit based on your race, sex, marital status, religion, age, national origin, or receipt of public assistance.
- You have the right to have reliable public assistance considered in the same manner as other income.
- If you are denied credit, you have a legal right to know why.

G. WHAT ARE THE FAIR CREDIT BILLING AND ELECTRONIC FUND TRANSFER ACTS?

These are laws designed to help protect you from billing or ATM errors. It is important to check credit billing statements and electronic fund transfer account statements regularly. These documents may contain mistakes that could damage your credit status or reflect improper charges or transfers. If you find an error or discrepancy, notify the company and contest the error immediately. The Fair Credit Billing Act (FCBA) and Electronic Fund Transfer Act (EFTA) establish procedures for resolving mistakes on credit billing and electronic fund transfer account statements, including:

- charges or electronic fund transfers that you, or anyone you have authorized to use your account, have not made;
- charges or electronic fund transfers that are incorrectly identified or show the wrong amount or date;
- computation or similar errors;

- failure to reflect payments, credits, or electronic fund transfers properly;
- not mailing or delivering credit billing statements to your current address, as long as that address was received by the creditor in writing at least 20 days before the billing period ended;
- charges or electronic fund transfers for which you request an explanation or documentation, due to a possible error.

The FCBA generally applies only to "open end" credit accounts like credit cards, revolving charge accounts (such as department store accounts), and overdraft checking accounts. It does not apply to loans or credit sales that are paid according to a fixed schedule until the entire amount is paid back, such as an automobile loan. The EFTA applies to electronic fund transfers, such as those involving automatic teller machines (ATMs), point-of-sale debit transactions, and other electronic banking transactions.

H. WHAT IS BANKRUPTCY?

When the colonists came to the land that would become the United States, many were victims of the same types of credit scams that are perpetuated today, except that the failure to honor ones debts in England in the 1700s would put a person in debtor's prison. If the debt could not be collected from land or personal property, then the sheriff would come and arrest the debtor and a judge would ultimately place that person in the prison.

When the federal constitution was formed, it did not include specific guarantees that individuals who were debtors could not be imprisoned for the debt. In fact, the use of "indentured servitude" as a means of repaying debt was more or less authorized by the constitution when it was framed to allow for slavery.

Over the next hundred years, each state generally included in its constitution the provision that a person could not be imprisoned for debt. The federal government recognized the wisdom of this approach, and in 28 USC § 2007, provides that no federal court may imprison a person for debt in any state with a constitutional prohibition on such imprisonment.

The federal constitution, however, in Article I, Section 8, Clause 4, does provide for Congress to have the power to regulate bankruptcies. Federal regulation of bankruptcies was thought to be important in order that citizens of one state could not use their laws to avoid paying citizens of another state.

Originally, bankruptcy was a means of making sure that all creditors were paid something. Over time, however, the purpose of bankruptcy has changed.

1. What Is the Purpose of Bankruptcy?

The purpose behind bankruptcy laws is the implicit recognition that if creditors extend too much credit to a person, such that the debtor cannot meet his or her obligations, the fault, if any, lies with the creditors who allowed the bankrupt person to get overextended. In many situations, particularly where the bankruptcy is brought about by hard times or medical costs, the statement is true. In other cases, people file bankruptcy to avoid their responsibility for debt. In either case, they are taking advantage of the chief purpose of the bankruptcy act, which is to "relieve the honest debtor from the weight of oppressive indebtedness."[6] The debtor who surrenders for distribution the "property which he owns at the time of bankruptcy" is given new opportunities "unhampered by the pressure and discouragement of preexisting debt."[7] So say the federal courts, and in saying have laid out the basic policy of bankruptcy. If a person honestly falls behind in his or her debts, and cannot exist and make the payments, the court steps in to relieve them.

a) When Should I Consider Bankruptcy?

Usually, only as a last resort.

There are three types of bankruptcy that a citizen can employ to relieve their financial obligations. Chapter 7 Bankruptcy is probably the one most familiar to the majority of Americans. In Chapter 7, the debtor surrenders all his property, with a few exemptions (books, tools of his trade, etc.) and the trustee in bankruptcy sells or disposes of these items and pays off creditors.

In Chapter 11, a form of bankruptcy primarily intended for businesses, a debtor is allowed to restructure his debt. If he owes $500 per month, and only makes $600 a month, the federal court may allow him to restructure his debt so as to get his business turned around.

In Chapter 13, called the "wage earner plan" by the courts and bankruptcy experts, a person who is in debt over his head and earning a monthly salary can restructure his debts by paying all of his money over to the federal court. The court gives back an allowance for food, clothing, medical care, and the like, and pays off the other creditors out of the stream of monthly payments it receives from the debtor. Chapter 13 plans normally run three to five years, and allow the debtor to keep certain items of property while repaying their loans.

---

[6]*Williams v. U.S. Fidelity & G. Co.*, 236 U.S. 549, 554-555.
[7]*Local Loan v. Hunt*, 292 U.S. 234, 244.

Depending on the financial situation, Chapter 7 or Chapter 13 is usually the best option for most debtors, but there are serious consequences to bankruptcy. It remains on your credit report for ten years. It becomes a matter of public record. In the short term, it can affect your ability to get credit and security clearances. Many people go through bankruptcy and turn around and receive credit cards from willing lenders within weeks. On the other hand, it can make it impossible for you to get certain jobs, can prevent you from owning your own home, and can have disastrous consequences for family members.

Sometimes people who know they are going to have to go bankrupt will pay off a debt they owe their mother or father before they file for bankruptcy. Unfortunately, the trustee for the government can go back to the person the bankrupt paid off and reclaim a portion of the amount, or all of it, to use in paying off other creditors or secured creditors.

The decision about what form of bankruptcy to choose is predicated on how bad the financial situation of the client is, and a seasoned bankruptcy attorney is necessary to advise a debtor on this subject. Often, a bankruptcy attorney will suggest that a debtor try a service like Consumer Credit Counseling to assist them with getting their debts paid off without the stigma of bankruptcy. In the past 20 years, Consumer Credit Counseling has worked miracles for countless thousands of consumers, and they are often an appropriate intermediate step on the way to bankruptcy court.

Since about 1990, bankruptcy filings have been automated, with the federal courts requiring forms generated by certain types of software. Bankruptcy lawyers have this software, but so do certain "paperwork preparing" companies that offer to prepare the forms for a fee much less than that of a bankruptcy attorney.

Just as with forming a business, the true value in having an attorney is not the preparation of the forms (although that is a major undertaking). Rather, the advice about what to do (and more importantly, what not to do) about certain debts before bankruptcy is filed is why an attorney is necessary. Because certain time periods can affect how debts are paid, an attorney is necessary to evaluate the claims of lenders and creditors.

2. What Are Consumer Credit Counseling Services?

In most situations, bankruptcy can be avoided by using a consumer credit counseling service. But beware. Many "debt management agencies" are no more than profit-driven companies that essentially function as a cross between a collection agency and a private bankruptcy trustee. They derive significant fees from their work.

For obvious reasons, consumers who use a debt management agency should use a truly not-for-profit agency in their home town. An agency that advertises on television is unlikely to be "not for profit" in the true sense of the word.

a) What Is the Effect of Bankruptcy on Small Businesses?

Perhaps the most telling effect of bankruptcy is the impact that it has on other persons and businesses. More than one business has fallen victim to a supplier's or buyer's bankruptcy.

If Joe's Home Health Care leases 20 oxygen concentrators from a leasing company, and that leasing company goes bankrupt, the trustee in bankruptcy has the power to "void" the contract with Joe's Home Health Care. It can essentially void the entire lease agreement and come pick up every concentrator Joe has, even if it is out in a patient's home. Joe is often powerless to stop this.

Suppose Phil is buying a house from Margaret under what is known as a land contract or a "contract for deed." In such a contract, the person who owns the property finances the property for the person buying it. Normally, the agreement runs more than 20 years, and a person solvent in 1990 might be insolvent by 2004, 14 years after the loan was originated.

If Margaret goes bankrupt, Phil may wind up losing his entire investment in the land because his rights to the land are found in the contract, and the trustee in bankruptcy has the power to void that contract and take the land. He can sell the land to someone else, and Phil loses his home and his investment.

When K-Mart Corporation went bankrupt, the persons who owned shares of its stock were left with a worthless investment. The bankruptcy more or less eliminated the requirement of the company to pay its shareholders anything. When the Savings and Loans went bankrupt in the 1990s, many an investor lost his life savings as a result.

Mary and Joe are a married couple who have not had a good run of luck. After six years of marriage, they decide to divorce. They own one vehicle, a 2004 Ford F-150. The truck is in Joe's name, but the court orders that Mary receive the truck. Joe is upset, and stops making payments. The finance company repossesses the truck. Mary says the truck is hers because the court gave it to her. Can Mary prevail?

In most cases, Mary can't win. Mary may have the title to the vehicle, but possession of the vehicle is now with the bank. The bank, when it issued a loan, placed a "security interest" on the truck, meaning that the loan is backed up by the truck as collateral. The bank can protect its collateral by seizing it, and in this case, selling it, even though Mary may have a divorce decree that makes the truck hers.

If Mary had declared bankruptcy, however, she might have been able to stop the repossession and get the truck back.[8] She would have been required to pay the back payments and keep payments current, because her lender has a "security interest" in property and is therefore a "preferred" creditor.

In short, bankruptcy law favors (1) the bankrupt person or business, and (2) any creditor who records a security interest in land or personal property. Secured creditors are paid first and paid the most from the bankrupt's property. Unsecured creditors (those who have things like credit cards or open accounts with the debtor) are paid pennies on the dollar, if anything at all.

While bankruptcy can be a godsend for the overextended debtor, it can wreak havoc on the small businessperson or the individual investor.

I. CAUSES OF ACTION

Sometimes, bad things just happen. They happen regardless of how careful a person is, and regardless of how lucky. Sometimes, things just happen, through no one's fault. When they do, there isn't much an attorney can do. Sometimes, however, things happen because people don't do their jobs, or because people who should use the highest degree of care in helping others, fail to use that degree of care. When that happens, when someone else is at fault for the bad thing that happened to you, you have a right to sue for compensation.

As I have said before, bringing a lawsuit is about compensation. It is not about hitting the lottery, getting rich, cashing in on a big award from a sympathetic jury, or screwing a company or business. It is wholly about compensation for injuries received.

In 10 years of practice, I have never had a client tell me that they really are glad something happened so they could get some money. In almost every case, a plaintiff will say to me, "if I could bring my mother back," or "if I could regain the use of my legs," and they finish that thought with "I wouldn't sue

---

[8]Mary can also get the truck back, in most states, by paying off the loan in full. This rarely, if ever, happens.

anyone." The fact is, when people get an award from a jury, that award is based on severe and often devastating injuries, and it can never make things "right."

The worst possible situation when you're injured is to be unable to pay for the care you need. Unfortunately, many people are in exactly that predicament. They are paralyzed, and cannot afford to have modifications to their house and car so that they can lead a fairly normal life. Or, they are saddled with hundreds of thousands of dollars in medical debt because the medical care that saved their life wasn't cheap.

It is truly unfortunate that so many people view lawsuits as a means to get rich. I have had people come into my office whom I thought manufactured a cause of action. I do not take those clients. Good lawyers don't.

It would be my fondest wish that you, dear reader, would never need a lawyer for anything. I would like nothing better than for you to live out the rest of your life without any injury or problem. But if you are injured, you need to know how to go about getting compensated, because the insurance companies won't tell you, and they surely will not deal fairly with you.

What do I mean by that? I mean that insurance companies have one job: protect the insured as cheaply as possible. If they can drive the cost of protecting the client down, they do so. The chief tool insurance companies have to do that is ignorance. They will lie directly to your face, telling you they have no liability. They will offer to pay a $50,000 claim with $5,000 and give you the impression you ought to be glad to get any money at all. In short, insurance companies have strong incentives, in order to remain profitable in a very tough business, to pay the very least amount possible.

In this section, we'll examine what a person can sue for when they are wronged by a company, an individual, or the government.

1. What Is Wrongful Death?

When the death of a person is caused by the wrongful actions of another person, the heirs at law have an action for wrongful death against those who caused the death. So, for example, when the pickup truck pulls out in front of the passenger car, and a mother of three is killed in the resulting collision, the driver of the pickup truck is liable for the wrongful death of the mother.

Wrongful deaths happen in motor vehicle accidents and product liability claims. For example, when the heater malfunctions and spreads carbon monoxide through the whole house, killing a father of four, the survivors have an action for wrongful death based on product liability. Where a drug is given in the wrong dose or through the wrong route, a claim exists. They occur in criminal situations, where a landlord fails to prevent an attack on a tenant by not replacing locks or lighting. In any situation where someone's death results from the neglect or intentional act of someone else, there is a potential wrongful death claim.

The only way to determine whether there is a wrongful death for which recovery can be made is to contact an attorney. The attorney can and will obtain records and evaluate the claim.

a) Who Can Bring a Wrongful Death Claim?

Unfortunately, not everyone can bring a wrongful death claim. In Missouri, heirs, children, siblings, and other relatives are in the class of persons who can bring an action. There are some plaintiffs in every state who are the "preferred" plaintiffs. In Missouri, for example, a child, parent, or spouse has the right to bring a wrongful death action, and they are in the "first class" of beneficiaries. If there is a member of that class and they won't bring a claim, no one else can bring a claim.

If there is no spouse, child, or parent, a sibling can bring an action, as can a nephew, or similar relative, but only under certain conditions. The best way to find out who has the right to bring an action is to consult an attorney.

2. When Can You Sue for Slander-Libel?

Slander and libel arise out of the publication of false statements to others. If someone defames you by telling untruths about you to others, that is slander. If they publish it in a newspaper, or stick a flyer up on a wall, that is libel. Either way, libel and slander are difficult causes of action which are disfavored by the Courts.

First, the constitution permits freedom of speech and freedom of expression. There is wide constitutional protection of the right to publish information, and even some false information can be protected. Second, the key element of a libel or slander case is damages, which is usually missing from the great majority of slander cases because, in most of those cases, people disbelieve the lie and do not act on it, leaving only hurt feelings on the part of the plaintiff.

A good slander case or libel case arises out of a false statement that causes such severe injury to reputation as to cause the loss of a job or negative effects in the community. For example, falsely accusing someone of child molestation, or being a child molester, causing that person to lose his job as a youth counselor or resulting in his wrongful incarceration would be a good claim for libel or slander if the libel or slander had neither a ring of truth nor a good faith basis.

Put another way, a person who sees suspicious behavior and who reports that behavior, may be privileged to report that behavior. He may be forgiven for getting things wrong if his intent was to protect a child. If the person leveling the accusation of molestation or abuse knows the person is not guilty, and makes the allegation solely to cause injury, there is a potential libel claim.

Each libel and slander case depends for its vitality on the strength of the individual assertions in the case. It is impossible to conjure up every potential situation where a libel or slander case would merit investigation and litigation. If you suspect you've been libeled or slandered, you should see an attorney immediately because most slander and libel causes of action have very short (one year or less) statutes of limitation.

3. Who Can Sue for Negligence?

When you or a loved one is injured as a result of negligence, defined as a failure to use ordinary care, you have a potential claim for a lawsuit. Although it is impossible to list every potential situation where negligence arises, if someone else is conceivably to blame for your injuries, the matter should be evaluated by an attorney.

Negligence generally means a failure to exercise ordinary care to protect others. For example, if a farmer has an uncovered well on his property, and he fails to fence it, or cover it, and your child falls into that well and breaks his leg, that is probably negligence.

Similarly, if a person leaves her property in a dangerous condition, for example, if she fails to fix a cracked board on her porch and someone falls through that board, she is potentially liable for negligence.

Negligence also arises, of course, in traffic accidents. Failure to yield, failure to signal a lane change, following too closely, and failing to stop for traffic signals are all examples of negligent conduct.

In addition to negligence, of course, the plaintiff must prove damages and causation. If a person runs a red light and doesn't hit you (but only scares you), that's not a case. On the other hand, if the person runs a red light and hits you, causing you to have a heart attack, that is negligence.

The best way to determine whether you have a claim is to see an attorney.

4. What Is False Imprisonment?

False imprisonment occurs in one of two situations: when someone's liberty is restrained by official action of a law enforcement officer, resulting in incarceration or imprisonment; and when someone is kept from leaving or detained as a result of the action of some third party. The key element of a false imprisonment claim is that the person restraining the liberty of an individual has no good faith basis for doing so.

Police officers normally have immunity from civil lawsuits for doing their job. However, when they purposefully violate the law and falsely restrain an individual, they may be liable both under the common law and under the constitution. False arrest or false imprisonment starts with knowledge on the part of the official that there is no good faith basis to believe that there is a need to restrain the liberty of the individual.

Recently, a "bounty hunter"—a person employed by a bail bonding company to chase down people who jump bail—came to the home of a man in Kansas City. The bounty hunter grabbed the man in his pajamas, cuffed him, and dragged him to a pickup truck. The man, an illustrator for Hallmark Cards, had a first and last name that was the same as that of a drug dealer in the Springfield, Missouri, area who had jumped bail.

The man was held in the back of a pickup truck and driven most of the way from Kansas City to Springfield before his lawyer was able to convince the bounty hunter that he had the wrong man. The bail bondsman, the bounty hunter, and the company that wrote the bond have all been sued for false imprisonment because the man was deprived of his liberty for several hours, driven away from his home in the dark of night, and threatened by men wearing pajamas and pointing guns at his head.

One of the more common places that false imprisonment lawsuits erupt is in the context of department store security personnel. One reason that cameras and security personnel have become so critical in most department stores is that the store wants photographic evidence of theft before it will empower its security officer to take action and arrest the offender.

The reason for this caution is found in the liability that attaches if the officer makes a wrongful detention by restraining a patron where there is no documented probable cause to do so.

5. What Is Outrage or Intentional Infliction of Emotional Distress?

The tort of outrage, or what is sometimes called intentional infliction of emotional distress, rests on the desire or effect of creating intense emotional distress on the part of the victim. Negligent infliction of emotional distress is also actionable, although in most cases the victim must experience distress so profound that he or she seeks medical attention for the problem.

It is hard to lay out the fact that would create a situation where someone would be liable for outrage other than to say there must be intense emotional distress, and the person causing it must intend to cause it.

In other instances, a person may sue for negligently causing emotional distress, but only where the person who claims injury has suffered a severe medical condition that is medically diagnosable, and was in the "zone of danger." For example, where the mother watches a driver run over her child, and then suffers a heart attack as a result of the stress, may be a situation where the tortfeasor is liable for Negligent Infliction of Emotional Distress.

6. Can I Sue for Products Liability?

Any time a product malfunctions and creates injury there is a potential product liability claim. Some of these are better than others. A lawnmower blade that disengages and cuts off the leg of a passerby is an extreme example of a good product liability claim, as is the case where a furnace malfunctions, causing carbon monoxide poisoning. A gun that fires when dropped on the ground, striking a child is another good example.

Product liability can be based on a dangerous and defective product, a negligently manufactured product, a negligently designed product, or, where the danger cannot be effectively eliminated by design and precaution, on failure to warn of the danger to consumers.

For example, in order for chlorine bleach to do its job, it has to contain sodium hypochlorite. The product cannot be made safe by different design. For that reason, in order to market the product, it must bear safety labels that say you can't mix it with ammonia and other cleansers. A bottle of bleach failing to have this caution on it creates a product liability claim.

Any time a person is injured as a result of a defective product (or even one that may not appear defective), a potential products claim exists and should be investigated.

7. What Is Premises Liability?

Premises liability includes any injury that occurs as a result of the dangerous condition of a person's property. For example, when a person falls down an unmarked elevator shaft in an abandoned building, premises liability exists. When a person falls because there is a gap in the sidewalk, premises liability exists.

Premises liability is also the branch of the law dealing with the situation where a landlord or business owner fails to protect a guest from injury inflicted by the criminal conduct of a third person. So, when the owner of a restaurant knows that he has been robbed three times after 10 p.m., but continues to remain open after that time without security, an injury to a customer in a holdup is a potential premises liability claim.

8. What Are Business Torts?

A business tort is an action brought by a business or merchant against another business or merchant. Any time a business engages in unfair competition or deceptive trade practices, it has the potential to hurt the business at which it is directing those practices. That business has the right to sue and recover the damages. So, when Company A has its representative say that Company B's oximeter does not work properly, or fails to give good readings, Company B may have a cause of action for trade libel. When Company A underprices their oximeters, taking a large loss on the units in order to drive Company B out of business, that is unfair competition.

There are hundreds of situations where one business can sue another for tortuous conduct, and far too many to go into here. However, when a business is harmed by the actions of another business, and those actions don't arise out of good faith competition in the marketplace (for example, stealing trade secrets or engaging in industrial espionage), those are business torts.

Violations of patents and trademarks are another form of business tort.

9. Can I Sue for Fraud and Misrepresentation?

Being taken for a ride in a business deal, or when buying a car, house, or other consumer goods, is never fun. Losing money, particularly lots of money, is not a good feeling. The law of fraud and misrepresentation is what keeps people who tell lies from profiting from their misdeeds.

There are nine badges of fraud in most states, but the thing that makes for a good fraud case is a situation where the person defrauded relied, and had the right to rely, on the representations of the seller. For example, when the builder tells the buyer of the new home that it has blown-in insulation in every room, and later inspection reveals that there was never any insulation blown in, the buyer may be permitted to rely on those representations and be able to recover the costs of repairs.

Generally speaking, fraud is a very difficult claim to make, but whenever there has been an attempt to steal money through artifice or deceit, that claim should be made.

Another issue to consider is whether the claim may be more properly made under a Consumer Protection Statute like a Merchandising Practices Act. In many cases, when there is a colorable claim of fraud, the best approach is to consider a cause of action under the Little FTC Act in your state.

J. IS DOMESTIC RELATIONS LAW IMPORTANT?

It is an ever-expanding area of the law, and rights and duties change frequently. Domestic Relations is the branch of the law dealing with relationships, and it covers situations where people are married, living together, and divorced. There are few hard and fast rules about domestic relations, but one thing is certain. In divorce and similar domestic relations situations, lawyers are essential to protect the rights of the parties. Lawyers are often said to be like nuclear weapons. If the other side has one, you need one. Unleashing them is unpredictable. And once they are set into motion, they often cannot be recalled.

Over the years, hundreds of people have called me for divorce help, even though they know I do not practice in this area. In each case, I have said, "hire a seasoned attorney." Sometimes people claim they want the "meanest SOB in the bar," to represent them in their divorce. This is seldom a wise choice because a lawyer who prefers to fight it out on everything is a lawyer who is going to cost a lot of money in the long run, usually without significantly better results.

Divorce is not for do-it-yourself kits, and it's not a time to pull punches.

Several years ago, a husband in a domestic relations issue called me for help. He was afraid his wife would run off with their children back to her native Ecuador, and he would never see them again. I helped him draft the paperwork to get an ex-parte order of protection. This special order is an injunction that requires the other parent to obtain access to the child only through certain means.

The man was conflicted, however, and still deeply loved his wife. She was a beautiful young woman, and quite manipulative. She was an excellent liar who could talk her way out of nearly any situation. She was also a mean and abusive person. She cooed sweetly into his ear that she would return and be a good wife if he would just drop the order of protection.

My advice was to retain the order. I explained that she could be lying. I told him that I had helped him once, out of an emergency situation, and that he now needed competent divorce help. He did not listen. He dropped the order, and she filed one against him the very next day, having the children seized from him by sheriffs in police cars who came with guns drawn because they had been told that he was armed and dangerous. The client had to give up all his firearms for the six months that the order was in effect, and his children suffered terribly in the intervening time until appropriate divorce counsel could intercede and solve the problems.

The moral of the story, and one he would tell you himself, is that you should hire a good attorney and take his advice, even if your heart isn't in it. If a divorce situation gets to the point where lawyers are involved, reconciliation is unlikely. But if it is going to happen, it will happen with or without the lawyers. So the better course of action is to get a lawyer and follow his advice. This is especially true for women who are in abusive relationships.

a) Orders of Protection and Spousal Abuse

One sad fact of a breaking marriage is that violence is often a side effect of the situation. People get violent and they act crazy, and the result is sometimes horrible. If you are in a relationship where you feel it necessary to terminate the relationship, an order of adult protection should be obtained from the courts at the first sign of any aberrant behavior or violence. These orders are universally available in all 50 states, and should be obtained whenever there is a threat of violence or harm.

b) Child Protection and Endangerment

Even though they are not guilty of anything more than being born, children assume, wrongly, that they are the cause of the divorce. Children require special attention, and both parties to a divorce must exercise care in how they deal with the other parent. They should not talk badly about the other parent even if they think that other parent is the Devil walking on earth. Instead, they should remember that the child is permitted and expected to love both parents, and that anything that harms that relationship harms the child.

Sadly, some parents aim their worst invective at the children in a divorce, and wind up harming them. When this happens, the same laws that protect spouses from abuse protect children, and an ex parte order of protection can be entered to protect them as well.

Sometimes there is a credible claim of abuse that arises out of a sincere desire to protect the child. In those situations the court will appoint a guardian ad litem (GAL) for the minors. The lawyer, who is independent of the lawyers who represent mom and dad, has a voice in determining whom he thinks would be better suited to raising the children, and gets to advocate on their behalf.

Sometimes spouses, for one reason or another, will make a claim of child sexual abuse in order to gain more favorable treatment in the divorce. For example, the wife may claim that the husband has been sexually abusing a minor child in order to obtain a more favorable divorce settlement. After all, a husband who is in jail is easier to divorce than one who is out and able to work.

Recently, a man won a $170,000 verdict against his ex-spouse for just this kind of conduct. The jury returned to him the amount of money he had paid for legal help to clear his name, as well as some punitive damages.

c) Divorce Law

Divorce law varies greatly from state to state. Generally a divorce granted in one state is valid in all other states, as is a marriage. There are sometimes temptations to go to another state in order to get a "quick" divorce. This is a temptation that should be avoided, particularly if the spouse does not agree. Divorce law is very different in each state, and going to a "quick divorce" state is never in anyone's best interest when there is real property to divide or child custody to determine.

How property is divided is a matter of state law and varies widely from jurisdiction to jurisdiction. Secure a good attorney to advise you. Under no circumstances should a do-it-yourself kit be used to do an "uncontested" divorce. In this author's view, there is no such thing.

K. KEY POINTS

- Privacy should be your number one concern.
- Do not give out your social security number to persons who do not need it to do their job.
- Consumer Protection Legislation is aimed at protecting you.
- Lemon laws are useful tools to help solve problems with new cars.
- The Federal Trade Commission has oversight responsibility to protect consumers from fraud.
- The FTC protects consumers from mail and email scams.
- In addition to the FTC, the state attorney general in your state will handle the "Little FTC" Act, which protects you against unfair merchandizing practices.
- The Truth In Lending Act is overseen by the FTC, and protects you from individuals or banks that do not provide all information to you when you seek a loan.
- Payday loans should be avoided because they frequently have interest rates of 400% or more.
- The Fair Debt Collection Practices Act is designed to protect consumers from abusive collectors.
- Creditors are not subject to the Fair Debt Collection Practices Act.
- The Fair Credit Reporting Act gives you certain tools to help you protect your good name and credit rating.
- The Equal Credit Opportunity Act is designed to ensure that consumers are not discriminated against in the issuance of credit.
- The Fair Credit Billing Act is designed to protect you against errors on your credit card statements.
- The Electronic Funds Transfer Act is designed to protect you against false or inaccurate ATM-based charges.
- Bankruptcy is a last resort method of dealing with credit problems.
- Bankruptcy should only be used after other methods (such as Consumer Credit Counseling) have failed.
- When someone else causes you injury, you have a right to sue.
- A right to sue is about obtaining compensation, not a windfall.
- You can sue for negligence if someone failed to use ordinary care to protect you.
- You can sue for product liability if a dangerous or defective product caused you injury.

- You can sue for fraud if someone cheats you out of money (but an action under the state Little FTC Act may be a better remedy).
- You can sue for Slander and Libel, but under certain circumstances only, and these lawsuits are very difficult to bring and win.
- You can sue for emotional distress caused intentionally or negligently, depending on whether you were injured or not.
- Domestic Relations is an important area of the law, and if you face divorce, remarriage, or problems with your spouse or children, you need competent legal advice.

L. SUMMARY

The civil law is there to help the average respiratory therapist. Just as a negligent therapist may find himself on the wrong end of a lawsuit, the competent and caring therapist may sometimes feel that the only way to vindicate his or her rights is to seek redress in a court of law.

The law is there to protect a therapist's investments, ensure access to credit, and protect them from scams and cheats. When a therapist is injured, or his family is injured, there are means to obtain compensation through the law. These should not be overlooked.

Finally, love may be blind, but marriage is an eye opener. More than 50% of all marriages end up in divorce. If divorce is a consideration, the party who retains legal counsel first, and who obtains good legal counsel, is the one that will have the most to show for it at the end of the proceeding.

CHAPTER 13

Surviving Litigation

"The only thing I expect out of lawyers is that they be back in their coffins by sunup."

F. Ross Johnson, former CEO of RJR Nabisco

A. INTRODUCTION

Litigation—the process of being sued for damages—isn't something you think about much during a regular day. If you live a righteous life, you probably think of it only when you read the news or watch television. But it has the potential to make a regular day into a regular nightmare. The purpose of this chapter is to prepare those who have never been through the ordeal for what happens in a lawsuit. Knowing what to expect helps take some of the fear out of the situation.

B. HOW DOES LITIGATION BEGIN?

In Chapter One, we discussed how a lawsuit is brought by an attorney after he completes an investigation. But for defendants, a lawsuit begins with a summons. It is a document that tells you that you are being called into court to answer for something you allegedly did. Along with the summons will be a "petition" or a "complaint" that spells out exactly what you did wrong, and what happened as a result. It normally arrives attached to a sheriff, the person designated in the court system to effect service of process on individuals and corporations.

Being served with a lawsuit can happen at any time. Suppose you're running to get to the next treatment that's due when your beeper goes off. The number is a hospital exchange with which you're not familiar. When you dial it, you hear "Human Resources."

All the HR clerk will tell you is that you need to come to the Personnel Department right away.

You hustle down to personnel, and instead of being greeted by the clerk, you find a sheriff who stands up when you walk in. He asks your name; you give it; and he says "these are for you." He walks out without another word.

At the top of the paper is the word "Summons" and below that some writing that sounds pretty scary. Unless you answer the allegations in the complaint within 30 days, someone is going to get a judgment against you for lots of money.

Welcome to the nightmare of litigation.

C. WHAT DO YOU DO WITH A SUMMONS?

There are two important rules about summonses. First, don't ignore one. Don't think the matter will just go away. It won't. Second, don't pick up the phone and call the lawyer who has sued you. Anything you say (borrowing a phrase from the criminal law now) "can and will be used against you." When you are sued, there is only one right response: contact an attorney for advice. If you have a malpractice insurance policy, you call the malpractice carrier and send them the summons and complaint (or petition) by fax. They will secure an attorney to help you.

If the lawsuit arises out of a traffic accident, contact your automobile insurer. They will find you an attorney. If you are sued for something unrelated to your work (a fall on your property, etc.), call your homeowner's or renter's insurance company. If you are not fortunate enough to have planned ahead (and you don't have insurance), you may be in for a very long couple of months.

1. How Do I Go About Securing Counsel if I Am Not Insured?

If you have been smart enough, and heeded the advice in this book, you've bought malpractice insurance or, if the case isn't about malpractice, you have homeowner's insurance or renter's insurance to protect you from the claims made in the lawsuit. If so, your insurance carrier already has a lawyer picked out for you, and will want to get the lawsuit papers so that they can get started on your answer. If you do not have insurance, then you need to hire an attorney to defend you. This will not be easy or cheap, but it will be necessary.[1]

---

[1]The law says you can defend yourself in court without a lawyer. The law also says you can do your own brain surgery.

Even if you have no insurance, frequently there is no reason to panic. Although you have been named in a lawsuit, it doesn't mean the other side will necessarily win. The other side is going to have to convince 12 people you did something wrong, and it isn't as easy as it sounds. But don't try to go it alone, without an attorney. If you have no insurance, find someone who practices malpractice defense, and make an appointment. Fees are generally negotiable; and even if they want $250 per hour, you can generally get them to take you, as an uninsured client, for $100 or less per hour.

2. What Inexpensive Steps Can I Take?

Demand that the attorney file a motion to dismiss if you were wrongly named. Sometimes plaintiffs' lawyers name everyone who touched the patient with the idea that if they do that, sooner or later they'll get the right person. Often, if you can show that nothing you did caused or contributed to cause the injury, or that you were incorrectly named, you can be dismissed from the lawsuit.

If the lawsuit cannot be dismissed, ask the attorney to invoice you regularly, and not to prepare any work or do anything until you approve it. Sometimes attorneys who work for the defendant "bill the file" and charge off expenses to files in order to justify their existence (this is especially common in large defense firms with hundreds of lawyers). A legal document should be drafted and revised only once. If it goes through multiple revisions, you should not pay for that because this is frequently a trick defense attorneys use to overbill for their services. Insurance companies frequently pay the bill without thinking twice about it. You should question everything.

3. What Is a Retainer?

A retainer is an unearned fee that is deposited with the lawyer in advance. When the lawyer earns that fee, he pays himself out of your retainer. Most lawyers will allow you to put down a retainer, an amount of money that will cover the first part of the case, and will bill you incrementally for the costs as they progress. In most cases, the larger the retainer, the larger the greed of the firm. A retainer of more than $1,000 for a new case is very high. But lawyers quit working when the retainer runs dry, so be very careful about paying too much or too often, and understand the hourly rates in advance. Insist on being notified every time the attorney makes a charge against your retainer. In some cases, it is the only way you'll know the attorney is actually doing something.

D. HOW DOES THE LAWYER-CLIENT RELATIONSHIP WORK?

If you hire an attorney, or if one is hired for you, you'll have an opportunity to meet and talk to the attorney fairly quickly. He will want you to do several things before the meeting. The most important, of course, is to read the complaint or petition and find out why you are being sued, and to write down as much as you can remember about what happened and when. For the purposes of this discussion, we'll assume that the lawsuit is based on malpractice claims, but the process would be the same if someone had broken an arm falling off your porch and was suing you for those damages.

1. How Can I Help My Lawyer?

Suppose you are claimed to have been negligent a year ago when you cared for Mr. Jones in the ICU. You vaguely remember Mr. Jones, but you do know that he died from acute asphyxia when a mucous plug developed in this endotracheal tube. Your recollection is that you had just come on during a morning shift when you were summoned to the ICU for the code. You bagged, suctioned, and finally extubated and reintubated Mr. Jones. Unfortunately, the damage had been done, and he died.

The lawsuit charges that you negligently allowed Mr. Jones to breathe un-humidified air, and failed to recognize the blocked tube in time to extubate and reintubate him.

You should go to medical records and review the chart, especially all your own charting, and should make lots of notes (on your own notebook—not in the chart) about what happened. You should not, of course, ever change anything in the medical records because the plaintiff's lawyer already has the records, and the changes you make won't show up on his copy, making you look guilty of record alteration.

You prepare a memorandum of all you know about the event and go to your lawyer's office. At this point everything you say to him, and indeed, the memoranda and notes you have made for him, are all privileged. That privilege cannot be broken except in the most unusual of circumstances. Even if you change lawyers later, your lawyer cannot say anything to anyone that would harm your case. It is permissible, and entirely proper, for your lawyer to know everything you know about the case.

The lawyer will want to ask you questions. She will read what you've written, and may ask you lots of tough questions about it. How do you know this? Are you assuming, or do you remember this for a fact? Where would I find this in the record? Did you make a note of this in the chart at the time? Who else was there? With whom have you discussed this?

2. What Must My Lawyer Do?

Your lawyer has to learn the law and the medicine in short order, and she has to learn enough to do a credible job of representing you. In addition, she has to answer the petition or complaint within 30 days, and she has to start gathering records and information from the other side. She will learn everything she can about the plaintiff, about the decedent, and indeed, about you.

She will want to meet with you several times, and she will send you letters letting you know what she has done, and why. At some point, she will schedule your deposition, and she will prepare you for it. She will ask you questions and prepare you for the onslaught of questioning that will come.

Your attorney will generally, though not always, work with the attorneys for other defendants. She will learn what they are going to say, and why they'll say it. She will help position the case against you properly. If it is in her best interests to work with the plaintiffs in order to get the case against you dismissed, she may do that.

Finally, she will take depositions. She will question the plaintiffs and their experts. She may ask you for help in poking holes in the plaintiffs' theory of the case. If the other side will not dismiss you from the case, she may move for summary judgment. Finally, if the judge rules that the case must go to trial, she will prepare the case for trial, scheduling your testimony and the testimony of experts who support you.

3. What Do I Do?

Your job is pretty much straightforward. You have to tell the truth about what happened. You can't shade the truth. Let's suppose you missed a ventilator check, or because of work load, got to it 45 minutes late. The patient later codes, and the allegation against you is that you didn't make that ventilator check, and that if you had, the patient would have survived.

If you missed (or were late with) the ventilator check, you have to say so. There is no right against "self-incrimination" in the context of malpractice. You can't simply refuse to answer the questions: you'll be held in contempt. So you testify truthfully. You admit that you missed the ventilator check. Your lawyer will never tell you to lie under oath, and a lawyer who does should be dismissed immediately and reported to the state bar. Your lawyer knows that it is always easier to defend the truth than to defend a lie. But just because you missed the ventilator check doesn't mean you're liable. There are always ways to defend the case on the issue of causation, as mentioned earlier.

If you did nothing wrong, but you know that someone else did, and you are asked that question, you have to testify truthfully, but you don't have to volunteer that answer. You cannot lie for someone else any more than you can lie for yourself. You don't have to volunteer information about anyone else, but you do have a responsibility to tell the truth as you know it.

You have to be honest with your lawyer, and you have to tell the truth in your depositions and at trial. If asked, you have to teach your lawyer about your job and about certain aspects of respiratory care that may not be obvious. You have to cooperate with your defense team. Those are just about all the responsibilities you have.

If a lawyer counsels you to lie, or asks you to shade the truth, you should discharge him. A lawyer who asks you to lie is suborning perjury and should be disbarred. You should discharge the attorney and report the misconduct to the judge and your state bar.

4. How Do I Prepare for My Deposition?

One thing you'll have to do is give a deposition (unless your attorney has the case dismissed). A deposition is a preview of your trial testimony, and requires you to tell the truth as you know it. A deposition allows the attorney who examines you (usually the plaintiff's attorney, but sometimes the attorney for any other defendant), to ask you all kinds of questions that may seem out of place.

For example, the plaintiff may ask to whom you are married and the name of your husband or wife. The attorney may ask where you live and whether you have children. Where do they go to school? Again, this may seem very personal and very intimidating because all parents want to protect their children.

But the answers you give help the attorney plan for trial. If a member of the jury works at the same school where your child attends, he or she may know your child or your family and that may make him or her less fair as a juror. Similarly, just as you don't want the plaintiff's cousin on the jury, the plaintiff doesn't want your mother-in-law on the jury (and you may not either, for that matter).

In a deposition, much of what the attorney asks won't be admissible at trial. For example, he may ask if you have been arrested for any reason. The attorney can't get the question or your answer into evidence, because only convictions can be admitted against a witness in most locations. However, by asking if you have been arrested, he may find information that will be admissible, and so he is allowed to ask. Of course, your counsel will object, but in most cases will instruct you to answer the question. As a general rule, however, you should follow your attorney's advice about whether or not to answer a question.

There is one time when your attorney will instruct you not to answer, and that is when the other lawyer asks you about anything your attorney has told you, or what you've told your attorney. This invades the lawyer-client relationship. But keep in mind, just because the person you're talking to is a lawyer doesn't always mean there is a privilege or a relationship.

For example, in one recent case in which I was involved, Greg, an attorney representing the nursing home, went out and spoke to a former employee who was not named in the lawsuit. The employee was not represented by Greg, and they did not have a lawyer-client relationship. The court could have instructed the witness to answer questions on this subject because there was no lawyer-client relationship and no privilege.

You may also be asked to bring things to a deposition, including things like records, reports, memoranda, letters, and correspondence. Listen to your attorney about what to bring, and never bring anything that your attorney has not seen first. Keep in mind that when the hospital and other physicians are also involved and have separate counsel, the fact that they are a defendant doesn't necessarily make them your friend. Listen only to your lawyer, and if another lawyer wants something, make him or her go through your attorney to get it.

Usually, your attorney will prepare you for your deposition by asking you questions and helping you understand the process. Do not **ever** give a deposition without an attorney present. If at all possible, even if called as a witness, you should go with an attorney representing you. This means an attorney representing only you, not one representing the hospital too. If you give a deposition unrepresented by counsel, you may wind up regretting it when you are later named as a defendant.

E. IS LITIGATION AS A FACT WITNESS DIFFERENT?

Yes. As a fact witness, you are there not to take sides or persuade the jury you are right, but rather, to tell very simply what you saw, heard, did, or witnessed. As such, you have one job: answer questions honestly.

Suppose instead of a summons to appear as a defendant, you're given a document labeled "subpoena" that requires that you show up for a deposition or for a trial. A subpoena is a lawful court order requiring you to show up and present testimony. It is not a voluntary document. The court can issue an order of contempt if you disobey the order to show up and give testimony.

A person receiving a subpoena is a fact witness. And witnesses have certain rights.

1. What Are the Rights of Witnesses?

A witness summoned to court must, in most jurisdictions, be paid a mileage fee for showing up and giving his testimony. In addition, he may be entitled to a witness fee of so many dollars per day. This witness fee won't be big, but it will be enough, usually, to defray the expense of parking.

A witness is also entitled to sufficient notice. In most jurisdictions, a notice that gives less than seven days time to prepare and respond is unreasonable. Unfortunately, you have to obey even a defective subpoena unless you or your lawyer file a motion to quash the subpoena.

Finally, a witness is entitled to be treated properly. No one may yell at you. No one may scream at you. No one may call you names. You may not be threatened or intimidated. You have the right to have an attorney present and with you when you are giving a deposition, and you should use this right. Normally the lawyer cannot represent you if you are summoned to trial to give testimony, but may advise you beforehand.

2. What Are the Duties of a Witness?

The witness has the duty to tell the truth. She must answer the questions put to her. A witness does not have to volunteer information.

I normally tell my witnesses that they should answer questions as briefly and directly as possible. My stock advice to witnesses is: "If you have to take a breath to answer a question, you're talking too much." As an example, if the question was "how did you get to the deposition," then the answer is "I drove." If they want to know what you drove, what street you came down, when you left, and where you parked, those are all different questions. The shortest most direct answer to a question is always the best.

3. Who Does Direct Examination?

The person who called you as a witness must examine you through what is called a "direct examination." In this examination, he cannot ask you leading questions (questions that suggest the answer) but instead, must ask you general questions and let you answer them.[2]

On direct examination, the witness is asked questions that are deliberately open-ended. For example:

Lawyer	*Are you employed?*
You	*Yes.*
Lawyer	*How are you employed?*
You	*I work for the hospital.*
Lawyer	*What do you do?*
You	*I am a respiratory therapist.*
Lawyer	*Can you tell me what a respiratory therapist does?*
You	*Yes.*
Lawyer	*What does a respiratory therapist do?*
You	*We care for the pulmonary status of all patients in the hospital.*
Lawyer	*Does that involve giving treatments?*
You	*Sometimes.*
Lawyer	*Did you give a treatment to Mr. Jones on 9/3/2004?*
You	*I gave Mr. Jones a number of treatments. Without the medical record to refresh my memory, I couldn't tell you what dates. . . . .*

As you can see, the therapist answering these questions answers only the question asked, and no more. When he is asked if he can tell the questioner what a respiratory therapist does, he says, yes, he can do that. The question "what does a respiratory therapist do" is another question.

This probably seems like gamesmanship, because in normal conversation we answer the question that questioners meant to ask, not the question they actually asked. But answering only the question asked is an important part of being a witness in any case. The attorney wants to establish a rapport with you. He wants you to forget you're answering questions under oath. He wants you to be comfortable. For that reason, he starts off with easy stuff

---

[2]This is different if you are a defendant. You can be examined, even on direct examination, with leading questions, because you are "adverse" to the other side. But as a fact witness, you do not have to deal with leading questions, and good lawyers won't let you answer those questions.

about where you live, where you work, and what a therapist does. If he can get you to answer the question he meant to ask, pretty soon he'll be asking "what happened then," and you'll be telling a story to him, instead of making him ask questions.

The reason lawyers tell you to be careful on every question is that every question matters. Every answer matters. You cannot relax. You have to keep the attorney narrowly focused on the subject by answering only the question he asks. If you strike up a conversation with him (which is what every attorney wants), pretty soon, even though you don't realize it, you'll be volunteering information that the attorney would not have thought to ask. The witness has to listen to the question and answer the question he or she is asked, not the question he or she wants to answer.

4. What if the Lawyers Ask the Wrong Questions?

Sometimes lawyers do that. Sometimes they ask you to tell them how a ventilator works, instead of how the ventilator malfunctioned. Anyone knows, in a malpractice case, that how the ventilator malfunctioned is more important than how it works. So instead of answering the question, you mistakenly answer the question you want to answer and give the lawyer ammunition to use against you:

> Lawyer   *How does the MA-1 ventilator deliver a breath to the patient?*
> Therapist   *It pumps it in, but that's not what happened here. What happened is that the exhalation valve came off and no one knew it because the alarm didn't sound.*
> Lawyer   *I see. Does that happen often?*
> Therapist   *Sure, all the time. That's the reason we use the low inspiratory pressure monitor instead of the one on top of the bellows, but we didn't have a battery for the one on Mr. Jones, and as a result, we were just supposed to watch it more carefully.*

The problem with this approach, however, is that the attorney will patiently ask you to answer the question he asked, because he has a plan to ask his questions in a certain way. The more information you volunteer, and the longer you take with explanations, the longer you will be on a witness stand. So allow the lawyer to do his job, and answer the questions he asks:

> Lawyer   *How does the MA-1 ventilator deliver a breath to the patient?*
> Therapist   *It pumps air into a small balloon in the exhalation valve. That closes the system and allows air to go down to the patient.*

Lawyer	I'm showing you exhibit 71, the exhalation valve; is this the balloon?
Therapist	Yes, that's the balloon.
Lawyer	Now what happens, Mr. Smith, if that balloon is broken or fails to inflate?
Therapist	The circuit never closes and the patient is never ventilated.
Lawyer	But the bellows in the assembly continue to go up and down, don't they?
Therapist	Yes, they do.
Lawyer	So, how would you know if this happened?
Therapist	There should be a low inspiratory pressure alarm that sounds.
Lawyer	That didn't happen here?
Therapist	No.
Lawyer	Why didn't it?
Therapist	Because the alarm didn't have a battery, and wasn't working.

The therapist is asked a series of more specific questions to obtain the answers the lawyer wants. The jury sees step by step what happened, instead of trying to grasp the therapist's answer that jumps right to the end. Of course, in the prior example, the jury follows along too, but the therapist looks like he is testifying for the plaintiff.

5. Can I Be Asked Leading Questions?

No, normally a witness may not be "led" on direct examination. In other words, a witness cannot be asked questions that suggest the answer:

Lawyer	You cared for Mr. Jones?
Therapist	Yes.
Lawyer	You gave him treatments?
Therapist	Yeah.
Lawyer	Those treatments were given at 2 and 6 p.m. on your shift?
Therapist	Yup, I think so.

In each case, the therapist isn't testifying, he is letting the lawyer testify for him. In this case, the questions can all be answered with a "yes." This is a leading question, and a leading question isn't proper on direct examination. Normally, an opponent will allow leading questions that don't matter if they are just to establish foundation. For example, "you work at the hospital," or "you're a registered therapist." Although those are objectionable, a savvy attorney isn't going to object because it saves the court time for those issues to be dealt with quickly. But when the questioning turns to the essential elements of negligence, or what went wrong, the attorney will object.

Sometimes a court will allow a lawyer to treat a witness as "hostile," which means they can be asked these kinds of leading questions. This happens when the witness is a defendant on direct examination, or when they are belligerent or refuse to answer questions without sarcasm or editorializing.

Since leading questions suggest the answer, the lawyer is allowed to testify through the witness, almost like a puppeteer.

Lawyer	*Permission to treat as hostile, your honor?*
Court	*Granted.*
Lawyer	*You were on duty the night of October 29th 1998 weren't you?*
Witness	*Yeah.*
Lawyer	*And you were assigned to ICU?*
Witness	*Yeah.*
Lawyer	*In your deposition, you told us you didn't like Mr. Jones and his wife. True?*
Witness	*I said I didn't like the way they talked to me.*
Lawyer	*Your Honor?*
Court	*Answer the question as either true or false Mr. Manetti.*
Witness	*True.*
Lawyer	*And you told us you weren't sorry to see him die, isn't that true?*
Witness	*True, but I didn't mean it the way it sounded.*
Court	*Young man, your lawyer can ask you about your statements and you can explain them later. Right now, if you please, answer Mr. DeWitt's questions.*

Unlike open-ended questions, the leading question puts words in the mouth of the witness. The witness isn't really testifying; the lawyer is. As mentioned, only when a witness is considered "hostile" or is affiliated with the opposing party may a lawyer lead them during direct examination. Normally, this technique is permitted only on cross examination. But on cross examination it can be a real ordeal.

One thing that is not allowed, however, is to argue with, or inject argument into a question or series of questions.

Lawyer	*You were on duty the night of October 29th 1998, weren't you?*
Witness	*Yeah.*
Lawyer	*And you were assigned to ICU?*
Witness	*Yeah.*

Lawyer	In your deposition, you told us you didn't like Mr. Jones and his wife. True?
Witness	I said I didn't like the way they talked to me.
Lawyer	You didn't say that you little snake. You want to look at your deposition?
Opposing Counsel	Objection, argumentative.
Court	Sustained.
Lawyer	You told us you weren't sorry to see him die, isn't that true?
Witness	True, but I didn't mean it the way it sounded.
Lawyer	You're lying. That is not what you said!
Court	Counsel. That's twice. There had better not be a third time.

A good attorney will protect a witness from an argumentative examination and questions like those in the preceding examples in both the trial and at a deposition.

6. How Do I Survive Cross Examination?

Cross examination is considered by lawyers to be the best engine for finding the truth. The seasoned trial lawyer never asks a question to which he does not know the answer; and more importantly, he never asks anything but leading questions on cross examination:

Lawyer	You just testified that my client, Mr. Smith, let the humidifier run dry on the night shift. Do you recall that testimony?
Witness	Yes.
Lawyer	Isn't it true that you delayed your rounds in the ICU for twenty minutes?
Witness	Yeah, but only because there was a code in ER.
Lawyer	That isn't my question. You admit, here, in front of this jury, that your rounds are supposed to start at 7:00 a.m., are they not?
Witness	Yeah.
Lawyer	And you didn't get to the ICU, by your testimony, until 7:23 a.m., correct?
Witness	Yes.
Lawyer	And when you got there, you found the Cascade humidifier empty, right?
Witness	True.

Lawyer	And your testimony is that Mr. Smith let that happen on his shift?
Witness	Yes. That's right.
Lawyer	You weren't there between 7:00 a.m. and 7:23 a.m., were you?
Witness	No. I was in ER.
Lawyer	So you don't know how long the Cascade was empty, do you?
Witness	No, but it must have been quite a while. There was no water in the tubes or anything.
Lawyer	You don't know, do you?
Witness	No.
Lawyer	It could have run dry at 7:01, couldn't it?
Witness	I guess that's possible.
Lawyer	Or it could have run dry at 7:15, couldn't it?
Witness	I don't know.
Lawyer	You don't know, or you don't want to take responsibility for it running dry on your shift?
Witness	I told you I don't know.
Lawyer	That's just the point. You don't know, but you're blaming my client, aren't you?
Witness	Yeah. He never does his job. I am in that ICU all the time covering for him.
Lawyer	Move to strike as unresponsive.
Court	Sustained. The jury will disregard that last comment.
Lawyer	The fact is, Mr. Jones, you don't know that the Cascade didn't run dry at 7:22, after you'd had 22 minutes to get there and refill it, but hadn't done it yet?
Witness	I told you I don't know.
Lawyer	You tried to get Mr. Smith fired over this?
Witness	I just told the truth.
Lawyer	You filed a disciplinary report with your boss?
Witness	I did.
Lawyer	Your former girlfriend has been dating Mr. Smith. You knew that?
Witness	I did.
Lawyer	And that's why you reported him, isn't it?
Witness	No. That had nothing to do with it. He is welcome to her.
Lawyer	That isn't what you told Mary Ellen Swank, is it?
Witness	I don't know what I told her.
Lawyer	If Mary Ellen Swank told this jury that you were out to get Mr. Smith, would you have any reason to quarrel with her?

Witness	*Heck yeah. I didn't care. We broke up months ago. And she's just lying to try to help him.*
Lawyer	*But the fact is, you never disclosed in your disciplinary report, or to your boss, that you didn't get to the ICU until 7:23 did you?*
Witness	*I didn't put it in the report, but my boss knew.*
Lawyer	*How did he know? You just said it wasn't in the report?*
Witness	*He knew.*
Lawyer	*Can you point me to a single piece of paper where you disclosed that to your boss?*
Witness	*He must have seen the medical records.*
Lawyer	*But you don't know that, do you?*
Witness	*It's a good guess.*
Lawyer	*But you don't know, do you.*
Witness	*No, I don't.*

Cross examination can be brutal, but a good witness doesn't fight with the cross examiner, because he knows that the good guys always get another chance, called redirect examination.

Lawyer	*You testified that you believed that the Cascade had been dry a long time when you got there. Can you tell the jury why you believe that?*
Witness	*Well, normally there is condensate that drops out in the tubes. Water has to be drained from the tubing if air is adequately heated and humidified. When I got to the ICU, there was no water in the tubes, no water in the water traps, and no hint of moisture in the circuit. From that I concluded that the Cascade had been dry for hours.*
Lawyer	*And what did you do?*
Witness	*I looked back to see what the 6:00 a.m. vent check said.*
Lawyer	*And what did it say?*
Witness	*Nothing. There was no check done, according to the check sheet. I left a blank, which Smith filled in that night when he came on.*
Lawyer	*And did he remember the settings?*
Witness	*He told me that "one vegetable is pretty much like the rest."*
Lawyer	*That's what he said?*
Witness	*Yes, and he said it just that way, that one vegetable is pretty much like the rest of them. He didn't like caring for chronic patients.*
Lawyer	*Now, you remember Mr. Carlton trying to suggest that Mary Ellen Swank, your former girlfriend, had suggested that you had it in for Mr. Smith. Do you remember that testimony?*

Witness	Yes.
Lawyer	Did you?
Witness	Only to the extent that I knew his negligence was hurting pa- tients. That's why I filed a report with my boss.
Lawyer	Do you care who he dates?
Witness	No.
Lawyer	How close were you and Mary Ellen?
Witness	We went out twice. She wasn't my type, and I wasn't hers. I in- troduced her to Smith.

The key to surviving cross examination is keeping your wits about you and trusting your lawyer to help you on redirect examination if the other lawyer scores any points.

7. How Should I Prepare for My Day as Witness?

How do you prepare for your role as witness? You study the records and reports, search your memory for details, review your proposed testimony with your lawyer, and then testify as honestly as you can. If you have to as- sume something, you tell the jury what you're assuming. If you would have to guess or speculate to answer a question, you tell the lawyer that. Above all, tell the truth, the whole truth, and nothing but the truth to the jury.

8. How Do I Comply with a Subpoena?

Sometimes a subpoena is a "subpoena duces tecum." That means that it re- quires you to bring not only yourself, but any documents requested with you to the place of the deposition. Sometimes a lawyer will call and ask you to produce the documents and tell you if you do, you don't have to show up for the deposition. If the matter involves a patient, and you do not have a med- ical authorization to release the information to the lawyer, you are ethically and legally bound to show up for the deposition and not release the infor- mation until you see a valid authorization. If the court orders the release, you can and should comply with the order, but otherwise, unless a court has or- dered the production of the records, you should never simply obey a sub- poena. Doing so is a violation of HIPAA.

9. When Should I Engage Counsel?

You should obtain counsel, as a witness or as a defendant, whenever you are going to be asked to provide testimony, or whenever you are sued for any reason. If you do not have a family lawyer, you should contact the local bar association for a referral to competent counsel in your area.

10. What Ethical Duties Do Lawyers Have When Dealing with Unrepresented Persons?

Although all lawyers are required to read and apply the Rules of Professional Conduct before being granted the privilege of the practice of law, some just never get it. Some lawyers will do anything to win, and that includes intimidation, threats, coercion, and sometimes outright lies.

Rule 4.3 of the Model Rules of Professional Responsibility requires lawyers to behave properly:

In dealing on behalf of a client with a person who is not represented by counsel, a lawyer shall not state or imply that the lawyer is disinterested. When the lawyer knows or reasonably should know that the unrepresented person misunderstands the lawyer's role in the matter, the lawyer shall make reasonable efforts to correct the misunderstanding. The lawyer shall not give legal advice to an unrepresented person, other than the advice to secure counsel, if the lawyer knows or reasonably should know that the interests of such a person are or have a reasonable possibility of being in conflict with the interests of the client.

The rules also require:

(a) In representing a client, a lawyer shall not use means that have no substantial purpose other than to embarrass, delay, or burden a third person, or use methods of obtaining evidence that violate the legal rights of such a person.

In addition to these rules, there are rules on what is called "ex parte" contact. That rule says:

In representing a client, a lawyer shall not communicate about the subject of the representation with a person the lawyer knows to be represented by another lawyer in the matter, unless the lawyer has the consent of the other lawyer or is authorized to do so by law or a court order.

This rule requires that a lawyer not contact a party he knows to be represented by counsel. This means that if the hospital is sued for malpractice, and you work for the hospital, the plaintiff's lawyer needs permission from your hospital's attorney (or from your attorney) before he may ethically contact you. In some states, this rule applies even after you leave the employment of the hospital, although in many states, it doesn't apply.

Before talking to any attorney about a case, it is always good to be represented by your own counsel.

F. SHOULD I BECOME A PROFESSIONAL EXPERT WITNESS?

To answer this question, you should really know something about the process.

Expert witnesses are a key part of the professional negligence system. While it may seem unseemly to testify against fellow practitioners for an error that anyone might make, experts are important because, by stating the standard of care and holding people accountable to that standard, they raise the standards in the profession.

For example, if a therapist has been culpably negligent, by leaving a non-rebreather mask attached to the patient's face but with the flow to the mask turned off, and the patient sustains real harm as a result, the therapist who did that is not someone who should be practicing. Would you want your mother, sister, or wife to be his next victim? Somewhere along the line, a fail-safe mechanism has failed. A department director has failed to identify or fire a weak therapist. A therapist has not been properly trained. By anyone's definition, a patient has been harmed, and the public image of therapists suffers as a result.

While expert witnesses uphold the standard of care, they do so at a personal price. They may not be as favorably regarded by other therapists, and they may find that they are the subject of derision for taking the job. And, there is the idea that they are aiding the "greedy trial lawyers." But there is a very good reason why very good therapists should seek out this kind of employment. It protects other therapists from frivolous cases brought as a result of erroneous testimony by nurses and physicians who do not understand the scope of practice of the therapist.

If a therapist is not available to review a case, a lawyer will ask a doctor. Since I've had doctors tell me in depositions that respiratory therapists shouldn't even carry stethoscopes (because they don't know how to use them), I believe a therapist who avoids the opportunity to opine on the standard of care for a therapist is probably doing his brethren a disservice.

And, of course, there is remuneration for services rendered. Most lawyers are willing to pay up to $100 per hour for a therapist to review records and issue an opinion as to negligence—and that applies even if there is no negligence. In other words, if it takes you three hours to go through the medical records and at the conclusion of that review, you believe the therapist didn't do anything wrong, the lawyer is obligated to pay you the witness fee ($300) because you are being paid for your opinion, not for a specific opinion that the therapist was negligent.

1. What Is the Role of Expert Testimony in Litigation?

The expert is a teacher. The expert, although hired by one side or the other, is not an advocate. His job is to talk about the science or the art of respiratory care, and not to offer testimony designed to support one side or the other. Even though he may hold opinions that one or the other of the defendants was negligent, this is an opinion that is based on facts, and is not an opinion based on advocacy. The expert's job is not to convince the jury, but rather, to teach the jury about a subject few will understand.

2. The Role of the Expert Witness as Advocate for Science

The expert's job at trial is to establish the standard of care. This begins with a recitation of his background. He must have sufficient knowledge, experience, and expertise in the area to help the jury understand the issues. Normally, an expert will discuss the studies they've done, their publications, and their extensive experience teaching other professionals.

The expert then discusses the standard of care in terms of what was done, what should have been done, and why that is the standard of care. He may then offer testimony that the defendant failed to meet the standard of care, based on the information seen in the medical record.

Cross examination usually goes to the expert's understanding of the facts involved. "If a fact you relied on turns out not to be true, Mr. Expert, what effect would that have on your opinion?" Often the expert is asked if he is getting paid, and how much he is getting paid. If the expert is from out-of-town, as most are in medical negligence cases, the net effect is to suggest to the jury that the testimony of the expert was scripted by one side or the other in exchange for money.

Good witnesses can avoid this by being honest about their opinions, never attempting to advocate, and by having a sound scientific basis for their testimony.

3. How Should I Prepare for Expert Witness Testimony?

An expert witness, once designated by the lawyer, will have to give a deposition. Often the cases settle after depositions, and the experts do not have to testify at trial, so a deposition may wind up being the most important testimony they give.

To prepare, the expert should read all prior depositions, particularly the deposition of the defendant, and should mark and highlight those portions that are significant. He should bring this with him to his deposition. A review of the medical records is essential. The expert must be completely familiar with all the important pages of the medical records, and should have those pages flagged that are critical to his opinion.

The expert should make a review of all the pertinent facts in the case, and those facts that, in particular, support his belief that a person either conformed to the standard of care or deviated from it.

If the issues are rare or novel, and the expert reads up in treatises or other volumes, he should mark those chapters and he should bring those books with him to his deposition so that, if asked, he may tell the lawyer what other experts buttress his opinion.

4. Will I Have to Give an Expert Deposition?

Yes, absolutely. And in federal court, you may have to write a report. The rules for a deposition for experts are not much different from the rules for anyone else. Answers should be short, should be responsive only to the question asked, and should be clear whenever possible. The witness should not answer questions that are poorly phrased or vague. The witness should not let the lawyer put words in his mouth.

Lawyer	*So, Doctor, in your opinion, this is a case where the Cascade was dry for perhaps as long as several hours, is that your opinion?*
Witness	*I would say at least one hour, to a certainty, and possibly two. Two hours is more a probability than a certainty.*
Lawyer	*And you think a therapist ought to check on the patient more frequently.*
Witness	*I don't know what you mean by more frequently. My earlier testimony is that a therapist should make rounds at least every two hours, and that hydration of the airway should be checked each time.*
Lawyer	*You disagree that four-hour ventilator checks are safe?*
Witness	*I didn't say that. In some cases, where nursing staff are sufficient to check on the patient's pulmonary status and have been appropriately trained, it may be possible to do every four-hour checks, but only in certain instances . . .*

The expert's job is to be precise, accurate, detailed, and not let the lawyer put words in his mouth. To do that, the expert has to be alert, and has to listen carefully to every question asked.

5. Will I Have to Go to Trial?

In some cases, yes. If the case does not settle, the next step is trial, and an expert at trial must be presented by the means shown above. The expert cannot be led by the party who offers his testimony, but he may be (and no doubt will be) led by the cross examiner.

Witness fees for experts usually include all travel and lodging as well as meals. Some experts bill in half-day increments to ensure that they are not called to trial and made to sit for long periods of time waiting to testify.

If an expert does not want to travel to trial and be presented live, he or she may ask the lawyer to have his or her deposition videotaped so that the videotape can be played for the jury. Most lawyers like to have their witnesses present live, but will often accommodate an expert if asked.

G. WHAT IS JURY DUTY AND WHY DO I CARE?

Among the rights all Americans possess is the right to a jury trial in a criminal or civil case. But the right to such a trial demands that jurors serve in this capacity, and jurors get very little pay, and even less recognition, for a great deal of work.

Having a driver's license, being registered to vote, and owning property all tend to make you more likely than not to be tapped as a juror. Some people never get called for jury duty, while others get called frequently and serve on two or three juries during their lifetime.

1. Who Is a Good Juror?

A good juror is someone who enters the jury box with a human experience and is willing to put aside biases and prejudices in order to reach a decision on the evidence submitted to him or her.

In other words, someone who has seen news reports of the murder, and who watched the police recover the bodies from the ocean in the Scott and Laci Peterson case, could still be a good and effective juror, so long as he or she was willing to put aside biases and prejudices in order to listen to the evidence.

There is a great deal of science, not all of it anything more than smoke and mirrors, that goes into picking a jury. Lawyers watch body language and rely on demographics to determine who might view a case in the most favorable light. They hire jury consultants to tell them whom to pick. Dr. Phil, of television psychotherapist fame, got his start by helping Oprah Winfrey pick a jury in her trade libel case in Texas. At the end of the day, however, twelve people and two alternates are impaneled to hear the case and render their opinion.

2. Should I Serve?

Therapists, nurses, doctors, lawyers—everyone gets called for jury duty at some point. Only those people who cannot avoid being present for work, like physicians and health care workers who work in short-staffed departments, should consider asking for relief from jury duty. This is because everyone has something to offer as a juror, so long as they are willing to be fair. If you are not capable of being fair, if you think that malpractice doesn't exist, or that anyone arrested by the police is guilty of something, then you should probably not serve.

Very few juries ever serve as long as the jurors in the Scott Peterson or O.J. Simpson cases. Most cases are wrapped up in a week, sometimes less. The service of the jurors on these cases is vital. The jury is the one great guarantee that neither the government nor the very powerful will use their power to abuse the people.

People often ask me how to get out of jury duty. If you desire relief from jury duty, in most cases all you need to do is show some compelling argument, like the need to take care of minor children, and you're relieved. But the question is not whether you can get off jury duty, but whether you should.

Therapists are smarter than the average population, and they have better reasoning skills. They are used to solving problems quickly, and are intuitive and creative. They are usually steeped in the scientific method. They make great jurors for those reasons.

There are few things that call for patriotism more than jury duty. A juror has to balance the power and majesty of the law against the rights of the defendant (either criminal or civil) and decide cases fairly and unemotionally on the evidence. I believe therapists are uniquely qualified to be jurors, and that they have an obligation to their fellow citizens to serve.

H. HOW IS THE LEGAL PROFESSION POLICED?

Every barrel of apples has one or two that have spots, and maybe a few more that are simply rotten to the core. The legal profession is no different. There are bad lawyers just the way there are bad policemen, doctors, and plumbers.

When a doctor does something bad, it can cost patients their lives. When a lawyer screws up, it can cost the client his or her life savings, or worse, ruin the one chance he or she had to hold a wrongdoer accountable.

The job of policing the legal profession rests with the state bar of each state, and of course, the federal courts have the right and duty to police members of the profession who litigate in federal court.

1. What Is the Chief Disciplinary Counsel?

In most states, a Chief Disciplinary Counsel—or lawyer prosecutor—is responsible for investigating complaints against members of the bar. The Chief Disciplinary Counsel (CDC) is a lawyer who is both a prosecutor and an investigator. He gathers the facts with respect to what an attorney did, and then determines whether additional investigation, or a complaint, is necessary.

Not every complaint is meritorious. Sometimes people have personality conflicts. But in other cases, lawyers go out of their way to treat people badly. When they do, the CDC's job is to make sure that they don't get away with it.

2. How Do I File a Bar Complaint?

A bar complaint can be filed by a citizen, another lawyer, or by a judge in a civil or criminal case. It is an allegation that an attorney violated the rules of professional conduct and did something that either hurt a client or was against the rules regulating the conduct of lawyers.

The most common form of lawyer misconduct, sadly, is stealing from the client. Unfortunately many lawyers will obtain money or property for a client, and steal it for themselves.

M.J., a solid trial lawyer in the Kansas City area, is one example. M.J. was a trial lawyer who was excellent at getting and settling cases. He was also a bit too fluent in spending money and getting himself deeper and deeper into debt. He began to settle clients' cases for hundreds of thousands of dollars, and pocket the money himself, forging their signatures to the releases and checks issued by insurance companies. Before it was over, he had stolen money not only from his clients, but from his friends and partners. He was caught, disbarred, and went to California to obtain a job with a computer company, his legal career in tatters.

M.J.'s story, however, is illustrative of what happens with some lawyers. They become so enthralled with the money they make, that they spend more than they get, putting themselves into bankruptcy if they're lucky, and into legal problems with the bar if they are not.

M.J.'s partners made good on all the claims brought against M.J., as a member of their law firm. The firm sustained serious losses of money for several years as it (and its insurers) paid out legal malpractice claims. Clients, who learned about the misconduct, fled the firm for other firms.

The second most common form of misconduct is simply not keeping clients informed about the status of their cases. Sometimes a matter will sit with a lawyer for months and the client will not hear a word. When that happens, the best thing that can happen is for the client to speak directly to the lawyer and ask for an update. If a lawyer will not communicate, however, the smart thing to do is to file a bar complaint.

3. How Do I Report Misconduct?

Lawyers are under a duty to report misconduct when they know of it. Thus, if a lawyer knows that another lawyer is doing something improper or unethical, he has a duty to report it. Very few do. The last person to tick off is a lawyer, and every other lawyer knows this.

Clients, however, are entitled to report misconduct when they merely suspect it, and they should. If an attorney will not return phone calls, will not meet with the client when the client wants to meet, or otherwise ignores a client's case, the client should immediately contact the state bar and file a complaint.

The earlier the state bar gets involved, the sooner and more favorable the result will be. If the case is settled or disposed of without your knowledge, or if the lawyer has simply dropped the ball, sometimes there are ways to get things set right if timely action is taken.

I. KEY POINTS

- Litigation begins with a summons and a complaint or petition.
- A summons is not something that can be ignored.
- Counsel should be hired immediately upon receiving a summons.
- If you have malpractice insurance, you can turn your petition, summons, or complaint over to the insurer and allow them to enter your appearance.
- Frequently, homeowner's insurance will cover a therapist for non-professional incidents (like falls on property).
- Attorneys are like plumbers; you can hire and fire them at will.

- An attorney should be selected on the basis of his expertise.
- Attorneys who defend lawsuits tend to bill by the hour.
- Attorney invoices should be scrutinized closely for billing errors.
- You can help your lawyer by reviewing records and providing him with a summary of what happened, and what you did, and why.
- You can ask your attorney to file a motion to dismiss if the case is brought against you wrongly.
- You need to be honest with your attorney.
- Your job is to tell the truth at trial and in depositions.
- Depositions are part of discovery, and attorneys can ask more in depositions than they can at trial.
- Your attorney's job is to explain the truth and craft your defense.
- An attorney who urges you to lie or shade the truth should be fired on the spot.
- Fact witnesses are different than parties, and may also be subject to a deposition.
- A fact witness is entitled to mileage and a witness fee if he is asked to provide testimony in a case.
- A fact witness, like any witness, is accorded courtesy by the lawyers, and no witness has to tolerate abuse.
- A fact witness has the duty to tell the truth as he remembers it.
- Witnesses are examined by direct examination (open-ended questions) unless they are hostile or affiliated with the defendant.
- A direct examination requires a witness to answer only the question asked.
- A cross examination requires a witness to respond even to leading questions.
- Leading questions suggest the answer and essentially allow the lawyer to testify for you.
- Expert witnesses help uphold the standard of care.
- Expert witnesses may be retaliated against by other professionals.
- There are good reasons to be an expert witness, but the most important is to protect other members of your profession from frivolous lawsuits.
- Expert witnesses receive fees.
- Lawyers are required to treat all non-represented parties with respect, and must be truthful with them.
- A lawyer may not take advantage of a person's ignorance.
- Expert witnesses have to give depositions and come to trial.

- Jury duty is an honor and a privilege.
- Lawyers are required to be loyal to their clients and to keep them informed.
- If a lawyer acts improperly toward a client, he should be reported to the state bar or to the Chief Disciplinary Counsel.

J. SUMMARY

The key to surviving litigation is knowing what to expect, and getting a good attorney. A good attorney can guide a therapist through the maze of litigation, and can help ensure that the therapist's assets and rights are protected. Understanding the process can ensure that there are no surprises for the therapist during the case.

Witnesses, defendants, and expert witnesses all have rights in the legal system. It is important not only to know what those rights are, but to understand the obligation that witnesses, and particularly expert witnesses, have to the legal system. The goal of the legal system is to find the truth, not to reach a certain result for one party or the other.

Attorney conduct is governed by rules set out by the state supreme court, and by the federal courts. If an attorney fails to live up to his professional responsibilities, those affected can and should report him to the bar.

CHAPTER 14

Criminal Law for Therapists

They that can give up essential liberty to obtain a little tempo-rary safety deserve neither liberty nor safety.

Benjamin Franklin

A. INTRODUCTION

Hopefully no therapist will ever need the information in this chapter. But it is possible that your spouse, your friends, or others you know may need this information. For that reason, I am going to provide a good explanation of what rights every citizen has when dealing with the police.

In this chapter, the police, fairly or unfairly, are viewed as the bad guys. That is because, with respect to the criminal law and an innocent person, they are the bad guys. A police officer gets no more (and no less) pay for impris-oning an innocent person than a guilty one. In most cases, police officers do not set out to put someone innocent into jail. But, police officers are human. If an easy explanation can suffice to close a case, and a more in-depth inquiry might produce conflicting information, too many police officers are willing to stop with the easy explanation. Unfortunately for most people, that means that your life and liberty are at risk.

Of course, I do not suggest that police officers, either as a group or indi-vidually, are bad, mean, or evil people. They are not. They are hard-working people who have the safety of their communities in mind. They want to get people who are dangerous off the streets. They have a difficult job, made more difficult by the courts, which often seem to be at cross purposes with them. Every so often there are one or two who are just bad apples.

For the purposes of the discussion that follows, it is important to remem-ber that everyone who is accused of a crime is considered to be innocent until proved guilty in a court of law. Every citizen, once accused, has the right to remain silent, to not provide evidence to be used against him, and to have a competent lawyer represent him. Unfortunately sometimes these rights are given little weight in the hunt for a convenient scapegoat for a crime.

1. A Tale of Two Cases

In 2003, I was called late at night by a friend. Her brother-in-law was in a St. Louis City jail. The friend, who was not prone to exaggeration, said that he had been attacked and beaten by the police for jaywalking.

Jaywalking, as far as offenses go, is pretty low on the list of serious crimes, and I could not believe that a principled officer of the law would clobber a citizen because he cut across traffic on foot. I called my friend's sister, and told her what to do to get her husband out of jail. She called back a few minutes later to tell me that he was out, and that she would be in my office on Monday morning.

When my new clients came in, the husband looked as though he had gone a few rounds with Mike Tyson (although, thankfully, both ears were still intact). He had clear finger-marks on his neck from where he had been choked into unconsciousness.

The clients told a story of going to a hockey game and walking back to their car. They crossed police barricades to walk across a street to their car and were ordered to the crosswalk by a filthy-mouthed police officer. After complying with the police officer's verbal orders, the husband maintained eye contact. The cop told him to quit looking at him, but the client, being angry, refused. He was thinking that the Constitution protected looking. Silly client.

The police officer, in front of his pregnant wife, came on the attack. He pinned the client and the client, not understanding what was going on, fought back. This drew two other cops who fought him into cuffs. They dragged him into the police station, smashing his nose into the glass door along the way.

They cited him for failing to obey an order of a police officer, and resisting arrest. These two misdemeanors would have made it hard for my client to ever be a teacher or get state employment had be been convicted.

I knew the clients well enough to know they were telling the truth. These were not hardened criminals making frivolous "police brutality" claims. I filed a complaint with the state board of discipline for police officers, with the St. Louis City office of Internal Affairs, and with the FBI (which investigates civil rights complaints—the clients were Caucasian, the police officer African-American). I pressed a serious attack on the charges, filing an entry of appearance, demand for discovery, and a notice to take the deposition of the police officer.

The city responded by offering to drop the charges in exchange for a waiver of civil liability. Because my client's ability to work was more important than civil damages, the clients agreed. The entire case against the client had been nothing but intimidation. The Internal Affairs investigation, however, did cost the police officer a promotion. The State Board closed its investigation after a year with no further complaints.

Here, the police officer was clearly wrong, and my actions were aimed at protecting the rights of the client. In the end, I would have happily taken the case to trial, but the client could not afford the risk of a conviction.

Sometimes, however, the law works quite well.

In 1997 I was asked to represent a man charged with promoting prostitution. The judge who appointed me to the case did not want the public defender to handle the case, so I took it. After discussing the matter with the prosecutors and examining the evidence, I concluded that the state had more than ample evidence to convict the client. Three of his former "business women" were planning on testifying against him. I urged him to plead guilty and take the deal offered by the state.

He refused, and we went to trial. His defense: the women were only having dinner with gentlemen who needed escorts while in town. His star witness: a woman who was—to be honest—homely. She testified that men paid her $300 a night to take her to dinner. This testimony is akin to someone saying they paid $175 for a McDonald's hamburger.

The client was convicted and sentenced to 25 years in prison.

My job, as the lawyer, was to do the best I could to protect the client's rights in both cases. In both cases, I recommended that the clients take the deal. In the first case, it worked out well for the clients who no longer go to St. Louis for anything. For the other client, the 25 years wound up being reduced to about 16 months of home confinement due to prison overcrowding.

The point to these stories is that lawyers don't know, when a client walks through the door, whether the client is guilty or not. They have to safeguard the clients' rights. In looking for a criminal lawyer, you should look for someone who understands this. A good criminal lawyer is one who will fight to protect your rights. And your rights are in jeopardy.

2. Are Therapists and Professionals Targets?

More and more therapists, nurses, and physicians are becoming the targets of overzealous prosecutors. While it used to be that a victim of malpractice might be able to file a lawsuit against a bad doctor or nurse, in some jurisdictions prosecutors have begun to prosecute care that they believe was criminally negligent.

In almost any jurisdiction, someone who is grossly negligent can be charged with negligent homicide. In other words, if he or she did not intend to cause harm, but simply were reckless, a therapist or physician could be charged with negligent homicide if their negligent act or omission caused or contributed to cause the death of the patient.

Serial murder suspects, like Efren Saldivar, are prosecuted as are nurses who are thought to be "angels of death." Anyone can have a bad night, and anyone can make an error, and as a result, anyone can become the target of a police investigation.

How that investigation proceeds, however, is as important as the outcome. Therapists are often willing to talk to police officers thinking that the police are not going to be unfair, and after all, they have nothing to hide. But, as a matter of policy, I never recommend that a therapist talk to a police agency of any kind unless and until he has a lawyer by his side.

B. WHAT ARE THE LEGAL RIGHTS OF SUSPECTS?

In the years before the United States was formed, citizens of the British Crown often did not enjoy the full panoply of rights to which they were entitled. They were called before judicial commissions called star chambers. They were not told of the charges against them. They were questioned, sometimes under torture, to exact confessions. Guilt was less important than punishment.

As the movie "Braveheart" showed, sometimes suspected criminals were tried by ordeal, rather than by a court of law. If a man were to cry out in pain or agony while he was being hung, drawn, and quartered, it was an admission that he was guilty, and deserved his punishment. If he did not cry out, he was found innocent, but having been hung by the neck, connected to horses who would pull his limbs off, and cut into quarters, he wasn't around to enjoy the apology from the government.

These abuses of the legal system led legal scholars and others to call for reforms, but those reforms did not find true expression until the United States Constitution was put to paper.

The Constitution, when it was written, did no more than set out the duties of each of the branches of the government, and the mechanism by which the document could be amended. There began a series of debates, often conducted by publication of treatises, on the wisdom of the constitution. These debates were later collected as the Federalist Papers, which to this day are an important historical reference for scholars who study constitutional law.

The constitution as it was originally drafted was found wanting because the founding fathers feared a strong central (i.e., federal) government. They wanted the powers invested in the states, and they wanted the federal government restrained from actions that would interfere with the states' powers. They also wanted to make sure that citizens retained important rights.

As a result, ten amendments we now refer to as the Bill of Rights were added to the constitution and ratified along with the document. The rights provide for freedom of speech, freedom of religion, the right to keep and bear arms, among others. The most important rights from a criminal perspective, however, are found in Amendments Four, Five, Six, and Eight.

Amendment IV.

The right of the people to be secure in their persons, houses, papers, and effects, against unreasonable searches and seizures, shall not be violated, and no Warrants shall issue, but upon probable cause, supported by Oath or affirmation, and particularly describing the place to be searched, and the persons or things to be seized.

The Fourth Amendment is designed to make people safe in their own homes and prevent government incursion where there is no reason to suspect a person of a crime. The Fourth Amendment is where the body of law comes from that governs search and seizure of criminal evidence.

Amendment V.

No person shall be held to answer for a capital, or otherwise infamous crime, unless on a presentment or indictment of a Grand Jury, except in cases arising in the land or naval forces, or in the Militia, when in actual service in time of War or public danger; nor shall any person be subject for the same offence to be twice put in jeopardy of life or limb; nor shall be compelled in any criminal case to be a witness against himself, nor be deprived of life, liberty, or property, without due process of law; nor shall private property be taken for public use, without just compensation.

The Fifth Amendment is a virtual mother lode of rights, providing that capital crimes must be presented by indictment, which is to say that unless a grand jury indicts a person for a crime, no such criminal act may be prosecuted and a capital (or death) sentence imposed.

It also preserves the right to protection from double jeopardy. Double jeopardy means that once "jeopardy" attaches (which means, once a jury has been impaneled to hear the cause of action) a person may not be tried for that offense again.[1]

The Fifth Amendment protects a person from being compelled to be a witness against himself in a criminal proceeding. This right is broadly interpreted to mean that a suspect does not have to give a statement to police and similarly does not have to testify in his own defense at trial.

The Fifth Amendment also provides for due process, which is generally thought to mean an opportunity to defend criminal charges through a fair process.

Finally, the Fifth Amendment provides that the government may not take private property for governmental use without just compensation.

Amendment VI.

In all criminal prosecutions, the accused shall enjoy the right to a speedy and public trial, by an impartial jury of the State and district wherein the crime shall have been committed, which district shall have been previously ascertained by law, and to be informed of the nature and cause of the accusation; to be confronted with the witnesses against him; to have compulsory process for obtaining witnesses in his favor, and to have the Assistance of Counsel for his defence.

The Sixth Amendment provides for a right to a jury trial in the state and district where the crime was committed, to be informed of the nature of the charges and to confront witnesses against him. In addition, it guarantees the right to compel witnesses to testify on his behalf for his defense, and to have counsel at his side during any criminal trial.

Amendment VIII.

Excessive bail shall not be required, nor excessive fines imposed, nor cruel and unusual punishments inflicted.

---

[1]The courts take a very narrow view on this score. When the state criminal court acquitted the Rodney King officers of assault, they could be retried on federal charges of denying King his civil rights because the elements of the crime of denying King's civil rights were different from the elements of assault for which they were initially tried.

The Eighth Amendment protects against cruel and unusual punishments, and against excessive fines and bail. The Fourth, Fifth, and Sixth Amendments control the process before conviction, whereas the Eighth is generally seen as a control of the punishments inflicted by the courts.

A careful reading of the amendments, however, quickly shows that the amendments were written and drafted to be applicable to the federal government only. The right to a jury trial, the right to counsel, the right to search warrant, all were provided for against the federal government; nothing prohibited the states from engaging in these acts.

The guarantees of protection afforded to citizens under the Bill of Rights were not made applicable to the states until the 14th Amendment was passed after the end of the Civil War. Only then were states required to grant equal protection of the laws to their citizens.

In the 1960s, a time that is now viewed as one of the most liberal times for the United States Supreme Court, Chief Justice Earl Warren presided over a United States Supreme Court that began to evaluate certain criminal law issues and provide for protections for individuals charged with crimes. The first in the long string of cases was *Miranda v. Arizona* 384 U.S. 436 (1966) (Appendix C-5).

In *Miranda v. Arizona,* a case that is now colloquially called Miranda, an Hispanic man was arrested for rape and robbery. Miranda, whose native language was not English, was kept and questioned non-stop for two hours in order to break down his will. He did not know he could have a lawyer. He did not know he could refuse to answer questions. In the end, the suspect confessed.

The confession was short-lived. Soon his lawyer claimed that the confession was coerced, and that Miranda did not get a fair shake. The case wound up in the United States Supreme Court, which decided that Miranda was not treated fairly. It began requiring police officers, when they placed a suspect in custody, to give the defendant a listing of his rights.

The Miranda Rights are simple. Anyone who has not been in a coma since 1966, or who has watched any television police drama, knows the recitation by heart:

- You have the right to remain silent.
- Should you give up that right, anything you say may be used against you in a court of law.
- You have the right to have an attorney present before any questioning. Should you wish to have an attorney, but cannot afford one, one will be appointed for you.

One right is frequently not provided to the suspect, even though it is spelled out in detail in the Miranda opinion. That right is the right to terminate questioning at any time by either asking for an attorney or indicating that you do not wish to speak to the police. Although not given as part of the Miranda rights, the right remains viable, and convictions do get overturned when police violate the rule.

Amazingly, hundreds of times a day suspects are read these rights, and hundreds of times a day suspects tell the police everything they want to know. Some give the police this information voluntarily. Some are coerced. Some are tricked. But the net effect is the same in most cases. The information provided is considered voluntarily given, and the evidence is admissible against them.

The Miranda rights, while an important subset of the rights of all citizens, are not a complete listing of suspect rights, which we will now examine.

C. WHAT PROTECTIONS EXIST FOR MY HOME?

In the days of the King, if the High Prosecutor wanted information to use against you he could simply direct the sheriff to kick down your door and seize it. If he came looking for evidence of theft, and instead found evidence of adultery, that was simply too bad for the suspect. The King's justice was harsh.

The Fourth Amendment, however, was meant to address this problem. When the police, or any federal or state law enforcement agency, want to obtain information or evidence against you, they must apply to the federal or state court for a search warrant.

A search warrant is a special type of court order that directs officers to search for the evidence of a specific crime in a specific way.

Suppose Joe is visiting Kaiser's Fine Jewelry one afternoon, and examines a pair of diamond earrings that his wife might like. Later, another person examines the same jewelry, but quickly palms it and leaves without paying. The clerk remembers the last person who looked at the jewelry was Joe.

The police come. They dust the cabinet where the earrings were stored for fingerprints. They find Joe's fingerprints on the glass. They now have the testimony of the clerk supported by physical evidence, the fingerprints, sufficient for them to say they have probable cause to believe Joe committed a theft by artifice or deception. They apply to the Court for a search warrant. They describe what they are looking for (diamond earrings) and the place where they think it might be (Joe's car, and his house). The police can now execute the warrant by going to the house and searching for the earrings. The police can search the entire house and car for these earrings. If, in going through the drawers, they find a drawer that contains marijuana, the discovery is incidental to their lawful search, and they can seize the drugs and prosecute for them.

On the other hand, suppose Joe has a swimming pool outside his house, and the pool has a separate cabana. The cabana isn't described in the search warrant. The police ask for permission to search. Joe says no. The police go there anyway and find a stolen grand piano. The piano is so large, and so different from what they were searching for, and found in a location other than the one requested to be searched, that there is no basis to claim the search was incidental, and therefore, the stolen piano probably won't be admissible.

Before a police officer may enter a residence, car, RV, or other possession and search it, he must either have permission, or he must have probable cause and a warrant.

So, for example, when a police officer stops a speeder for speeding, and writes him a ticket, the detention during that period of time is custodial, and the police officer cannot ask questions without giving a Miranda warning. But, if the police officer suspects that the driver is carrying drugs, she may hand over a ticket to the driver and then say "do you mind if I search your car?" If the driver gives permission, anything the police officer finds is admissible. If the driver does not give permission, the police officer must have an independent basis to request a search warrant, since writing the ticket and issuing that ticket terminated her probable cause for the speeding offense.

Sometimes police, either in combination with a traffic stop, or when confronting a suspect on the street, must first determine if the suspect is armed so as to protect themselves. In *Terry v. Ohio,* 392 U.S. 1 (1968) (Appendix C-8) the Supreme Court specifically provided for an exemption to the warrant requirement under these circumstances. The Court said that in the circumstances of a given case, where a reasonably prudent officer is warranted in believing that his safety or that of others is endangered, he may make a reasonable search for weapons of the person he believes to be armed and dangerous, regardless of whether he has probable cause to arrest that individual for crime or the absolute certainty that the individual is armed.

D. WHAT ARE MY RIGHTS IF MY VEHICLE IS STOPPED?

Usually, if a police officer suspects that there are drugs in a vehicle, he will ask early on for permission to search. If that request is denied, the officer may elect not to write a ticket, and may elect to arrest the subject for the speeding instead of giving him a ticket. The arrest requires that the vehicle be towed; and before it can be towed, the police officer must make an "inventory search" of the vehicle in order to protect himself from a later claim that he took something from the vehicle. During this inventory search, any contraband will most likely be found.

On the other hand, if the suspect says no, the police officer may call out a drug dog to do a "sniff" of the car. A dog sniff is not considered to be a search of the vehicle by most courts. If the dog "hits" on the vehicle, the officer has probable cause for a search warrant.

For a person who is not carrying anything unlawful, the smartest approach to a request to search is to allow the officer to conduct the search. For someone who is carrying on unlawful activities, the best approach is to refuse and take your chances with a search warrant. Of course, the far better choice is simply not to engage in criminal activity.

What happens, however, when the state obtains evidence against a suspect by violating her rights under the Fourth Amendment? What remedy does the suspect have, since the evidence, having been found, is now asserted as the basis for arrest? In *Mapp v. Ohio*, 367 U.S. 648 (1961) (See Appendix C-7) the United States Supreme Court held that evidence which is unlawfully obtained is inadmissible. The Court said:

> *Today we once again examine . . . constitutional documentation of the right to privacy free from unreasonable state intrusion, and, after its dozen years on our books, are led by it to close the only courtroom door remaining open to evidence secured by official lawlessness in flagrant abuse of that basic right [to be free from unreasonable search and seizure], reserved to all persons as a specific guarantee against that very same unlawful conduct. We hold that all evidence obtained by searches and seizures in violation of the Constitution is, by that same authority, inadmissible in a state court.*

E. HOW DO I INVOKE MY RIGHT TO COUNSEL?

One of the most important rights a citizen has is the right to be represented in a criminal setting. If a suspect can't afford to hire a lawyer at $150 to $200 per hour, then the government may appoint a lawyer to represent him. In some states, the lawyer is the public defender. In other states, the circuit or district court will appoint a lawyer to defend the citizen. In the federal courts, the lawyer is almost always a public defender, unless the federal public defender has a conflict of interest, in which case the court may appoint a local attorney to represent the suspect.

The Sixth Amendment, however, guarantees access to lawyers; it does not actually guarantee that a lawyer will be provided by the government to defend you. This right, another offshoot of the Burger Court, arose from a case called *Gideon v. Wainwright*, 372 US 335 (1963) (See Appendix C-6), where a federal prisoner wrote out his plea for relief under the doctrine of habeas corpus in pencil and sent it to the U.S. Supreme Court. The court appointed a young lawyer named Abe Fortas—who was later appointed to the Supreme Court by President Johnson—to press the case for prisoner Gideon. Gideon was charged in a Florida State Court with a non-capital felony. He appeared in court without funds and without counsel and asked the Court to appoint counsel for him. Because the felony wasn't a capital offense, this request was denied on the ground that the state law permitted appointment of counsel for indigent defendants in capital cases only. Petitioner conducted his own defense about as well as could be expected of a layman; but he was convicted and sentenced to imprisonment. Subsequently, he applied to the State Supreme Court for a writ of habeas corpus, on the ground that his conviction violated his rights under the Federal Constitution. The State Supreme Court denied all relief. The Supreme Court held that the right of an indigent defendant in a criminal trial to have the assistance of counsel is such a fundamental right essential to a fair trial, that Gideon's trial and conviction without the assistance of counsel violated the Fourteenth Amendment.

In most cases, the public defender scrutinizes peoples' assets to determine whether they can afford a lawyer. If they can make bail, in most cases, they are not eligible for a public defender and they must find and pay their own attorney. The public defender assumes that the criminal with $1,500 for bail could have just as easily used that money to pay for an attorney.

Of course, just because a person has a right to an attorney, doesn't mean that they have to exercise that right, and lots of folks represent themselves (though rarely adequately) in criminal proceedings. Just because you can represent yourself, doesn't mean you should. Most people can cut their own hair, but the result is rarely something attractive.

F. SHOULD I INVOKE MY FIFTH AMENDMENT RIGHTS?

There are hundreds of people in jail today who did not invoke this important right, and almost every one of them would give anything to have the chance a second time. The Fifth Amendment provides that no person shall be compelled to be a witness against himself. The right to remain silent, and the right to not have the silence used against the suspect, is considered sacred under United States law. If you are questioned about anything by an official police agency, you should never answer questions until you have consulted with an attorney.

A suspect who is arrested for theft, but who will make no statement to the police, may not later be described as uncooperative by the police. The state can make no reference, direct or indirect, to the suspect's exercise of the right to remain silent. A prosecutor cannot say, in closing argument for example, that "the defendant had the opportunity to testify, and he did not. He could have told you what happened, but he didn't." Such a statement would be a comment on the right of the accused to remain silent, and as such, would be improper.

It is instructive to look again at what happened in the Efren Saldivar case for an illustration of the reasons why therapists must always exercise the right to remain silent, especially if they are not involved or not guilty. In the Saldivar case, the police would have had nothing to go on if Saldivar had said simply "I do not wish to talk to you." Doubtless the inquiry would have ended right there, because the police had no case.

But once Saldivar started talking, the police were able to build a case. Saldivar sank his own boat. Had Saldivar remained silent, he might have lost his license, and might well have lost his job, but he would never have gone to jail.

1. How Do I Invoke the Right to Terminate Questioning?

Everyone has the right to tell the police that they do not want to be questioned, and/or that they do not want to be questioned without a lawyer. Once a suspect makes a definite statement that he wants a lawyer, or that he wants questioning to stop, the state cannot continue to question or pressure him to submit to questioning.

Innocent or guilty, the only smart thing to do when confronted by police officers or federal agents about any matter is to simply refuse to give any information. While the federal agent can arrest you for giving false information to her, she can't arrest you for not talking to her. You have no obligation or duty of any kind to communicate with the police or federal agencies.

Once you have invoked these rights, the only way police can question you is if you ask to see them. No one ever walked down a jail cell hallway with hands shackled and said "gosh, I wish I had said some more things to that cop." But the opposite is clearly true.

2. Can I Get Bail?

Because the criminal justice system is designed around the concept of "innocent until proven guilty," every person accused of a crime has a right to reasonable bail. Bail is normally an amount of money or property put down by an accused (or others on his behalf) in order to secure his return for trial.

Bail is a promise. In exchange for giving the court a sum of money, the person accused of the crime can be set free until he or she is convicted by a jury or pleads guilty to the crime. The person granted bail promises to appear. If that person does not appear, he or she forfeit their bail.

The amount of bail depends, in large measure, on the seriousness of the offense. For a crime like shoplifting, a judge might well let an accused out on his or her own recognizance. In other words, his or her word to return is all the security the Court requires.

For more serious felonies, like robbery, larceny, theft, etc., the court may demand more money. Sometimes a court will set a bond at $10,000, and tell the accused he or she can post 10% of that amount with the court. In that situation, the bailee simply gives the court $1000 cash, and is permitted to leave the jail. However, if he or she defaults—if he or she fails to show up for court or for a scheduled hearing—the entire bail amount is forfeited, and he or she becomes liable to the court for the full amount of $10,000.

Bail bondsmen operate as sureties. Their job is to take the risk that the accused will not show up at trial. They extract a fee from the accused, usually at least 10% of the bail amount, and that money is forfeited to the bondsman. The bondsman posts a $10,000 security bond with the court, which is a contractual promise to pay $10,000 if the court orders the bond forfeited.

The bondsman is now responsible to ensure that the accused shows up for trial. If he doesn't, the bondsman may hire a "bounty hunter" to track that person down. The relationship between the bondsman and the bonded person is contractual, and generally gives the bondsman the right to to kick down your door and drag you to jail in your underwear if you jump bond. Bounty hunters are, for the most part, brutal people who enjoy the power they have. If you fail to honor your promise to appear, you can expect to deal with them, and they are not regulated in the way that police officers are in most jurisdictions.

The Eighth Amendment guarantees that bail not be excessive, and that fines and penalties not be excessive. A fine of $10,000 for jaywalking would be unconstitutional as would bail for a speeder in the same amount.

For very serious offenses like murder, capital murder, rape, felony murder, or manslaughter, the prosecution may seek remand. Remand means the prosecutor wants the accused held in jail until the time of his trial because he is either (1) a risk to flee the jurisdiction, or (2) a danger to the community.

Usually the prosecution either gets what it wants directly (remand) or gets the equivalent, in that the court orders the person held in lieu of $500,000 in bail. In that situation, the court may require that the cash amount be posted instead of a surety bond. When that happens, the practical effect is to guarantee that the accused will remain in jail.

G. WHAT TACTICS DO POLICE USE IN QUESTIONING?

Thank God we have police. There are some very bad people, and the police get rid of them for us. When the police are messing with the drunk down the street, they are our friends; however, when they are knocking on our door, they are the enemy. Any time a police officer shows up asking questions, you should hire counsel. This is because, as stated earlier, the police have an incentive to close the case, not necessarily to pursue justice.

1. Do Police Officers Care About the truth?

Most cops will tell you they only want the truth, but what they really want is a case closed by conviction. The problem is that cops don't write down everything you tell them. When the witness says "I can't be sure, but I think the guy was wearing brown pants and a white shirt," the police write down "brown pants, white shirt." They do not write down the part about not being sure. That information hurts their case. Similarly when the witness says "I didn't get a good look, but the guy looked a lot like that Tony DeWitt character," the cops write down "Tony DeWitt."

Within a few minutes of arriving at the scene of a crime, a good cop has a theory about how it went down. If there is a murder of a husband or wife, in most cases it is the spouse of the victim who first merits suspicion. If the early facts support that, other evidence and other theories of the case may be ignored and other leads disregarded. The search for the truth quickly gets changed into the quest for a convenient explanation and a quick end to the case.

One of the criticisms leveled against the police officers in the Laci Peterson case is that they never pursued a suspect other than Scott Peterson. The defense used this to suggest that others committed the crime. Sadly for Peterson, the jury didn't believe Scott Peterson because he had been such an artful liar to so many different people.

2. Why Should I Remain Silent if I Didn't Do Anything Wrong?

Why is it so important to remain completely silent when questioned? If people are truly not guilty, can they hurt themselves by saying it? Yes, and they frequently do.

The best illustration of why you should never talk to the police without an attorney is found in the movie My Cousin Vinny. The hapless Ralph Macchio is talking with the sheriff who leads him through his trip to the store. Macchio is thinking that he is in trouble for shoplifting a can of food, and when the sheriff finishes, he says "And then you shot the guy."

"I shot the guy," Macchio asks? He says it again, clearly as a question: "I shot the guy?" His voice rises an octave as he asks this question.

But what happens in court? When the sheriff testifies, he says, in a flat monotone, that Macchio said "I shot the guy."

The sheriff's testimony was technically true, even though the inflection and tone of the suspect's answer were completely different.

There is never, ever any time when it is to your advantage to speak to the police without an attorney. This is the only unbreakable rule in this book.

3. Do They Really Use Good Cop and Bad Cop?

Yes. All the time. At the risk of sounding like a broken record, it is never a good idea to talk to police without an attorney present. Only bad things can come of talking to the police. Nothing good can come from it. When a police officer says "if you don't have anything to hide, there's no reason not to talk to us," the proper response is that "there is no reason to talk without an attorney at my side to make sure my rights are protected."

Cops play games. One cop is angry; the other is gentle and kind. You can trust him or her to be your friend, help you through this. But, of course, if you don't talk, he or she can't help you. Even if you've seen every cop movie ever made, when it happens to you, the coercive nature of the questioning and the mannerisms of the people involved quickly cause you to gravitate toward the cop who is your "friend" in this. Therein lies the danger!

This is all gamesmanship. The job of the police officer is to close a case and arrest a suspect. It is not, under any set of circumstances, to help one suspect over the other. The job of the police is to put bad people in jail. If the police believe you are bad, you are headed to jail.

Sometimes a police officer will simply lie. Police officers are allowed to lie to suspects, and sometimes, courts even encourage the act. A cop may say "we have a witness who saw you mail the letter," when in fact they have no such witness. The unschooled will simply confess. What's the difference if they have a witness? Yet, if they thought for a moment, they might realize that even if the witness did see you mail a letter, it doesn't mean it was the letter.

It is for precisely this reason, that police officers frequently use deception and trickery, that you must never be questioned without a lawyer by your side.

4. "We Can Clear All This Up . . ."

Another favorite tactic of police is the "we can eliminate you as a suspect if you talk to us" ploy, or the other more common question, "will you help us clear this up so we can all go home?" When the police are talking about going home, they are talking about them going home, not you. They have a new residence in mind for you.

5. What Should I Do if Questioned by the Police?

Clearly you should never talk to a police officer alone. You should always have legal counsel at your side. If you cannot have legal counsel there, do not engage in any conversation. This is true irrespective of whether you are considered a suspect or not.

Don't underestimate the power of silence, either. When you tell the cops that you don't want to be questioned, they won't talk to you anymore. But that doesn't mean they won't talk. They are apt to talk about how the courts are going to deal with the person who committed the crime, about how courts are more lenient when people talk, and the like. The fact is, when you ask for a lawyer it doesn't mean that you necessarily have a written guarantee that they are going to call one for you (or get you a public defender).

Instead, what is likely to happen is that they'll simply leave you alone while you wait for your attorney. From their perspective, the longer it takes to get an attorney there, the better. They use the power of silence, and the coercive effect of being held in handcuffs and cut off from the rest of the world, to their advantage.

The way to deal with this is to have a relationship with an attorney before anything bad happens. If you know an attorney, and can deal effectively with him or her, you should keep his or her card in your wallet at all times. One never knows when the police will come knocking.

6. Am I a Target?

Frequently, lawyers will ask "is my client a target of this investigation?" If the answer is no, the lawyer is more willing to let the client talk. If the answer is yes, the conversation never happens.

Sometimes the government won't say if you're a target. If they won't say, then you are a target. That may not always be true, but it's the only safe way to behave.

Keep in mind that if the police call you to an appointment at 8:00 a.m. after you've worked a night shift, you have the right to have the interview conducted at a place and time of your choosing—usually your attorney's office—and to know the subject of the interview. If the interview involves a patient, or medical records, you should have a right to seek a court order prohibiting the interview.

Usually, police try to choose the time and manner of questioning. They position themselves between the door and you in a rather pathetic attempt to control you. They may not be able to lawfully detain you, but when you consent to talk to them, and they use these coercive tactics, it is for a reason. The reason is: it works.

7. Am I Being Asked to Testify Against a Former Patient?

In many cases, you can be made to testify against a former patient. For example, you have no doubt seen drunk drivers in the Emergency Room. You can be called to testify to what you saw, etc. You cannot be called to testify about what the patient told you in confidence unless the Court orders you to do so. You must assert the patient privilege and answer only after the Court orders you to answer the question.

H. WHAT ARE THE LEGAL RIGHTS OF VICTIMS?

It is unfortunate, but true, that your odds of needing the information in this chapter are more likely to be on the side of victim than accused criminal. Health care personnel are routinely victims of crime, in part because criminals know or think that they have access to drugs.

Crime affects everyone at some point. I do not know many people who have not, at some point, had a brush with the system as victim. In the past few years, the law has changed with respect to victims. In many jurisdictions, victims are now entitled to restitution from the convicted criminal. Even when the crime is "victimless" like prostitution or drug possession, criminals are made to pay into the victim compensation fund in order to make sure that those whose lives are shattered by crime get some help in rebuilding those lives.

If you are a victim of crime, report it. If someone steals your bicycle, or your leaf blower out of your yard, report it to the police. It is doubtful that the item will be recovered, but often a quick report will result in a quick apprehension. When that happens—and it does happen from time to time—the system works well.

All too frequently, however, crime victims are afraid to report major crimes like rape, robbery, and the like, because they fear being victimized a second time by the criminal justice system. The recent criminal charges filed, and then dropped, against Kobe Bryant are an example. Bryant may or may not have been responsible for criminal behavior, but he was denied his day in court to prove that because the victim dropped the case. The reason was, of course, the fact that in vigorously defending his rights, Bryant had the power to emotionally and psychologically rape the victim a second time through rigorous cross examination and exploration of her other sexual history. Of course, there are many who believe that the entire episode was no more than a shakedown of Bryant for money; and it must be remembered that Bryant was not only not convicted, but the charges were dropped, denying him an opportunity to defend his good name.

Recently Bryant's attorney, Pamela McKinney, talked to the Kansas City Metropolitan Bar Association. She told the lawyers that her biggest problem in the case was not her client or the facts, but the way the media pushed at every turn to reveal some additional and salacious facts. Often the media do not serve victims or the accused very well in this regard.

1. Must Police Keep Me Informed?

One of the first rights a victim has is to know the status of his or her case. If the police make an arrest, the victim has a right to know who was arrested, and to learn what evidence (in general, not in specific) that the prosecution has.

2. Can I Participate in Trial?

In addition to general notification, the victim has a right to participate at trial, and in some states, a duty to do so. The victim must testify about what happened, and will need to face cross examination by the defendant's counsel. The prosecutorial team will assist the victim in preparing for trial, and will help guide the victim through the process.

3. Can I Be Heard at Sentencing?

If the accused is found guilty, the victim has the right to participate in sentencing by providing victim impact testimony. Victim impact testimony sets forth the impact of the crime on the victims. The state is entitled to show that the victim's life has been changed, and what the effect has been. Victim impact testimony is common in murder and rape prosecutions, but can be given in any felony or misdemeanor case.

4. Will I Get Notification of Release or Parole?

Unless the criminal merits the death sentence, at some point the convicted criminal will be either paroled or released from prison. When that happens, the victim is entitled to know when and where he will be released. The victim is also entitled to be present and give testimony in any parole hearing and to make his or her voice heard on the subject of probation or parole.

I. KEY POINTS

- The police are generally not bad people, and generally, they want to keep us all safe.
- Police become bad people when they try to convict those who are not guilty.

- If you are truly not guilty, the police are still not your friend, no matter how much they may try to tell you that they are.
- There is only one unbreakable rule in criminal law: don't say anything to anyone other than your attorney until you have had an opportunity to talk to your attorney.
- Everything you say that helps you will be forgotten; anything that hurts you will be engraved in stone.
- You have a right to be free from unreasonable searches.
- You have that right as much in public (walking down the street) as you do in your home.
- The police have a right to frisk you on reasonable suspicion alone.
- Police need a warrant to search your car or your home.
- Police need a search warrant to come into your house and execute an arrest warrant on someone staying there.
- Police are more interested in convictions than truth.
- Do not ever give up your right to remain silent.
- Always invoke your right not to be questioned until an attorney arrives.
- Anytime you think about talking to the police, think about the movie My Cousin Vinny and what happened to Ralph Macchio in that movie.
- Just as criminals have rights, victims have rights too.

J. SUMMARY

The Constitution of the United States, and each state constitution, provides certain basic rights for all who are accused of crimes. Among those rights are:

- The right to counsel.
- The right to terminate questioning.
- The right to remain silent.
- The right to have searches conducted only by search warrant.
- The right to bail in a reasonable amount.
- The right to a reasonable fine or penalty if convicted.

If you take nothing else from this book, remember that there is never a time when you want to be questioned in any criminal proceeding without an attorney, and anything and everything you say will be used against you.

CHAPTER 15

Finding Legal Representation

*Lawyers are the only persons in whom
ignorance of the law is not punished.*

Jeremy Bentham
18th Century Legal Scholar

A. INTRODUCTION

Lawyers are like nuclear weapons. When the other side has one, you need one. Once launched, they are impossible to recall, and you don't want to be on the receiving end of one because they frequently cause massive destruction. So goes conventional wisdom.

But the fact is that sooner or later you are going to need a lawyer to help you deal with the issues in your life. You are going to need that help, and the goal of this chapter is to help you understand how to go about finding good representation.

B. WHY DO I NEED A LAWYER?

Other than your family doctor, whose care and compassion are necessary to see you through harrowing medical ordeals, your family lawyer should be your most important business relationship. A family lawyer can help you with your personal needs (e.g., setting up your will, providing counsel on purchases, etc.) and when you need a specialist for a particular problem, he will know whom to call.

Unfortunately, just as people who are healthy don't go see a doctor, people who don't have legal problems never think about whom they'll call in the event of a serious problem. They then find themselves getting a call at 2:00 a.m. from the jail. Their son, their husband, or their next-door neighbor is in jail on a drunk driving charge and needs a lawyer right away.

Even worse, not having had a prior relationship with a lawyer, their first inclination is to pick up the phone book and start looking for the guy who has the biggest ad and who promises the most with respect to the area of law they now require. If Mr. Ima Shyster, Esq., promises in the yellow pages to "fight hard to get you justice," and the ad touts his reputation as a fine lawyer and excellent advisor, there is probably good reason to suspect that the lawyer is neither a fighter nor a justice seeker, but more likely, someone who makes money on generating a lot of leads and provides little, if any, help. The fact is, good lawyers don't need to advertise.

Richard, a truck mechanic, has two convictions for driving while intoxicated. If he gets a third conviction he could lose his license for ten years and, possibly, serve up to three years in state prison. When he is released from jail he finds Dale, an attorney whose yellow pages advertisement says he focuses on defending drunk driving cases.[1] Dale demands a $2,500 retainer. Richard pays it.

Three weeks later, Richard meets with Dale. Dale now has the prosecutor's file, including the Intoxilizer results, and advises Richard that he can delay trial for more than a year if it appears he is going to trial. He then tells Richard that there is a possible defense that he could explore, but that it will require additional money. Richard pays another $2,000 to avoid the potential conviction. More importantly to Richard, until he is convicted, he won't lose his license. The attorney begins to engage in what lawyers call E&D tactics: Evasion and Delay.

A year and three months later, the lawyer calls Richard and advises him to plead guilty. He is pretty sure he can arrange it so he will only get three or four weeks in jail.

"What about that defense?"

"Can't prove it," the lawyer says. Incredibly, he can show Richard no evidence that he has evaluated this defense, but states he has talked with experts. He can't name those experts, however.

A review of the court file shows that the lawyer has simply filed multiple and repetitive motions for continuance, and hasn't done anything to advance the case. Now, after more than a year without doing anything but filing continuances, the lawyer wants Richard to plead guilty in order to avoid jail

---

[1]People often wonder why lawyers say they "focus their practice" or "confine their practice" to representing a specific kind of client. This is because in most states there is no separate bar examination or separate set of credentials available to designate people as "specialists" and a lawyer whose signature isn't dry on his license is considered, in most states, to be as qualified as Johnnie Cochran in defending or prosecuting any particular case.

time. Since he is not going to trial, Richard asks for his additional $2,000 back. The lawyer refuses, saying he has already done the work.

Richard made a classic mistake. He thought that the yellow pages advertisement was indicative of the kind of representation he would get. If, in fact, he had checked out the lawyer with the state bar, and with other lawyers, they would have advised him to use someone else.

If Richard had a family lawyer, someone he could count on to help advise him in a tough situation, he could have found a competent attorney who does defense work and who would have disposed of the case on more favorable terms.

Family lawyers are important in the way that primary care physicians are important. A primary care physician knows you, your medical history, and your likes and dislikes. She advises you on keeping fit and avoiding illness, and has the leg up on diagnosing you when you come in sick because she's seen you well.

Similarly, the family lawyer knows the important details of your life and relationships. He knows your next of kin. He knows your wishes. If you've taken the time to draft wills and powers of attorney to provide for care when you are disabled, he has these on file and can forward them to the appropriate authorities. The bottom line is that the family lawyer can be a resource for help when you do not know where to turn.

C. WHAT ABOUT PERSONAL INJURY MATTERS?

Ellie gets a call from the school. Her daughter Claire was hit by a car while on a field trip. She is in serious condition. Over six months, Claire goes through six operations including one to repair damage to both her hips. Her medical bills total $112,000. She calls the driver's insurance company, and they offer her $50,000 to settle her claim. Claire needs an attorney to help her get compensation from the driver's insurance company. Ellie doesn't have a family attorney, so like Richard, she goes to the telephone book.

Ellie calls attorney P.R. Imadonna to help her. Appearing on the back of the telephone book, Mr. Imadonna boasts multi-million dollar recoveries and "no fee unless we recover for you."

Ellie visits, signs a contract, and six weeks later Mr. Imadonna is telling her that he won't handle her claim, but that another attorney from Chicago, more than 800 miles away, will be handling her claim for her.

If Ellie is smart, she'll discharge Mr. Imadonna and find an attorney in her jurisdiction who routinely handles personal injury cases. Mr. Imadonna is what lawyers call a "finder." He has no significant legal skills of his own. He merely advertises, finds great cases, and then "refers" them to seasoned trial attorneys in other cities so as to assure a good referral fee and a large recovery. Mr. Imadonna has no vested interest in Ellie's case because he makes his money by having large numbers of referral fees from lots of other lawyers. He is like a re-marketer. He buys cases on the open market, and repackages them for attorneys who specialize in that area of the law.

If Ellie or Richard had previously formed a good relationship with their own local lawyer, a phone call to that lawyer would probably have produced a response like "I don't do that kind of case, but I know who does. I will set up an appointment for you and get right back to you."

Good attorneys know the true experts in their field the way that family doctors know which neurosurgeon to refer to in a crisis; by following their clients' causes of action with the referral attorney, they earn any fee paid to them by the client. If the client needs medical authorizations notarized on a Saturday, it's the family lawyer, working with the larger firm handling the personal injury action, who handles that paperwork. When the case comes to trial the jury doesn't have to take the word of "out-of-towners," but can rely instead on their own local lawyer who sits with the referring attorneys and advises at critical parts of the trial such as jury selection.

Shysters like Dale and Imadonna don't actually earn any fee, and shouldn't actually be paid one.[2] That doesn't mean they don't try to collect a fee; it just means that courts are usually hostile to such fee claims.

D. HOW DO I GO ABOUT SELECTING COUNSEL FOR SPECIFIC TYPES OF CASES?

For the sake of argument, let's say you've not read this chapter until today, and today you have a specific need for a specific lawyer in a specific area of the law. How do you go about finding out which firms are good, and which firms are bad? The answer is, you do a little bit of research.

1. How to Pick a Good Business Lawyer

If you have a small business, and you need to find a good business lawyer, the easiest way to find a good one is to call similarly sized businesses in your

---

[2]Most state bar associations have fee dispute resolution. If a lawyer charges what the client feels is an unfair fee, the state bar will help resolve that issue at no cost to the client.

community, and ask to speak to the chief financial officer or CEO. Find out from them whom they use for their legal services. After about six or seven calls you will begin to find a consensus as to which firms do the most business work.

Once you've found a firm, look them up in the phone book or elsewhere. Firms with flashy advertisements and claims are good firms to avoid. A law firm that has to advertise, in most cases, has to advertise because it has not established a reputation of service among the business community.

When you call for an appointment, ask to speak to the partner who handles the area of law with which you need assistance (e.g., defending product liability claims). Set up a meeting and ask the questions set out below in the Interviewing Counsel section. If you are satisfied with the answers, ask about the retainer policy. Under what circumstances will you be billed? Does the firm offer transactional billing (meaning, for example, will you charge me a flat fee, rather than an hourly fee, to defend or handle a certain type of case)?

Most importantly, trust your gut instincts. If you have the feeling that your pocket is about to be picked, get up and leave. Don't hire a lawyer you don't like and trust just because he has a great reputation. A great reputation may simply mean that people are too intimidated and afraid of the lawyer to say anything.

2. How to Pick a Good Criminal Defense Lawyer

If you watched the news on television, or followed the O.J. Simpson case in the media, you know that some criminal defense lawyers spend as much time promoting themselves as defending their clients. This is an unfortunate consequence of the fact that the media, rightly or wrongly, sets out to make defense attorneys either angels or demons depending on their view of the particular case.

Mark Geragos is an accomplished trial attorney, but he has spent more time defending his clients in the media than in the courtroom. And while a good public relations offensive is often a smart move in a high profile case, after watching him on television, I would most likely not hire him to represent any client of mine. This is partly because the most dangerous 10 feet in America are the 10 feet between any television camera and Mr. Geragos.

The criminal law, particularly that of the non-serious or first-time offender, is not particularly complicated or difficult. In most criminal cases the only cases that get filed are the ones in which the evidence is overwhelmingly in favor of conviction. In most federal and state jurisdictions, a prosecutor won't bring a case unless she is 95% certain she can get a conviction.

Consider the case of L.L., a 28-year-old woman arrested for DWI. Although I normally do not do any criminal defense work, I agreed to represent this woman as a favor to a friend. In our first meeting, she told me that she had been parked on the side of the road when the Sheriff's officer pulled up. She had not had the car turned on. She was not driving. She did not understand how she could be arrested for DWI.

I got the arrest report. It told a different story. L.L. had been clearly intoxicated, unable to stand up, let alone walk a straight line, and the videotape of the arrest captured more four letter words than a contemporary rap song. The videotape also captured the exhaust plume from the car.

The Intoxilizer measured L.L.'s blood alcohol content at .145, almost twice the legal limit of 0.08. This would not be a difficult case for the prosecutor to prove.

As is almost always the case, the issue was not so much whether I could get the client's case dismissed or thrown out—there were no procedural or technical errors. The question was, what could I do?

The client worked for the state of Missouri as a clerk, and as a state employee, a conviction on even a misdemeanor would result in a job disqualification. In Missouri, for certain jobs, it's "DWI, say goodbye." So, the issue was whether I could get the client a suspended imposition of sentence or SIS. In an SIS, the court holds the file and suspends the imposition of any sentence for the time of probation. If the client completes the probation period without any violation, the suspended sentence is never imposed and the case is dismissed at the end of the probation period. No criminal record (for purposes of the public record) results.

What was needed was a negotiation where I could convince a prosecutor to give her more favorable treatment. After a couple of calls, lots of pleading, and a little whining, I was able to get a recommendation for SIS, which the judge later imposed.

Unfortunately, some people think they need a pugilistic My Cousin Vinny approach for such matters. They want to hire the meanest, nastiest lawyer at the courthouse. This is seldom wise. In almost all criminal matters, the best negotiator, the best communicator, is the lawyer to have.

In picking a defense attorney, the best way to determine a person's competence is to determine how many similar cases he or she has taken and defended over time. If a lawyer has tried seven or eight similar cases, he may be competent. If he has no experience, he should not be hired. If he suggests that the best way to approach the case is to fight every issue out with the prosecutor, you may have a lawyer who is simply going to churn out paperwork and bill you by the hour without providing you with any real relief.

The crime reporter at the newspaper will know who the most seasoned criminal lawyers in your town are, even if you don't. Bail bondsmen may also give you names. Bondsmen frequently have referral arrangements with lawyers and get referral fees from lawyers for sending them clients.[3] In that instance, the lawyer may not be the best, he may simply be the one who needs clients the most.

More important than the referrals of friends and neighbors, you need to meet with the lawyer and determine whether she is the best person to represent you or your family member. Pay attention to the lawyer's office and surroundings. A lawyer in a cheap office without a secretary is a struggling lawyer. She is going to be more likely to simply be interested in the fee rather than the case. Is the lawyer professional? Does she greet you properly? Does she have a professional-looking office? Lawyers who operate in shoddy conditions are always to be avoided.

3. How to Pick a Good Plaintiff's Lawyer[4]

The worst way to pick a lawyer is by responding to a television advertisement. A lawyer who advertises is a lawyer who has to advertise in order to get clients. In most cases, this means that the firm is either not well known, or, in the alternative, is simply trolling with a large net looking for the bigger fish.

There are lawyers who promise to deliver excellent representation, but whose real job is simply to find clients with good cases so they can refer these clients on to other more seasoned attorneys.

For example, one law firm, whose name will remain anonymous, uses an 800 number and large television and telephone book advertising to get clients in the door. If the case is of a particular type, a product liability case involving guns for example, the case is sent to one law firm where the lawyers have handled numerous similar cases. If the case involves medical negligence, it is sent to a firm that does primarily medical negligence work.

The law firm, before it sends these clients to the other law firm, signs the clients to a 45% contingent fee contract. That contract provides that,

---

[3]It is absolutely unlawful for an attorney to pay any non-attorney for a case referral.

[4]Note: If you live in Missouri, Kansas, Iowa, Arkansas, or Illinois, you can skip this section and call me: 888-717-7575.

on resolution the client will pay the lawyers 45% of the proceeds. But the way the contract is calculated, which is not readily apparent to the client, makes the fee closer to 50% or 55%. If the client had simply tried from the beginning to find a firm specializing in this area of the law, the result would have been much less expensive for them:

Television Firm	*Plaintiff's Firm*
Fee Provision: 45% of total	*Normally 40% of total*
*How calculated: on **total** recovery*	*How calculated: on **net** recovery*
Settlement: $100,000	*Settlement: $100,000*
Expenses: $20,000	*Expenses: $20,000*
Fee calculation: 45% of 100,000 is a fee of $45,000. Client pays firm $45,000 plus $20,000 in expenses and has net recovery of $35,000.	*Fee calculation: Net recovery is 80,000. 40% of 80,000 is $32,000. Client pays a total of $52,000 to law firm, and receives a total of $48,000.*
Main firm gets 75% of fee, TV firm gets 25% of fee.	*Referring attorney gets 10% to 15% of fee from Plaintiffs firm.*

A family attorney would not have signed up the case, but rather, simply sent the client to the Plaintiff's firm, who would have taken a much smaller fee, and paid back a much smaller referral fee to the family lawyer.

A good plaintiff's attorney rarely charges more than 40% for all services. Some firms charge a sliding scale; for example, their fee is 25% if the case can be settled before filing an action, 33% after an action is filed but before trial, 40% if settled after trial, and 50% if the case has to be defended on appeal. These firms have some incentive to quickly file cases and press for settlement only after the trial has started. They may not act on that incentive, but a straight 40% contract is much better for the client.

If you do not have a family attorney, look for an understated ad in the telephone book. Lawyers who use multiple colors, boldfacing, and who scream that they will "fight for you," are rarely seasoned trial counsel. Focus instead on law firms that have small but tasteful ads and who represent plaintiffs only.

Another good way, of course, is to ask other family members and friends. Talk to them about the lawyers, and whom they would select. Sometimes attorneys have a good reputation for a particular kind of case (e.g., probate) and not a very good reputation for others (divorces). The opinions of other persons are very important in helping you determine whether this lawyer is for you.

4. Should I Check the State Bar?

Absolutely! The final step, of course, is to check with the State Bar and determine whether the lawyer has ever been disciplined. If an attorney has been disciplined by the state bar for an offense related to honesty, ethics, or the like, it is a good idea not to hire her.

Several years ago, two St. Louis attorneys, one of whom was a classmate of mine in law school, were disbarred by the Missouri Bar for a gross violation of the lawyer-client privilege. They took sensitive information learned in representing a car manufacturer and used that information to help plaintiffs sue that manufacturer. The Missouri Bar found the conduct reprehensible, and ordered the attorneys disbarred. Only three years later both attorneys were on the front page of the *Missouri Lawyer's Weekly* with a huge verdict in a personal injury case.

How does someone go from goat to hero in such a short time? Simple: the client most likely didn't know about the lawyer's past, and smooth salesmanship and promises of wealth were all it took to convince the client to sign the contract. Your state bar can tell you whether any attorney has been convicted of ethical violations and been publicly reprimanded, censured, suspended, or disbarred. You need to learn this information because sometimes lawyers continue to sign up cases without a license, counting on being able to bring those cases to a close once they have obtained reinstatement.

Always check to make sure that your lawyer is in good standing with the state bar before hiring her.

E. ARE THERE DIFFERENCES BETWEEN BIG FIRMS AND SMALL FIRMS?

Big law firms (75 lawyers or more) tend to be money and billing driven, not client or case driven. The larger the law firm, the larger the overhead and the greater the likelihood that these lawyers will do everything possible to increase your bill. Unless you are General Motors Corporation, or some similar corporate entity, you rarely, if ever, need a law firm with that many lawyers running around. The best size for most small businesses is the 10- to 20- lawyer firm that specializes in the area of the law that you need. A law firm of this size is capable of meeting your needs without being so large that it has a need to pay the overhead with your case.

For individual plaintiffs and defendants, a law firm of three to ten people is probably just right. Bigger Plaintiff's firms tend to be volume driven. They rely on multiple small cases to make their money, and may not deliver good customer service. Of course, the single most important factor determining whether to hire a lawyer is how he deals with your questions and concerns.

F. HOW DO I GO ABOUT INTERVIEWING COUNSEL?

When a lawyer is interviewed, it should be just like hiring an employee. The lawyer may begin by jumping right into what went wrong, why you're there to see him, and gathering facts about you. Put on the brakes.

Until you know that this lawyer is the right lawyer for you, you should first interview him and find out whether he is. You need to know not only the lawyer's background, but what he will expect of you and what he will expect to do for you. The lawyer will want to know about your case. That isn't important, however, until you know something about the lawyer.

Begin by asking general questions about the lawyer's background:

- Where did you get your law degree?
- What was your class rank?
- How long have you been in practice?
- How long have you been with this firm?
- What is your primary area of interest in the law?

Lawyers are not used to being asked such questions, and may respond, initially, a bit defensively. Ignore this. You are employing a lawyer to work for you. You have a responsibility to yourself to ensure that the lawyer you hire is one who can get the job done. You're going to pay a fee; you should know what you're buying.

If you feel comfortable with the lawyer's answers, then move into the general facts of your case, and what you need done (e.g., "I have a neighbor who is trespassing. I need to get an injunction. Before I give you the facts, I need some additional information from you.").

Now you need to ask:

- How many cases like mine have you handled?
- Do you have expertise in this area?
- Tell me about your expertise.
- What was the most difficult case of this kind you ever handled?

- Is there anyone else more qualified in this firm or some other firm to handle this matter for me?[5]
- Tell me why you think you are qualified to handle this case.
- Is there anything I should know about you before I hire you that you haven't told me so far?
- Have you ever been disciplined by the State Bar?

Only if the lawyer answers these questions frankly and honestly should you proceed to reveal your confidences and place your trust in him or her. Lawyers don't like to be on the hot seat. They don't like talking about themselves. They don't like admitting, for example, that they were in the middle 50% of their law school class. They don't like admitting that they've never handled an injunction before.[6] They may especially dislike the last question if they have a disciplinary record. Still, it's wise to find out what kind of legal mind you're hiring.

Your lawyer is your agent. You will be bound by whatever he does on your behalf. If he tells your opposing counsel that he is going to settle the case for $50,000, even if he has no authority to do that, you may still (in some jurisdictions) be bound. If he misses a deadline, then you've missed the deadline. If he makes an admission to the judge, it's the same as your having made that admission.

It is vital, therefore, to have a lawyer with whom you can feel completely comfortable and are willing to trust.

If the lawyer offers you a contract for employment of attorneys, remember that the contract was written to benefit her firm, and her personally, and not to benefit you. It is not a contract that is in any way designed to assert your rights. Instead, it is a contract that is designed to secure as much for the lawyer as possible. Read it carefully.

G. HOW SHOULD MY LAWYER-CLIENT RELATIONSHIP BE STRUCTURED?

It is important for you to remember, and for your lawyer to remember, that he or she works for you. They do not work for your insurance company (even if the insurance company hired them to defend you). They work for you. They owe a duty of loyalty to you. They are required to put your interests and

---

[5]If a lawyer acts offended when you ask this question, it is time to leave. An attorney with your best interest at heart will want you at the best firm possible.

[6]Just because the lawyer hasn't handled an injunction doesn't disqualify him if he knows how to do it and can do it properly.

needs ahead of their own. If they cannot do this, they cannot properly represent you.

Irrespective of whether they are defending you in a criminal matter, or prosecuting a wrongful death matter, they have an obligation to treat you with respect, answer your questions, return your phone calls, and keep you informed about the status of your case. If they fail to do this, they are failing in their professional responsibilities.

Keep in mind that if your case is valuable (for example, you have a wrongful death claim that could exceed $1,000,000), the law firm very much wants to represent you. That is the time to negotiate about fees, expenses, and the like. Even though a law firm may present you with a form contract that specifies how they will calculate their fee and ask you to sign it, you can line out provisions you don't like, initial them, and make a counterproposal to the firm. If you think 40% is too high, tell them you will pay no more than 35%; and if that isn't good enough, you'll take your case somewhere else.

Most of the time, attorneys want to handle your case, and they want to do it in the worst way. They will happily knock down their contingent fee. It is better to have 35% of a $10,000,000 case than 0% of any other case. If the firm won't knock down its fee, then refuse to sign, and tell them you'll have to talk to other firms. In most cases the willingness to walk out will get you a lower fee.

Always get any arrangement, whether it is for a flat fee in a criminal case, or for a contingent fee in a plaintiff's case, in writing. Don't write a check until the agreement is on paper and to your liking. Insist on seeing and approving a contract. The law in most states requires that any contingent fee contract be in writing. Flat fee contracts are not required to be in writing, but should be for your protection. Anytime a flat fee is stated, you should insist on having the lawyer spell out that this includes trial, appeal, and re-trial if necessary. Failure to do so can result in bad outcomes.

This is especially true with solo practitioners. The $2,500 paid in August won't seem like much of an incentive to try your case in February, when the lawyer has spent the money and gone on to other things. For this reason, it is very important with any solo practitioner to make sure that he will carry the case through to the end, and that he will hire and compensate any additional legal talent you need. When a lawyer negotiates a flat fee, he has an obligation to live up to it. Insist that he hold your fee in his trust account until the case is finally disposed, and that he take his flat fee only at the end of the case. Get this agreement in writing.

If you are not properly treated, if you are not kept informed, remember that lawyers are like plumbers and electricians, and they can be hired and fired at will.

H. KEY POINTS

- You should have a good family attorney.
- Attorneys are like plumbers and electricians; they can be hired and fired.
- If you sign a contract with an attorney, that contract binds you even if you fire the attorney later on. So be careful about what you're signing.
- Interview counsel before hiring them. Ask what they've done, where they've done it, and what results they've obtained. Results speak louder than recommendations or promises.
- Avoid lawyers who advertise on the back of the phone book.
- Avoid lawyers who are mean or disagreeable. If they are mean or disagreeable to you, they are probably not going to pursue your case diligently.
- Get any agreement on fees in writing.
- Check out any attorney with the State Bar before signing any contract.

CHAPTER 16

The Ethical Rules of Health Care

The ideals which have always shone before me and filled me with the joy of living are goodness, beauty, and truth. To make a goal of comfort or happiness has never appealed to me; a system of ethics built on this basis would be sufficient only for a herd of cattle.

Albert Einstein

A. INTRODUCTION

Ethics is a difficult concept to explain and write about because everyone has different views about ethics. Ethics are first and foremost what moral and ethical codes require us to do. Ethics are directive, in the form of "thou shalt" and "thou shalt not." They are absolute, and they are situational. Most importantly, they overlap and they have internal conflicts.

Some have quipped that having a lawyer write about ethics is like having an atheist write about religion. But lawyers are themselves bound by a strict ethical code. That ethical code is designed to first protect the public. In considering a course of conduct, attorneys are taught to first determine whether the course of conduct will harm or potentially affect their client.

For example, if an attorney has defended a hospital in a medical malpractice case, he cannot later prosecute such a case against that hospital because the hospital, as a former client, is entitled to believe that he will safeguard their secrets. The attorney must refer that case on to another attorney.

In health care, ethics are often less easy to distill to a set of rules. The goal is to first protect the patient and do no harm. But often the line between harming the patient and helping the patient is fuzzy at best.

This chapter tries to illustrate the conflicts in health care ethics and ways a seasoned therapist might try to reconcile health care's conflicting positions.

B. IS ETHICS EVER CLEAR?

Sure, when there is a choice between right and wrong, right is always the correct choice. When there is a choice between wrong, and more wrong, or less wrong, or when the principles of right and wrong are difficult to fashion, the answers are much more difficult.

It is easy to answer the question: "is it ever ethical to steal from a patient?" The answer is a clear and resounding no. But if the question is: "should you ever accept a gift from a patient," that is a more difficult question. Under normal circumstances, the rule would be equally unequivocal: no. But sometimes circumstances have a way of making ethical rules and guidelines much less clear.

Consider the patient on life support who has no realistic hope of recovery. Ethical and moral rules tell us that we cannot take active measures to end that patient's life. That would be euthanasia. But every day of the patient's existence is painful for the patient and his family. Our goal in health care is to relieve pain and suffering. Can we let our concern for the living transcend our responsibility to the dying?

In ethics, as in law, there are very few clear and easy cases, and many murky grey areas. Often the only thing we have to guide us is our own internal conscience and our own willingness to be guided by it.

Religion and belief systems play an important role. Judeo-Christian theology generally teaches that we should do to others that which we would want done to us. Almost every other form of religious belief, including the Islamist, Buddhist, Confucian, and Native American belief systems have some version of that principle built into their rule-based systems.

This is not an accident. Even from ancient times, those with wisdom understood that modeling proper behavior to others led to proper behavior being returned. And, of course, the opposite is true too. When you do violence, you most often receive violence in return.

1. How Does One Develop an Ethical System?

An ethical system starts with an understanding of right and wrong. Everyone has this understanding intuitively. Ethics is the art of taking your behavior and your actions toward the right and away from the wrong.

The second step is to develop principles that will enable you to guide your behavior when stress and circumstance can cloud judgment and reason.

As an attorney, I have a very clear rule-based ethical guideline in the form of rules laid down by the Supreme Court of the state where I practice. As a therapist, you have ethical rules laid down by your state board and, if you are a member, by the AARC.

The ethical guidelines for patient care personnel revolve around one central theme: the patient comes first.

C. WHAT IS "PATIENT FIRST"?

At the heart of all patient ethics codes is the idea that we put the patient first. This is sometimes called an Aristotelian First Principle.

1. What Is a "First Principle?"

St. Thomas Aquinas was both a great theologian and great legal theorist. In his book on law, St. Thomas lays out the first principle that underlies all of law: the first principle of law is to do good and avoid evil.

The same could be said about ethics in health care. The first principle is to do good and avoid evil. All ethical principles are bound together with this glue.

In patient care, the first principle manifests itself by placing the patient above other concerns, so long as in placing the patient first we do not engage in anything evil. We first "do no harm" because what we do is aimed at improving the patient's condition. We only take other positive action when we know that it won't harm the patient.

2. Is There an Ethical Duty to Elevate the Patient?

Patients are not people who make clinicians work; they are the reasons for the clinicians' work. Some patients are disagreeable. They are ugly to caregivers and staff alike. They act inappropriately. Some are clinically insane or demented and cannot act in a proper manner. All of these patients must be treated the same way we would treat our mother or grandmother if she were our patient.

A therapist's job is to elevate the patient into the position of boss. The patient is there providing you a job. His welfare is your chief concern. If a therapist is to act ethically, he or she must first elevate the patient to this position of importance.

When a patient is important to us, it is easy for us to do the good work that we normally do. When a therapist "does good" he does so by performing his tasks competently, efficiently, correctly, and only for the good of the patient.

3. Can I Use the Golden Rule As an Ethical Yardstick?

Yes, and in fact, you should. In almost every belief system, as noted earlier, there is a universal theme: do unto others as you would have them do unto you. In very nearly every ethical situation, the issues can be resolved if this dictate is properly applied.

The injunction to do unto others only that which you would have them do to you is a proper ethical yardstick for evaluating what a therapist should do in a given situation. Everyone has gut instincts that tell them that something is either right or wrong. A therapist should learn to go with those instincts and trust them.

One of the most dangerous powers a therapist can have is the power to rationalize conduct. Almost anything can be rationalized if a therapist tries hard enough. I once had a therapist tell me, "It was right for me to ask the patient's mother out on a date after I recognized that she was single, because I would be a good influence on her kid."

This statement, of course, was pure rationalization. There is no data supporting the supposition that the therapist would be good for the child or her mother. This was simply what the therapist wanted to believe. His conduct in doing so placed the hospital in a precarious position. He had to be disciplined because of his failure to keep his personal and professional lives separate.

As a general rule, if you would have to paint your behavior in terms that are less blameworthy, then you probably shouldn't be doing it.

4. How Important Is "Do No Harm?"

It is vital to the ethical foundations of patient care. It is the rock upon which the profession—indeed, all medical professions—are built.

The "avoid evil" aspect of patient care ethics is frequently found in the Hippocratic oath's proscription against giving bad medicine or doing harm. "First, do no harm" is the watchword that every rookie therapist, nurse, and physician learns. It is better to do nothing than to do something harmful.

5. What Constitutes Harm?

Harm, of course, is a relative concept. After surgery, it hurts the patient who must cough. We do not like to inflict pain, but coughing is important to ensure against atelectasis and other problems. The greater good wins out.

Similarly, when we make the patient cough, we are not doing harm, we are preventing a larger harm, in much the same way as we are doing when we draw an arterial blood gas. Of course, if we do not follow the rules and procedures developed to ensure patient safety when we perform these tasks, we may create a situation where harm is the ultimate result. It isn't the blood gas that causes harm; it's the failure to do the Allen's test first. It isn't the nebulizer treatment that causes harm; it's the bacteria in a four-day-old nebulizer being sucked into the lungs.

In fact, the single most common form of harm that befalls any patient in the hospital arises not from intent to do harm, but from intent to do as little as possible. Laziness, in all its ugly forms, is most often at the heart of patient harm. You know this from your own experience. Nosocomial pneumonia arises, in 90% of the cases, from a failure to follow proper handwashing technique. The failure to wash hands, or wash them properly, has its root cause in laziness and a lack of professionalism.[1]

Very few clinicians will actively engage in conduct that is aimed or designed to harm a patient. Instead, they simply take short cuts. Instead of actually measuring the dynamic and static compliance on the ventilator, they look at the numbers they charted last time and chart them. The patient doesn't look any different; the ventilator doesn't sound any different. What harm can there be?

Instead of measuring the FIO2 with an oxygen analyzer, they write down 45% and circle it showing that it was analyzed at that level. Instead of getting a fresh set of weaning parameters, they let the patient sleep and use the parameters from the day before, because in their opinion, "this patient isn't getting any better."

Any time a clinician places his need for ease over the patient's need for good solid clinical care, that clinician causes harm, even though the harm may be too small to measure. It may not cause a problem, because many times there is no change in the FIO2, there is no change in the compliance numbers, and there isn't any change in the weaning parameters. But not

---

[1] I recognize that time is frequently a challenge for therapists, and they cut corners where they can. Patient safety is never the right place to cut corners.

measuring those parameters and falsely charting that you have is causing long-term harm because it is seldom the first error that causes harm.

When we start substituting our good for the good of our patient, we make it easier to stop acting on the patient's behalf all the time. It becomes easier to tolerate mistakes and error in ourselves and in others; and over time that has the effect of greatly reducing the quality of the care being delivered.

In fact, the most serious harm that comes from cutting corners is a decline in your level of professionalism and a willingness to accept shoddy work from others because "who are you to criticize?" It is a slippery slope to stand upon, and when you take that first step down the path of laziness, when you first start substituting your convenience for the good of the patient, you are on the road to ethical perdition.

6. Are There Ethical Duties Relative to Preventing Harm?

The most important ethical duty a therapist has with respect to preventing harm is to do his or her absolute best every day, and at no time to accept anything other than the best for the patient. This is hard. It means, sometimes, that you'll miss lunch. It means that an 8-hour shift will become a 16-hour shift on a Saturday when you really wanted to be home because, unfortunately, someone else called in sick. It means doing more than you have to, and enforcing your code of ethics rather than simply doing what is easy.

To me, a therapist who refuses to do things the easy way is a hero. I know a man like that. James Jeffcoat, RRT, a therapist who practices in San Antonio, Texas, used to practice at a hospital that required therapists to "stack" treatments. He was asked to give multiple nebulizer treatments at one time as a policy of the hospital. Not only was this a terrible policy, a policy that went against the standards of care of the profession and the white paper issued by the AARC, but more importantly, Jim knew it was wrong. It was the wrong way to treat the patients.

Other therapists just did what they were told. Not Jim. He did what he knew to be the right thing. He missed lunches, didn't take breaks, and worked faster than other therapists. He came in early, and he left later, and while he was there, at that hospital, every patient got 100%.

Eventually the strain was too much. Jim left the hospital and went to Texas so he could practice as he was trained to practice. But for many years, even though it wasn't easy, Jim Jeffcoat was a hero who put his patients first.

Jim also didn't suffer fools easily. If a therapist didn't know what he needed to know, Jim either taught him to do better, or filed complaints against those he knew weren't doing what they were required to do. He demanded, both through his direct work in the hospital, and his work in his state society, that the professionals he worked with act like professionals.

The ethical duty to do no harm can be summed up easily. Do everything that is necessary to meet the standard of care. If you work somewhere that this isn't possible, it is time to quit and find somewhere you can.

D. IS MAINTAINING CONFIDENCES AN ETHICAL DICTATE?

Another important ethical duty is the duty to maintain the patient's confidences. Patients don't want everyone knowing what is wrong with them. They want to know that the information you give them will remain confidential.

1. Must I Adhere to a Patient's Wishes with Respect to the Patient's Own Family?

The therapist owes a duty to the patient. She does not owe a duty to the patient's family. If the patient's family wants to know what is going on, and the patient doesn't want them to know, then the patient's wishes control, not those of the family.

Sometimes this is difficult, particularly where the patient may have a communicable disease that makes testing family members imperative. Even though the therapist may feel a commendable obligation to help the family, she cannot reveal confidential information.

2. What About the Rest of the World?

Clearly the therapist has a duty to keep clinical information secret from the rest of the world. Sometimes clinicians breach this duty for money, for example, by taking pictures of their famous patients in hospital rooms and selling these pictures to the media. Therapists who breach the patient's right to privacy are unethical, and should be disciplined by the state board and by the NBRC.

3. How Do Ethical Duties Impact Legal Duties?

A therapist's ethical duty to the patient is different from his legal duty. A therapist present in the ER when an intoxicated patient is brought in may be summoned as a fact witness at the criminal trial. If so, the therapist has an ethical duty to refuse to testify, citing the privilege afforded to medical communications.

It may be that the judge will order the therapist to testify. If he does so, the therapist will be compelled by the judge to testify, and must tell what he knows. But an ethical therapist will refuse when asked, even in court, because the privilege imposes an ethical duty that is larger than the legal duty to testify imposed by the Courts.[2]

Therapists, physicians, nurses, psychotherapists, and others have been sent to jail for refusing to testify on ethical grounds. Although this is laudable from a strictly ethical perspective, it is the view of this author that if the court orders a therapist to testify, then the therapist should testify, having discharged his ethical duties by reciting the privilege.

4. Am I Bound by the Ethical Codes of Professional Organizations?

If you are a member, you're bound.

In addition to the ethical concepts, principles, and practices that a therapist learns in school, there are professional codes of ethics governing the members of various professional organizations. The American Thoracic Society, American Association for Respiratory Care, and American College of Chest Physicians all have their own ethical rules.

a) AARC Code of Ethics

The AARC is the predominant professional association for respiratory therapists in the United States. The AARC maintains a code of ethics to which all therapists are expected to adhere. The AARC's code of ethics states:

AARC Statement of Ethics and Professional Conduct:

In the conduct of professional activities the Respiratory Therapist shall be bound by the following ethical and professional principles. Respiratory Therapists shall:

Demonstrate behavior that reflects integrity, supports objectivity, and fosters trust in the profession and its professionals. Actively maintain and continually improve their professional competence, and represent it accurately.

---

[2]Court orders, however, should be obeyed.

Perform only those procedures or functions in which they are individually competent and which are within the scope of accepted and responsible practice.

Respect and protect the legal and personal rights of patients they care for, including the right to informed consent and refusal of treatment.

Divulge no confidential information regarding any patient or family unless disclosure is required for responsible performance of duty, or required by law.

Provide care without discrimination on any basis, with respect for the rights and dignity of all individuals.

Promote disease prevention and wellness.

Refuse to participate in illegal or unethical acts, and refuse to conceal illegal, unethical or incompetent acts of others.

Follow sound scientific procedures and ethical principles in research.

Comply with state or federal laws which govern and relate to their practice.

Avoid any form of conduct that creates a conflict of interest, and shall follow the principles of ethical business behavior.

Promote health care delivery through improvement of the access, efficacy, and cost of patient care.

Refrain from indiscriminate and unnecessary use of resources.

b) AARC Role Model Statement

In addition to a Code of Ethical Conduct for therapists, the AARC has released additional documents dealing with professional responsibility. They include the Role Model Statement and Statement on Diversity. The Role Model Statement says:

Role Model Statement

As health care professionals engaged in the performance of cardiopulmonary care, respiratory therapists must strive to maintain the highest personal and professional standards. In addition to upholding the code of ethics, the respiratory therapist shall serve as a leader and advocate of public health.

The respiratory therapist shall participate in activities leading to awareness of the causes and prevention of pulmonary disease and the problems associated with the cardiopulmonary system. The respiratory therapist shall support the development and promotion of pulmonary disease awareness programs, to include smoking cessation programs, pulmonary function screenings, air pollution monitoring, allergy warnings, and other public education programs.

The respiratory therapist shall support research to improve health and prevent disease.

The respiratory therapist shall provide leadership in determining health promotion and disease prevention activities for students, faculty, practitioners, patients, and the general public.

The respiratory therapist shall serve as a physical example of cardiopulmonary health by abstaining from tobacco use and shall make a special personal effort to eliminate smoking and the use of other tobacco products from the home and work environment.

The respiratory therapist shall strive to be a model for all members of the health care team by demonstrating responsibility and cooperating with other health care professionals to meet the health needs of the public.

c) AARC Statement on Diversity

The AARC's Statement on Diversity is short and to the point:

The AARC is committed to the advancement of cultural diversity among its members, as well as in its leadership. This commitment entails:

- *being sensitive to the professional needs of all members of racial and ethnic groups,*
- *promoting appreciation for, communication between, and understanding among people with different beliefs and backgrounds,*
- *promoting diversity education in its professional schools and continuing education programs, and*
- *recruiting strong leadership candidates from under-represented groups for leadership and mentoring programs.*

In addition to these resources to guide therapists, the AARC has an on-line educational program on professionalism, which can be found at: http://www.aarc.org/resources/professionalism/index.asp.

5. What's the Legal Risk in Not Knowing My Ethical Duties?

Let's suppose you are a therapist who is also a member of the AARC. Let's suppose you are in a managerial position, and you opt to hire a white therapist over a more qualified Hispanic therapist. The Hispanic therapist sues.

Let's suppose your rationale for hiring the other therapist is that you wanted to maintain a workforce that is representative of the community, and the therapist who has sued you is "unrepresentative."

A good trial lawyer will impeach you with the AARC's Diversity Statement. For example:

Lawyer   *Isn't it true that the AARC is your professional organization?*

Therapist   *Yeah.*

Lawyer   *Isn't it true that the AARC is committed to being sensitive to the professional needs of all members of racial and ethnic groups?*

Therapist   *Uh, I guess?*

Lawyer   *Are you aware of the AARC Statement on Diversity?*

Therapist   *Uh, no.*

Lawyer   *And you consider yourself a professional?*

We've picked a situation that we hope would never occur to illustrate the point; however, the point could easily be demonstrated in a medical negligence trial if the therapist was accused of performing a nasotracheal intubation even though he was not certified to do so. The AARC's ethical rule regarding a therapist's duty to perform "only those procedures or functions in which they are individually competent and which are within the scope of accepted and responsible practice," would be a serious hurdle for the defense to overcome.

E. HOW CAN I RESOLVE ETHICAL CONFLICTS?

Irrespective of whether there is a code of ethics for your professional organization, or whether there is simply a hospital mission statement to guide you, a therapist is sure to face ethical conflicts in her practice.

1. How Do I Go About Recognizing a Conflict?

The first step in resolving an ethical conflict is recognizing that one exists. And sometimes, that's difficult to do. If a family member asks you to go to the cafeteria and get a bottle of diet soda, it may not seem like something that presents a serious ethical issue. But, if after doing that, they insist on buying you a soda too, that may come close to receiving gratuities.

The really dangerous slippery slope of gratuities is not the potential that someone will give you money, but rather, that they will expect different or better service from you because they have compensated you. This creates a problem when there are other patients with more serious problems than the patient who now demands your attention on the basis of the gratuities. If the gratuities cause you to breach your duties to the other patients, that is a serious ethical issue.

It is for this reason that you should never place yourself in this position. And, of course, you should never inadvertently create a problem by suggesting that getting caught taking gratuities could cost you your job. You increase the risk, by saying something like that, that the patient will simply find other ways to compensate you. The far better response is "I don't mean to hurt your feelings, but that is an absolute no with me. Thank you, but no."

Likewise, it goes without saying that you should never enter into any kind of personal relationship with a patient. Several years ago, a very young therapist who worked for me was sent to the pediatrics unit to do an ECG on a patient. The patient was only two years younger than this 19-year-old student therapist, and when the therapist recognized that he was attracted to the woman, he should have immediately called for someone else to do the ECG. Instead, he performed the ECG, and, as the woman sat naked from the waist up, he asked her if she would like to go out with him.

It never occurred to this therapist that the patient was in an untenable position with respect to being exposed to a man who might take an interest in her. Although apologies were made, the therapist eventually wound up leaving the hospital because of the ethical breach. It was a tough lesson for him to learn, but better learned as a student therapist than later as a credentialed practitioner.

A far more dangerous situation exists when a therapist is affected by events in the patient care areas, and lets that affect his objectivity. It is important to keep a safe clinical distance from patients; and when a patient becomes a cause instead of just another patient, it may be wise to recognize that this creates an ethical conflict. When a therapist's personal feelings are caught up in his or her clinical decision-making, that is the time when the poorest decisions are made.

If a therapist is troubled, for example, by the care being administered to a patient, and the reason for his concern is that the patient is brain dead and should be allowed to die, it is important to recognize when that concern is such that it might affect your patient care. If the therapist finds himself not giving his best to that patient, perhaps in the hope that the patient will pass away, he is walking down the same ethical hallway that Efren Saldivar walked down when he decided to euthanize patients at Glendale Adventist.

Every therapist has a conscience, and that conscience should be your ethical guide. If what a patient, physician, nurse, or fellow therapist is doing, or is asking you to do comes close to being the wrong thing, that's a warning bell. Your conscience knows when you are coming close to that line, and you have a duty to listen to that voice inside yourself that urges you to pull back.

Recognition of ethical issues is not difficult if the therapist simply uses this rule: "If what I am thinking of doing, or considering doing, were to be published on the front page of the newspaper tomorrow morning, would I be proud, or ashamed?"[3] If the answer is ashamed, you've just recognized an ethical conflict.

If a therapist recognizes an ethical conflict, the next step is to find a way to resolve it. The simplest resolution may be to take a break from that patient's care. In other cases, it means bringing the problem to the attention of the chain of command.

2. Is the Chain of Command Responsible for Ethical Issues?

If there is an ethical breach in the department, the chain of command in the department is ultimately responsible.

Every therapist knows that the boss does not want to be bothered with small things. However, an ethical issue is not a small thing. If you have a concern about a situation that affects you, and you believe you are in an ethically difficult spot, the proper thing to do is to raise the issue with the supervisor and chain of command.

---

[3] When the story on Efren Saldivar broke, every therapist shared in the shame he brought on the profession. Remember that feeling, if you were fortunate enough to live through it. It is a good indicator of what unethical behavior can bring to you, your institution, and your family.

Usually, that means telling the boss that you cannot care for a patient because of clinical detachment problems, or otherwise. For example, several years ago a patient who happened to be a very good friend of my wife was admitted to ICU. I was called up to intubate the patient, and fortunately the patient did not need intubation after cardioversion. As soon as the emergency issue was decided, I passed off the patient to my supervisory staff because I could not care for him. He was too close a friend, and my detachment was seriously compromised. When the patient died several days later, I was spared the price of personal involvement, namely, guilt.

If you have such an issue, your supervisor should know about it, and the sooner the better. The sooner she knows, the sooner your boss can bring in other individuals to help address the ethical issues.

3. What Are Ethics Panels?

These are groups of involved clinicians who meet to discuss whether (and in some cases, how) to withdraw life support, and other sensitive ethical issues.

When a patient is in a vegetative state, and decisions must be made to withdraw or withhold life support, the proper forum for the discussions about those issues is an Ethics Panel. Normally such a panel involves all the caregivers, and the family, who work through the ethical questions with regard to continuation of obviously futile care. Ethics panels provide comfort for the family, and support for the clinicians who must face difficult choices in the care of their patients.

4. What Is the Ethicist's Role in Clinical Practice?

Some hospitals, particularly university hospitals, now have ethicists on staff to advise physicians and health care workers on the ethics of a particular situation. If an ethicist is available, therapists should feel free to use him or her whenever possible.

Ethicists can often ask the questions that need to be asked. They can pinpoint the issues and advise as to the best course of conduct. They are always a welcome addition to the health care team when a patient presents with end-of-life issues.

5. What Is the Interaction Between Ethics and Law?

In most cases a therapist who acts legally and properly also acts ethically. In most cases a therapist who acts ethically also acts legally. The relationship between a strong code of ethics and a strong adherence to the law is important in health care. Therapists who desire to skate near the outer limits of the law risk falling through the ice of uncertainty, just the way the therapists who dance on the wrong side of ethical lines soon find themselves dancing to discordant music.

Lawyers are proper advocates and advisers on things legal, but not always on the ethics of a situation. Lawyers generally do not understand the dynamics of health care, and they understand the relationships between patients and their families even less. A lawyer is, by default, an advocate. His job is to push for a victory for his side. He is a hired gun brought in to fight a single battle. As a result, the issue of whether an action or choice is legal is always a different question than whether a choice is ethically correct. It is perfectly legal for the surgeon to send lavish gifts to the cardiologists who send him the most patients. It may not be ethical, however, if those gifts are designed to buy a recommendation that is not in the patient's best interest. And if you ask a lawyer about that question, he can only answer the legal issue, not the ethical issue.

For these reasons I recommend access for all therapists and all hospital personnel to an ethicist. Ethicists are the proper people to resolve ethical issues and provide guidance on ethical issues.

F. KEY POINTS

- Ethics arises from the first principle: do good and avoid evil.
- In medical ethics, the principle can be expressed in short hand as "first, do no harm."
- The best ruler in making ethical measurements is the "golden rule."
- The AARC has a code of ethics that dictates professional standards for therapists.
- It is important to be aware of the AARC ethical code.
- Recognizing ethical conflicts is the first step toward remedying them.
- One way to recognize a conflict is to apply the "front page" rule: if what you did showed up on the front page, could you show your face in public again?
- It is the duty of every therapist to practice ethically.

Index

Aquinas, St Thomas, 463
Arrest, resisting, 428
Assault, ability of clinicians to commit, 205
Defined, 203
  distinguished from battery, 204
  intent as an element, 204
  lack of physical contact, 204
Assumption of the risk, defined, 252
  how proved, 253
  knowledge of danger, 53
  surgical error and, 254
  voluntary assumption of, 253
Assumptions, as the mother of all lawsuits, 287
At Will Employment, defined, 84
  history of, 84
  individual states, 85
attempt to injure, as element of assault, 203
Attorney, right to assert, 433
  unethical acts, 406
Attorney-Client Relationship, explained, 404
  Structuring, 457
Attorneys fee, must be in writing, 458
  comparison of, 454
Attorneys, acts as agents bind client, 457
  advertising and, 454
  differences between firms, 455
  duties during questioning, 443
  record of discipline with State Bar, 455
Autonomy, defined, 33

B

Back Pay, as remedy for discrimination, 153
Background checks, in employment, 184
Bad Faith, defined, 77
  in health care cases, 77
Bail, bounty hunters, 439
  for felony crimes, 439
  when allowed, 439

Baker by Thomas v. General Motors Corp., 93
Bankruptcy, as last resort, 385
  attorneys and, 386
  Chapter 11, 385
  Chapter 13, 385
  Chapter 7, 385
  effect of family, 386
  effect on small business, 387
  effect on stockholders, 387
  filing, 386
  fresh start, 385
  generally, 384
  power of US Trustee, 387
  preferential payments, 386
  purpose, 385
Battery, ability of clinicians to commit, 205
Defined, 204
  need for physical contact, 204
  wrongful touching, 204
Bigots, no room for in organizations, 177
Bill of Rights, generally, 15, 27
  criminal law and, 431
  applicable only to federal government, 433
  extended to state action by 14th Amendment, 433
Billing, and documentation, 268
Blessing Hospital, 184
Bona fide occupational qualifications (BFOQ), 157
Borderline employees, recognition of, 180
Bowman v. McDonalds, 216
Branches of government, 15
Breach of Duty, what constitutes, 218
Briefs, appellate, 25
Burden of Proof, 19
Burden shifting, in discrimination cases, 183
Business invitee, defined, 261
Business lawyer, selecting, 450
Business torts, generally, 394

I

M

Y

Z